"Dr. Bock and Nellie Sabin have made a valuable contribution . . . *The Road to Immunity* should be in every person's home health library. It will be used a thousand times."
—Gary Null, Ph.D.

GET WELL AND *STAY* HEALTHY—BEGIN TODAY!
Did You Know . . .

A high-sugar diet may suppress the immune system and accelerate aging

Safflower oil, the most unsaturated vegetable oil, can hurt the immune system

Substances found in the liver of the Greenland shark are helpful for cancer patients undergoing chemotherapy and radiation

Cysteine, an amino acid, can help the body excrete toxins

A Chinese herbal approach called *fu zhen* can help recurrent or chronic viral illness

Shiitake mushrooms not only taste good, but they stimulate the release of interferon

Milk thistle and other botanicals can help the liver heal and detoxify

Oxygen therapies boost energy and aid cellular repair—and can be as simple as deep breathing

Medications, including birth control pills, can increase the need for certain nutrients

Take the path to glowing health . . .
THE ROAD TO IMMUNITY

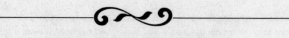

THE ROAD
TO
IMMUNITY

HOW TO SURVIVE AND THRIVE
IN A TOXIC WORLD

KENNETH BOCK, M.D.,
and NELLIE SABIN

POCKET BOOKS
New York   London   Toronto   Sydney   Tokyo   Singapore

This book is intended solely for informational and educational purposes. Please consult a health care professional before making any significant lifestyle changes, and seek appropriate medical advice if you have any questions about your health.

The case histories in this book are true, but I have made many changes to conceal the identity of the individuals. I have changed names, life circumstances, and even gender to protect the privacy of my patients.

An *Original* Publication of POCKET BOOKS

POCKET BOOKS, a division of Simon & Schuster Inc.
1230 Avenue of the Americas, New York, NY 10020

Copyright © 1997 by Dr. Kenneth Bock and Nellie Sabin
Foreword copyright © 1997 Bernard D. Raxlen, M.D.

All rights reserved, including the right to reproduce
this book or portions thereof in any form whatsoever.
For information address Pocket Books, 1230 Avenue
of the Americas, New York, NY 10020

Library of Congress Cataloging-in-Publication Data

Bock, Kenneth Alan.
    The road to immunity : how to survive and thrive in a toxic world
/ Kenneth Bock and Nellie Sabin.
        p.   cm.
    Includes bibliographical references and index.
    ISBN: 0-671-54507-8
    1. Immunity—Popular works.   2. Health.   I. Sabin, Nellie.
II. Title.
QR181.7.B63   1997
618.07′9—dc21   97-18169
                                                                       CIP

First Pocket Books trade paperback printing October 1997

10   9   8   7   6   5   4   3   2

POCKET and colophon are registered trademarks of
Simon & Schuster Inc.

Text design by Stanley S. Drate/Folio Graphics Co. Inc.

Printed in the U.S.A.

*For our children, Alicia and Jordan, Eleanor and Schuyler,
in the hope that this knowledge will help strengthen their immune systems
to meet the challenges of the coming years.*

Acknowledgments

❧

There are many things I knew I wanted to accomplish during my lifetime, but writing a book was not on my list—until recently. I was led in this direction by my clinical work with patients, and by the need I saw for this information to be written in an understandable and practical way.

I could not have accomplished this project without the help of many people. I would like to thank my agent, Angela Miller, who saw the value in this work and who introduced me to Nellie Sabin, my collaborator and partner in this project, without whom this book never would have succeeded. This project required a great deal of time and effort, and I feel fortunate to have found someone like Nellie, who is so thorough and conscientious, and with whom I found working to be so easy and enjoyable. Also thanks to Claire Zion for her vision, and to Leslie Stern, my editor, for her support and her readily available assistance to help make this book a reality.

I also would like to thank my friends and colleagues, among them: Neil Orenstein, Ph.D., for his generous help with research; Jesse Stoff, M.D., for his kindred support; Dan Kinderlehrer, M.D., for his deeply appreciated assistance with the chapter on healing; Thomas Hesselink, M.D., for his exhaustive research into the mechanisms of oxidative medicine; and Moira Shaw, my spiritual sister, for her inspiration in creating the 50/50 work and her generous assistance in integrating that work not only into this book but into my clinical practice as well. Moira's work has been extremely helpful on deep levels for my family, friends, and many of my patients. Thanks also to my dear friend Vicki Weissler, O.M.D., who so graciously shared her vast knowledge of acupuncture, healing, and stress management with me, and for her enthusiastic help with these aspects of the book. I also would like to acknowledge Barbara Brennan, who introduced me to the deeper aspects of healing and to the Pathwork, which has given me incredibly valuable insights into living fully and accepting life on its terms.

It is a privilege to be able to thank my early mentors in the field of nutritional medicine, including Jeff Bland, Ph.D., Sid Baker, M.D., Leo Galland, M.D., and Michael Schacter, M.D. Many thanks to Russell Jaffe, M.D., Ph.D., for inspiring me with his brilliant treatise on immune system defense and repair. Thanks also to Charles Farr, M.D., Ph.D., and Robert Rowan, M.D., for their pioneering work in oxidative medicine; to William Rae, M.D., for his help in the field of chemical sensitivities, immune dysfunction, and, more recently, energetic medicine; and to Len McEwen, M.D., for his discovery of enzyme-potentiated desensitization, as well as Butch Schrader, M.D., for his unceasing work to further the development of EPD in the United States. Linus Pauling, Ph.D., genius and pioneer, always inspired me by standing up for what he believed in and searching for underlying truths, wherever that search led him.

I am indebted to Lynda Thompsett, for her transcribing and typing, and to Chris Welch, for designing the Immune System Profile. I particularly want to thank my many patients, most especially those whose stories are included in the book, but also the many others who have taught me the value of listening. From my patients I have learned of the essential need for openness, acceptance, and partnership in the healing relationship.

Writing a book is harder than I ever imagined, and I am indebted to friends and family for their support, including my brother and partner, Steve, for his love and help when it was needed; my lifelong friends Kenny Solomon and Cary Bayer; and my dear friend David Marell for his helpful perspectives during our weekly breakfast meetings. I am grateful to my parents, Nora and Fred, for their unconditional love and heartfelt support.

Mostly I must thank our families—my wife, Marian, and my children, Alicia and Jordan; and Nellie's husband, Bob, and their children, Eleanor and Schuyler—for enduring the countless hours that we had to spend away from them while working on this project. I recognize their hardship, and am deeply grateful for their understanding, love, and forgiveness.

—KENNETH BOCK, M.D.
April 1997

Contents

———— ❧ ————

I

YOUR BEST DEFENSE
UNDERSTANDING THE IMMUNE SYSTEM

II

THE IMMUNE SYSTEM EMPOWERMENT PROGRAM

A COMPREHENSIVE APPROACH TO STRENGTHENING YOUR IMMUNE SYSTEM

4 MODERN LIFE AND IMMUNE SYSTEM OVERLOAD

III

FINDING YOUR WAY BACK TO HEALTH
ESSENTIAL STEPS TOWARD WELL-BEING

Foreword

❧

The trumpeting media do not let a day go by without declaring authoritatively that a particular health risk (high cholesterol, hormone-fed animals, contaminated water, polluted air, among others) contributes absolutely to the dreaded scourges of cancer, heart disease, or neurological deterioration; only to be followed the next day by the news that a certain nutrient, hormone, or lifestyle change can provide us with youthful longevity. While it is welcome news that sickness is controllable and preventable, it is difficult for us to keep up with the bewildering explosion of legitimately researched information even while we disregard the unproved nonsense. Illness can be avoided. Wellness can be ours, but how?

When we want to feel our best or when we are ill and seeking solutions, the choices can become confusing and overwhelming. As patients, we need a "bridge," a physician-guide who can intelligently span and integrate traditional and holistic medicine. Dr. Bock's *The Road to Immunity: How to Survive and Thrive in a Toxic World* is such a "bridge." It comes directly from his clinical experience (shared with that of his brother and partner, also a family physician) of more than fifteen years of close observations of patients, therapeutic successes, and long-term follow-up. As a holistically oriented, board-certified family physician, he defines his operational paradigm as "progressive medicine."

Dr. Bock's integrated concepts govern his work and are widely explained in this thought-provoking book. Here you will find no hyperbole or need to exaggerate untried claims. Patient successes, described here in the case studies, speak for themselves and they clearly illustrate examples of his system of thinking. Dr. Bock presents a new taxonomy of illness, different from what is learned in medical school and ordinarily followed by most doctors. The new diagnostic grid overlays the often puzzling symptoms that confront him daily (and those of us who practice similarly) and have bedeviled his patients and other specialists.

Dr. Bock recognizes that the body needs to be nourished on a cellular level, in order to maintain a healthy homeostasis. He also recognizes that nutritional supplementation can not only help to prevent illness through appropriate preventative maintenance, but can also be employed therapeutically.

As a physician healer, Dr. Bock pays close attention to details; looking for clues, avoiding a snap diagnosis, and appreciating the total complexity of the patient's problem. Listening skills are central to initiating the healing process. Time, the most precious commodity in a physician's working day, is generously allotted by Dr. Bock to each patient's problem. For him this time-bound intimacy is the essential foundation of the healing experience, without which all other therapeutic interventions would fail to achieve their desired results.

Beyond exerting every effort to help his patients physically, Dr. Bock recognizes the healing effects of love, openness, and acceptance. He believes in the balance between the physical and the spiritual, which is an essential ingredient for immune-system health. Healing, he states, requires personal change—sickness is not just something to get over. Illnesses, especially chronic illnesses, may have meaningful impact on our lives and affect us in ways we never imagined. In other words, we need to heal ourselves. In my field (neuropsychiatry/complementary medicine), I am of a like mind with Dr. Bock's comments that counterproductive thought patterns based on a distorted belief system will interfere with our health and may keep reemerging until distortions and misconceptions are cleared. When we finally align ourselves with our deepest truth, healing at all levels becomes possible.

The information in this book is authentic and grounded, as opposed to being excessively hyped, which tends to be the case in the "anything goes" wellness market. Two years were spent writing this manuscript. It is therefore indicative of the thoughtful, careful intelligence of this highly committed physician. This book is nothing less than a blueprint—a manual guide for the new progressive alternative medical model, which is fast becoming accepted as an integral part of the mainstream health-care system. Dr. Bock embraces his profession with passion and enthusiasm that are inspiring and persuasive.

I often share with my patients a quote from Leonardo da Vinci that I think is appropriate here:

> Good practice is when the doctor, together with an understanding of the patient's nature, also understands what union is, what life is, what constitutes the temperament and thus health. When these have been well understood—he will also understand their opposite. And when this is the case he will know how to heal.

If you, as the educated reader, are interested in how a rigorously trained physician integrates holistic concepts and techniques into a dynamic medical practice, then you have a pleasant journey ahead with Dr. Bock as your guide on "the road to immunity," taking the first steps in knowing "how to heal."

—Bernard D. Raxlen, M.D.
May, 1997

THE ROAD
TO
IMMUNITY

Introduction

❧

Why does one person get a cold, but the next person doesn't—even though both were exposed at the same time?

Why does one person get cancer, but the next doesn't—even though the body is fully capable of destroying cancer cells?

Under the old medical paradigm, we were all victims waiting to be sabotaged by the next virus or bacteria that came along. This approach to health dates from Louis Pasteur's experiments with bacteria in 1862. Under the germ theory of infection, when we got sick, we blamed the agent that made us so.

Most people have heard of Pasteur's lifework. He is famous for battling bacteria and infectious diseases by means of pasteurization and vaccination. However, few people know that on his deathbed Pasteur realized that all his life, his efforts actually had been misdirected. *"Le germe n'est rien,"* he said; *"c'est le terrain qui est tout."*[1] [The microbe is nothing; it is the soil that is everything.] After his lifelong pursuit of germs, Pasteur realized too late the importance of *host resistance.*

We now know that sickness is selective; it requires our body's cooperation. Because we are only as healthy as our defenses, the new medical paradigm is self-defense. Good health is maintained through immune system strength and immune system balance.

You don't need to get sick just because your colleague came to work with the flu or your children brought colds home from school. People who have a vigorous immune system can resist many illnesses and therefore lead fuller, happier lives than people whose immune system is weak.

As a physician with a busy medical practice that emphasizes health and well-being, I see patients every day whose immune systems have been weakened. After years of studious inquiry, plus years of clinical experience and observation, I have developed the Immune System Empowerment Program, which can be used by everyone to strengthen and maintain a healthy, balanced immune system.

Your immune system may be weakened if you show any of the following symptoms:

- Persistent fatigue
- Frequent colds or bouts of the flu
- Chronic or recurrent infections
- Any acute infection

- Chronic congestion
- Recurrent headaches
- Cognitive problems (for example, memory loss or difficulty concentrating)
- Neurological problems (for example, numbness or tingling)
- Joint swelling or pain
- Muscle pain and/or weakness

The Immune System Empowerment Program has helped many people recover from these kinds of problems, and it can help you as well. The benefits of improved health include:

- Increased energy, vitality, and enjoyment of life
- A dramatic reduction in episodes of illness
- Reduced need for drugs (fewer prescriptions and/or lower doses of medications)
- Lower medical bills
- Reduced need for surgery

The basic Immune System Empowerment Program (for people who are well or whose immune system is moderately stressed) does not require a doctor's assistance. The enhanced Immune System Empowerment Program (for people who are sick) offers treatment suggestions for patients to discuss with their physicians, as well as guidelines for locating an open-minded physician should you need one. In this way, the program has something to offer everyone.

MY TOOLBOX

As a holistic physician, I utilize a wide variety of healing therapies. My Immune System Empowerment Program is grounded in solid medicine, but also includes some unconventional therapies with which most doctors are not familiar but which are nonetheless safe and effective. To get my patients healthy (and to keep them that way), I recommend a combination of traditional medical practices (for example, medications or surgery when absolutely necessary), natural healing therapies (including a sound diet, vitamins, nutrients, herbs, homeopathy, and acupuncture, among others), and emotional support (such as stress management and psychotherapy). These treatments are most powerful when used simultaneously. Together they help the body heal itself.

I believe that alternative and traditional medicine are best used together. Used separately, they can be inadequate, even harmful. We once had an eight-year-old patient at our health center who had been treated homeopathically for Lyme disease. By the time he was brought to our office, he was experiencing eye muscle paralysis and double vision. He desperately needed antibiotics, and fortunately responded rapidly to intravenous treatment. This patient had been treated exclusively with an alternative therapy at a time when traditional treatment was needed.

On the other hand, it is very common for me to see patients whose immune systems have been abused by course after course of antibiotics, resulting in complications that are sometimes severe. Because their immune systems have been disrupted, these patients often have chronic yeast (candida) problems or allergies, and their intestinal flora often has been knocked out of balance. I usually recommend natural therapies to rebalance their intestinal flora and to rejuvenate their immune system.

Physicians today are not trained in preventive medicine. The focus of their education is disease, not health. For this reason, many doctors fail to ask their patients the right questions and also overlook extremely helpful healing therapies. For example, most doctors underestimate the importance of nutrition, even though research and plain old common sense lead us to the conclusion that all of the cells in the body are influenced by what we eat. In their zeal to make a diagnosis and to prescribe pharmacologic treatments, most physicians tend to forget that we are made up of trillions of cells, and that we function only as well as our cells function. Cell function can be enhanced or depressed according to the materials our cells have to work with. This is why our general state of nutrition plays such a vital role in our general state of health, and why a healthy diet and certain supplements are vital parts of my program.

We now know that our emotional state, too, influences cell function. Emotions are translated by the body into chemical messengers that cells use to communicate, especially immune system cells. These "conversations" can lead to responses that are beneficial or harmful to our health. No program for good health would be complete without attention to the way in which emotional well-being can translate into physical well-being.

Good health is more than the absence of illness. Restoring full health requires not only treating any disease or medical condition that is present, but also stimulating the body's natural healing abilities by rejuvenating and rebalancing the immune system.

HARNESSING THE IMMUNE RESPONSE: MEDICINE FOR THE NEXT MILLENNIUM

The body wants to be well. Our immune system, fantastically intricate and highly sensitive, is in a state of constant vigilance against abnormal cells. It is capable of instantly recognizing threats within the body and of using several different means to eradicate them. Some of these threats are external in origin (for example, a virus); some arise internally (for example, cancer cells). With incredible accuracy, the immune system can target these potentially harmful agents and neutralize them.

Still on the medical frontier are cures that will be based not on directly attacking bacteria or viruses or cancer cells, as most current therapies attempt to do, but on empowering the immune system to launch its own attack. Researchers are coming to recognize that orchestrating an appropriate immune response may be the most powerful treatment of all.

Although a "strong constitution" is due in part to heredity, our immune strength is directly influenced by certain choices we make. By choosing to protect and nourish our immune system, we can harness the body's innate power to heal.

PROTECTING AND STRENGTHENING THE IMMUNE SYSTEM

The typical modern lifestyle ravages the immune system. There are many reasons why. Every day we are exposed to all kinds of pollutants and toxins, including smoke, chemicals, and heavy metals. We eat too much bad food and not enough good food. We are casual about what we put into our bodies—including over-the-counter drugs, prescription drugs, and recreational drugs—and we are often stressed, lonely, isolated, insecure, and fearful. The immune system is rugged enough that we can get by under these conditions for years, even decades. However, all these factors eventually take a heavy toll. Insult piles up upon injury until one day we get sick.

Fortunately, we can reverse much of the damage we've done over the years, starting with some simple strategies. Take me, for example. I am exposed to all kinds of illnesses every day. With two offices to maintain, many patients to care for, and a family with young children, I'm extremely busy and I generally don't get enough sleep. This is not a lifestyle that is conducive to good health. However, I seldom get sick because I've put myself on my own Immune System Empowerment Program. I take several different kinds of vitamins and nutrients every day, I try to eat well, I avoid substances I know are harmful, I love my work, I exercise and practice stress management, and I make a point of spending time with my family.

These are not difficult steps to take. All of us can do a great deal to strengthen our immune system. We can start by shielding it from unnecessary strain or damage and by providing it with the nutrients it needs: fresh air, clean water, healthful food, and love (yes, love is a nutrient). It is important to use a comprehensive approach that strengthens the immune system on all fronts—a total program for immune system health. All the vitamins in the world will not keep you well if you make unhealthy lifestyle choices such as smoking or eating poorly. This book will show you how to survive and thrive in an increasingly toxic world.

PROGRESSIVE MEDICINE

When I see sick patient after sick patient, most of whom have already visited other doctors without getting better, I realize that the medical establishment is not doing a good job of keeping people well, and that something else is needed. It has taken me many years of serious study and inquiry to integrate a variety of effective treatments, both traditional and alternative, into what I call *progressive medicine*. Progressive medicine includes proven therapies ranging from the judicious use of antibiotics to the five-thousand-year-old practice of Chinese herbal medicine to the latest bio-oxidative therapies.

Let me give you an example of progressive medicine in action. My patient Karen already knew her diagnosis when she came to see me. She was exhausted, her throat hurt, and tests indicated some irregularities in her liver function. Her doctor told her she had mononucleosis and that she should go home and rest—standard medical advice for mono because there is no treatment to directly combat the Epstein-Barr virus, which causes it. Karen was appalled. A professional dancer, she had an extremely important audition coming up that she felt she absolutely could not afford to miss.

Ordinarily a patient like Karen—who actually had mono-hepatitis (liver inflammation due to the virus that causes mono)—could expect to "rest" for four to six weeks or even several months before she could hope to approach her previous energy level. At our Center for Progressive Medicine, Karen was treated with intravenous vitamin C, nutrients, and special herbs for liver support—treatments designed to help her immune system rally. She made a full recovery in two weeks, trained for her audition—and got the part.

These treatments are not new, or crazy, or risky. They are tried-and-true therapies that we use every day to help our patients regain immune system strength. They are not yet especially common, but I expect someday they will be.

I see many, many patients who are at their wits' end because they know they are sick, but they have been told by medical specialists that their problems either are not significant ("Be thankful you're not worse") or are in their head. The fact that modern laboratory procedures do not reveal any particular illness for these patients does not mean they are healthy.

Many of my patients suffer needlessly for years because their condition lies just outside the parameters of traditional medicine. Many have hidden allergies, chronic yeast problems, chronic Epstein-Barr infection, and subtle nutritional and metabolic imbalances. There are many other bona fide medical conditions that traditional doctors are slow to accept and diagnose, including environmental allergies, chemical sensitivities, chronic fatigue immune dysfunction syndrome, chronic Lyme disease, and reactive hypoglycemia. I never heard much about these problems in medical school, but they have been discussed in alternative medicine circles for years.

I'm a doctor. I want people to be healthy. Because I can't stand seeing so many people unnecessarily sick, I decided to write this book. In it I will share with you what I have learned about maintaining the immune system balance that is so vital to our health—the balance within.

READ THIS IN GOOD HEALTH

This book is divided into three parts:

- Part I is required reading for understanding how the immune system operates. Awareness is the first step to empowerment.
- Part II explains the basic Immune System Empowerment Program that I devised for my patients. This program is useful for anyone in any state of health and does not require a doctor's assistance. It is basic enough to help everyone but flexible enough to accommodate individual needs. Rigid protocols can't possibly be good for everyone because we are all biochemically (and emotionally) unique.
- Part III is for people who are ill. It enhances the basic Immune System Empowerment Program and contains important advice about how to find a good doctor, how to get the correct diagnosis, and how to get well. After you read Part III, your next visit to the doctor will be different. You deserve to get what you need from your doctor, and this book will show you how.

Patients come to our health centers in Albany, New York, and in rural Rhinebeck, New York, from as far away as Canada, California, and Florida. Some have stayed in touch via phone consultations after they moved thousands of miles away, even to other countries. This is personally rewarding, but more important, it shows how much people need the kind of progressive medicine we offer at our health centers. Patients come to us as sick as can be, having exhausted many other approaches, and *they get better.*

It is tremendously satisfying for me to watch my patients recover their vitality, sometimes after years of illness. They go back to school or work, they start exercising again, they mend their relationships. Older patients feel and act ten years younger. Best of all, our patients stay well. Some have chronic illnesses that will never go away, but we are able to achieve improved health for them while we search for new therapeutic approaches that may ultimately help them even more.

This book is the result of twenty years of clinical observations and experience, but it also brings you the most up-to-date medical information available. Every day I reconsider the treatment options I have at my disposal. Is there anything I haven't tried that might help one of my patients? Is there a new approach I could add to my medical arsenal? I am constantly on the lookout for new theories and protocols. Over time I have been able to sort out the new ideas that are worth pursuing from the worthless fads and schemes that have always shadowed medicine. I try to stay ten years ahead of the game so that I can pass along the latest breakthroughs to my patients and to you.

The human body and the human spirit are resilient. Starting now, you can boost your immune system for lifelong health.

I

YOUR BEST DEFENSE

UNDERSTANDING THE IMMUNE SYSTEM

READ THIS FIRST

The next three chapters provide an introduction to the immune system and how it works on a cellular level. It's important to read these chapters for an overview of immune system health before jumping to Part II, the Immune System Empowerment Program.

Chapter 1, Progressive Medicine, explains why I became a holistic physician and how I developed my program for immune system health. Chapter 2, The Immune System Kettle, introduces general concepts that are essential in understanding how the immune system protects our health and appreciating how our systems of defense and repair can be overloaded. In Chapter 3, Immunology 101, you'll learn exactly how every day your immune system fights the good fight against viruses, bacteria, toxins, and other threats to optimal health, and why maintaining immune system balance is so critical.

We now know that sending our immune system into battle rested and fully equipped can have a tremendous effect on the outcome of each skirmish. By the time you finish reading Part I, I hope you'll be galvanized into action and ready to implement the Immune System Empowerment Program. As you'll see, doctors may be able to help you get healthy, but only you can keep yourself that way.

Chapter 1

❧

PROGRESSIVE MEDICINE

If everyone is thinking alike, then no one is thinking.
—BENJAMIN FRANKLIN

I didn't start treating Mrs. N. for Lyme disease until 1986. Mrs. N. had come to me two years before with an unusual combination of symptoms that various physicians had not been able to treat successfully. A rheumatologist suspected her joint pain was due to rheumatoid arthritis, but she had not responded to treatment. A dermatologist had not helped her skin rash; a neurologist had not relieved her headaches or explained the numbness in her fingers; and her family doctor had found no cause for her constant weariness. He referred Mrs. N. to a psychiatrist, recommending that she consider antidepressants—an idea Mrs. N. found alarming.

I found Mrs. N. to be a cogent, coherent, spirited woman. She was also scared. "Dr. Bock," she said quietly at her initial visit, "I am certain that I have some kind of illness. I know some people develop symptoms because of what is going on in their mind, but before I became ill I was really quite content. *Now* I'm worried."

On Mrs. N.'s chart I noted "atypical neurological disorder." True, she was feeling somewhat down, but in her circumstances, who wouldn't? Could it be true that her problems were "all in her head"?

Testing revealed a subtle thyroid imbalance, which we corrected; chronic candidiasis, which we treated; and various allergies, which we identified and dealt with. Mrs. N. began to feel somewhat better—but still she was not well.

My job is to help people get and stay well. In a situation like Mrs. N.'s, the idea that I don't have the answers is unacceptable to me. Patients like Mrs. N. force me to become a medical detective. An "atypical" diagnosis or a patient who isn't responding to treatment can lead me down any number of paths. Over the years I have attended countless conferences and lectures, read innumerable texts and articles, and exhausted a myriad of avenues of research looking for clues that would help me help my patients. My patients have obliged me to constantly expand my body of knowledge, to find out more about diseases and disorders and to research alternative therapies that might be effective.

By 1985, Mrs. N.'s condition had improved but she was still ill. I then started thinking seriously about Lyme disease, an affliction that manifests itself in a baffling variety of symptoms. Lyme was not a new disease at that time, but the spirochete that causes it had just been discovered by Dr. William Burgdorfer in 1982, and the disease was starting to gain more attention in the medical literature. I had never seen a case of Lyme arthritis in medical school, and there had been no significant discussion of Lyme during my rotation in rheumatology, so the disease was new to me. However, it seemed plausible that Mrs. N. might have it. Mrs. N. lived in Connecticut, an area endemic for Lyme. When I tested Mrs. N. for Lyme, her results came back positive. I started her on an aggressive treatment of intravenous antibiotics, simultaneously taking steps to make sure her immune system was supported during this taxing process (more about this later).

Mrs. N. got better. Almost all of her various symptoms responded to treatment. After her underlying problem—the Lyme disease that had escaped diagnosis for years—was correctly determined, her "atypical neurological disorder" suddenly made sense.

Mrs. N. was thrilled. "Every day I feel better!" she exclaimed, looking more radiant than I had ever seen her. The problem clearly had never been simply "in her head."

I'm a board-certified medical doctor, and I value every course I ever took in medical school. I do believe, however, that there is more to practicing good medicine than what you are taught in medical school. There is certainly more to practicing good medicine than treating each symptom with ever stronger medications, and falling back on the idea that the patient is somehow at fault when conventional medical protocols fail. And fail they will—because they are outdated.

Looking back on my medical career, I now can see that I was always interested in integrating different realms of thought into a comprehensive whole. When I went off to medical school in 1975, however, I had no idea how many years it would take me to become a holistic physician, nor did I realize that I would acquire some of my most valuable information far from any lecture hall.

MEDICINE BY THE BOOK

I knew right away I wasn't going to fit in at the University of Rochester medical school. This was 1975. I had long hair, I was a vegetarian ("So you eat brown rice, Mr. Bock?"), and I had sixties values about politics, spirituality, and communal living. In addition, I'd taken a circuitous route to medical school. At the University of Buffalo I'd majored in American Indian studies, thinking maybe I'd be an ethnobotanist. After I'd finally decided to follow in the footsteps of my older brother, Steve, and become a doctor, I'd taken all my premed courses in one year.

I received an excellent, though solidly traditional, education at Rochester. It was a conservative, very demanding school. I studied around the clock. I wanted to learn—and I also wanted to prove that a person outside the traditional mold could make a good doctor.

For the first two years of med school, you sit in vast lecture halls for hours, then go study for hours. You see only academics—teachers and other students—and the occasional cadaver. There's not a lot of levity, but you get through it.

For the next two years, medical students put what they've learned into action by doing clinical rotations in different specialties. Then you get to exchange information with nurses, patients, and doctors practicing clinical medicine.

Looking back, I realize that Rochester served me well in three essential ways. First, I learned basic facts and procedures that I've used every day since. Second, I learned excellent research skills—which I've relied upon heavily as I investigate and evaluate alternative therapies. Finally, Rochester was particularly strong in psychiatry and psychosomatic medicine at that time. My training there in examining the social and environmental conditions surrounding illness helped shape my holistic approach to medicine.

For all these strengths, however, medical school had some serious weaknesses, some of which I was aware of even then. There was only one course on the immune system, and just one three-week course on nutrition that turned out to be really nothing more than an introduction to gastrointestinal physiology. I knew I wanted to learn more about nutrition, so I started reading about it in my "spare" time. Many people scoffed at this. Most doctors are woefully uninformed about nutrition and the vital role it plays in overall health.

The more I found out about nutrition, the more I learned about preventive medicine. This, too, was a subject we didn't hear about in medical school. Instead, we were very busy learning which drugs to use for what conditions.

After four years, it was time to decide what kind of doctor I wanted to be. Specialists pick their favorite body system and settle into practice for life. Back in 1640, mathematician and philosopher René Descartes proposed that the study of the human body be broken down according to the body's different systems. This was an extraordinary concept at the time, and for the 350 years since Descartes we have been able to further and further refine our understanding of how the body's various systems function. However, I knew I wanted to focus on how the body functions as a whole. All the delicately balanced systems of the human body are interdependent in ways we are just now beginning to understand. Teasing them apart is valuable, but does not show us how to treat the whole—just as shattering a clock reveals its inner workings and gears, but tells us nothing about the nature of time.

I chose to become a family practitioner—an all-purpose doctor. That way I could continue to integrate everything I was learning about nutrition, preventive medicine, and traditional medicine and how they affect all the systems of the body. I also liked the idea of having close, ongoing relationships with patients that would last over time, instead of seeing patients only on a crisis basis.

My next step was a three-year residency at Lancaster General Hospital in Lancaster,

---

COMMONLY ASKED QUESTION NO. 1:

What is nutritional medicine?

On my business card, underneath my name, it says "Preventive and Nutritional Medicine." Nutritional medicine recognizes the importance of nourishing the body on a cellular level in order both to prevent and to treat illness and to achieve optimal wellness. Although only a small minority of physicians would say they practice nutritional medicine, the reality is that we all eat, and we all consist of trillions of cells that need to be properly nourished. Nutritional medicine takes each of our own biochemically unique nutrient requirements into account.

Dr. Linus Pauling coined the term *orthomolecular medicine* back in 1968. Orthomolecular (literally, "correct molecule" or "right molecule") medicine is based on the concept that nutrient deficiencies are expressed as illness, and therefore treatment should consist of varying the concentrations of natural chemical substances that are normally present in the human body, thereby restoring proper balance to the body's systems. Under the orthomolecular model, arthritis would not be treated with anti-inflammatory medications because it is not caused by a deficiency of aspirin, and anxiety would not be treated with psychotropic drugs because clearly it is not caused by a deficiency of Valium.

Pennsylvania. This is where I finished my formal education, doing more rotations and gathering more clinical experience.

Jeffrey, one of my patients during this period, was quite upset. He was experiencing anxiety attacks. Sometimes he'd feel shaky and his hands would tremble. His heartbeat was rapid, and he was subject to sudden sweats. "Sometimes," he confessed, "I'm afraid I'm going a little crazy."

I proceeded carefully with Jeffrey and ruled out any serious illnesses, as I'd been trained to do. The results of his blood tests all came back normal, and an EKG indicated nothing wrong with his heart. By now I was confident that Jeffrey's problems were psychiatric in nature, so I prescribed Valium to ease his mind.

I was on solid medical footing doing so. This was completely typical of what a family practitioner would do in those days—and what many doctors still do. Family practitioners screen for any apparent illness, referring patients to specialists as needed. Once an illness has been diagnosed, a doctor has a game plan to follow that has been set forth in the medical textbooks. As Emanuel Cheraskin, M.D., D.M.D., puts it, "The name of the game is the name." Once you have the name of the condition, you know what drugs to prescribe. If the first drug doesn't work, you step up to a stronger one. This regimen does not vary from patient to patient, except insofar as people respond differently and can experience different side effects.

If no illness is apparent, or if the patient is complaining of symptoms that affect all (or at least multiple) systems of the body, doctors frequently assume that the patient's problems are emotional. I know now that sometimes they are—but many times they aren't. We never learned in medical school the extent to which different physical problems can cause psychiatric complaints. It never occurred to me that Jeffrey was not going to feel any better.

ALTERNATIVE MEDICINE

In my third year of residency, I attended a conference that changed the way I practiced medicine. At this conference, nutritionally oriented doctors were discussing chronic candidiasis (yeast infection), immune dysregulation (when a patient's immune system does not return to normal after a viral illness), and other conditions I'd never heard about in medical school. I knew I had to keep learning about these kinds of illnesses. They were real, they were important—and they weren't in any of my medical books.

This began my insatiable interest in, and attendance at, nutritionally oriented conferences. These conferences were ahead of their time in terms of medical acceptance, but they were just in time for some of my patients. I'm not impulsive by nature, but I learned not to wait for a new development to be discussed in a "refereed" medical journal before taking it seriously. Most physicians regard *The Journal of the American Medical Association* and *The New England Journal of Medicine* as gospel, to the point where they overlook treatments and conditions that aren't mentioned in these publications. However, there are many other good journals (such as the *American Journal of Clinical Nutrition*) that are not read nearly as widely, yet provide much useful information. Frequently it takes five to fifteen years (the medical "lag time") for subjects that first appear in these other journals to reach the most prestigious publications.

My residency in Lancaster came to an end in June 1982. This was a critical juncture for me. I was now a fully trained family practitioner. Should I practice what I already knew—or find an environment in which I could learn more about alternative medicine?

The decision was difficult, but I opted to give up the security of what I knew and join a busy holistic practice in New York State. There was a lot happening in medicine that I knew little about, and I owed it to my patients to learn more.

In the beginning, I followed the physician in this practice from examining room to examining room, listening and watching. Imagine my surprise when who should greet us one day but Jeffrey, my patient from Lancaster. Still not feeling better, despite his Valium, he had gone searching for an alternative physician who might be able to help him. I was shocked. Jeffrey was shocked to see me, too.

The doctor listened carefully to Jeffrey's complaints and asked a few questions I hadn't thought to ask. Jeffrey revealed that his symptoms were worse when he was hungry and hadn't eaten, and he admitted that yes, he did frequently crave sweets.

Jeffrey had reactive hypoglycemia—another disorder I hadn't heard about in medical school. His treatment consisted of many recommendations I hadn't heard much about in medical school, either, including dietary modification and nutritional supplements. In addition, the doctor told Jeffrey to gradually cut out the Valium, confident that he would be able to do this without much difficulty now that he was being appropriately treated for his underlying condition.

Jeffrey left the office feeling hopeful and looking greatly relieved. I finished the day feeling humbled but also inspired. How many other diagnoses had I missed because I'd never heard of them? I hoped not many—and I vowed never to miss a case of hypoglycemia again.

Every day the doctor I worked with diagnosed hypoglycemia, candidiasis, food allergies, chemical sensitivities, and other illnesses with which I was not familiar. He prescribed intravenous vitamin C, herbs, vitamins, and other treatments that were new to me. And whatever he was doing, it was working. Many of his patients improved dramatically from one office visit to the next.

Medical school had taught me a great deal about the two powerful guns in the armamentarium of traditional medicine: drugs and surgery. Until now I had limited my practice of medicine to these two spheres. Now I was adding many additional treatment options to my "little black bag," forming a more comprehensive arsenal. Moreover, I was learning that coordinating several healing approaches was more beneficial to the patient.

I had always been a good listener, but now I was learning just how closely a doctor needs to listen to his or her patients. I realized that the extensive psychiatric training I had received at Rochester was playing a more important role in my ability to help patients than I ever could have imagined. I learned to listen carefully, suspending all judgment, as patients chronicled their problems. I learned to honor their complaints, paying close attention to details, looking for clues to the cause of their distress. I learned not to be too quick to offer a diagnosis in complex cases.

In postgraduate medical training, we were taught to arrive quickly at a diagnosis, give a prescription, and move on. Now I was seeing how important it is to note and evaluate *all* of a patient's symptoms, even the minor ones, no matter how long this process took. Sometimes it is the odd bit of information that makes the difference in determining a correct diagnosis.

I had also been taught in medical school that one kind of germ caused one set of symptoms. I was having to rethink this approach, too.

Doctors are something like the proverbial blind men surrounding the elephant. Grabbing the elephant's knee, one blind man declares, "This animal is large and leathery!" Grabbing the elephant's tail, another says, "Not at all—it is thin and bristly." Holding the tusks, the third blind man states with conviction, "Surely you jest. This creature is nothing but bones." Mrs. N., my patient with Lyme disease, had many physical complaints. Each specialist could see a different illness in her symptoms. What got lost somewhere along the line was the big picture—seeing all of her symptoms in context.

Most of the patients who came to this holistic practice had already been to traditional medical doctors and had already received the standard medical therapies I had learned about in medical school. I found this very sobering. If we couldn't help these patients get better, who would? On the other hand, it was exhilarating to see desperately ill people start to feel better, to have hope again. When I saw a cancer patient who had been given six months to live, but who was taking over 100 grams of vitamin C a day (an absolutely huge dose, one that is rarely attempted) and was still going strong two years later, it opened me up to what is really possible and how magnificently our immune system can take care of us when we take care of it.

At this point in my medical career I was not satisfied with traditional medicine, which I knew was too limited, but I wasn't yet comfortable with alternative medicine. I felt as if I were standing in a doorway between the two approaches. Behind me was a carefully circumscribed room illuminated with bright light; before me was darkness lit by stars of possibility. The only way out of this dilemma was to learn everything I could about the best alternative medicine had to offer. So I set about studying with each of the other practitioners in the office.

The chiropractor was a true healer, very compassionate, always mindful of each patient's comfort level with different treatments. The massage therapist had healing hands and showed me the power of "hands-on" healing. The nutritionist was expert at mapping out a dietary approach to managing all kinds of health problems, including hypoglycemia, diabetes, yeast sensitivity, heart disease, and cancer. The naturopath used diet, herbs, and supplements to heal his patients.

The patients who came to this holistic practice learned how to manage their own ongoing care. After receiving an in-depth analysis of their needs and sensitivities, they learned what foods to eat and to avoid, what supplements to take, and what problems to watch out for. As time went on, they needed less and less medical attention. I realized that in medical school we had been so busy learning how to treat acute health problems that we never learned about preventive medicine.

There's at least one reason why. Preventive medicine has seismic economic implications. Sickness is expensive, and therefore profitable for doctors, drug companies, hospitals, and the rest of the health care industry. Keeping patients healthy and teaching them how to be responsible for their own good health undermines this whole structure.

Realizing I had a lot to learn, I immersed myself in alternative medicine, pursuing what I could see were valuable options for my patients who had conditions that had eluded traditional medicine—illnesses that were difficult to diagnose and treat. I kept going to conferences and spent a lot of time reading at night. It was a challenging, exciting, rewarding year. Eventually, however, the inevitable occurred. Just as I had run up against the confining edge of conventional medicine, I now ran into the far side of alternative medicine.

Some of what I observed at the holistic practice just seemed too subjective to me. For example, I have never been entirely comfortable with applied kinesiology—the practice of testing a patient's tolerance for various substances by checking for muscle response as the patient holds one item at a time. Some people swear by kinesiology, but to me at that time the results were not reproducible enough. (Interestingly, I recently met a respected German physician who appears to practice applied kinesiology in a way that is very effective and reproducible. The time I spent in his office with him and his patients renewed my interest in this field.)

There were other, more important issues as well. All members of this practice took a dim view of antibiotics. The naturopath could not prescribe them and would never recommend them, period. The physician could prescribe them but rarely did. Even more problematic was the fact that no one had admitting privileges at the local hospital. The practice was a little world unto itself.

There was no doubt in my mind that my patient Luis needed to be hospitalized for intravenous antibiotics. He had a whopping case of pneumonia, and oral antibiotics weren't helping. But because I didn't have admitting privileges to the hospital, I had to refer Luis to a doctor he didn't know, and I was unable to monitor his recovery. I could not see Luis through the best treatment that "straight" medicine could offer him.

I saw no reason to forsake everything I had learned in medical school. Now I knew what kind of medicine I wanted to practice.

PROGRESSIVE MEDICINE

Alternative medicine received its name from treatments that people tried when all else failed. Therefore, alternative medicine is defined not only by what it offers, but also by what it does not. It is a limited approach to healing.

Complementary medicine uses nutrition and herbs to complement traditional medicine. It, too, cannot stand alone.

Progressive medicine is a unifying approach to health care. Progressive medicine combines the best of traditional medicine with the best of alternative medicine. Progressive medicine is not "alternative" or "complementary" medicine; it is *good* medicine.

In November 1983, I opened up the Rhinebeck Health Center with two other physicians, one of whom was my brother, Steve.

We moved immediately to get admitting privileges to the local hospital and to become an integral part of the medical community in Rhinebeck. We developed a reputation as rather conservative alternative physicians. It did not take long to build up a busy practice. The health center clearly filled a need. We emphasized natural, noninvasive, nontoxic treatments as much as possible, and we went to great lengths to discover underlying illnesses or conditions that had previously eluded detection. Patients were looking for something more, and they came from far and wide.

Not everyone was happy with us. One of my patients who came in with acute wheezing was very annoyed with me when I prescribed an asthma inhaler. She said disapprovingly, "I thought you were a *natural* doctor!"

I couldn't force this asthma patient to use an inhaler, even though it was clear to me that she needed immediate help getting oxygen into her body. Most of my patients aren't that rigid, and I try not to be rigid, either. Pure philosophy doesn't cure anybody. Generally my patients and I try to accommodate each other's preferences.

Medicine is a partnership, like a dance between doctor and patient. Listening is the key. What is the patient looking for? What are his or her expectations? What does he or she need from me? With what treatments is he or she comfortable? Not everyone comes to my office ready to use an inhaler or happy to take Chinese herbs. So we start slowly and build up mutual trust. It's senseless for me to sit behind my desk and give recommendations that a patient isn't going to follow. "Patient compliance" is necessary for healing to begin, but patient compliance often begins with doctor flexibility.

Sometimes I feel as if I'm leading my grandmother out onto the dance floor. Do we start right off with a rumba? Of course not. Will we ever do the rumba? Well, why not?

Each human being is unique, physically and spiritually. This is one reason why "cookie cutter" prescriptions cannot work for everyone. I closely monitor how my patients are responding to treatment, fully aware that what works for one might not work for the next. Traditional medicine, in my view, still does not offer a sufficiently individualized approach to healing.

I'm not really practicing "conventional" family medicine anymore. People with simple medical problems can get that type of help elsewhere. The patients who find their way to me usually have complex problems that have eluded diagnosis and treatment. Often their immune systems are overburdened. For some patients, I'm at the end of the line.

I'm happiest when I can solve a medical mystery or go one step further treating someone who is ill. In this way, my patients have been my teachers. Many of my patients have been told by doctors—well-respected physicians with high-level positions at hospitals and medical colleges—that nothing more can be done for them and that they must learn to live with their symptoms.

Often there *is* more that can be done, but only if the patient is willing to set aside this discouraging diagnosis and to be open to new possibilities and points of view. Starting to look for the underlying cause of their symptoms is like beginning a journey. Sometimes the route is uncertain, but the destination—good health—is always clear.

When I'm stumped, it's easy for me to *admit* "I don't know," but it's not easy for me to stop there. I continue to push the envelope, looking for new ways to help the immune system regain its essential balance. I know the answers are out there. Just because we haven't accessed them yet doesn't mean they don't exist.

I am reminded of Irene, a patient of mine who had been given the diagnosis of irritable bowel syndrome (IBS), a catch-all term that is basically just a description of symptoms. Having ruled out any serious illnesses, her gastroenterologist told Irene she should be happy that her symptoms were not caused by, say, colon cancer.

Irene was not content with this diagnosis and wanted to exhaust every avenue before resigning herself to IBS. "I've heard that you've helped other people with chronic problems," Irene said. Her voice was calm, but she was sitting very straight, her back rigid with anxiety. "I never used to have these problems before—so is there a chance they'll go away again?"

At our health center, we discovered that Irene had low stomach acid, which in turn led to her intestinal problems. By correcting her stomach acid balance, we were able to completely reverse her symptoms. Her problems did indeed go away.

I knew about low stomach acid, but I didn't realize how common it is until I attended a medical conference in which the presenting physician observed that up to 20 percent of the clinical population, especially the elderly, has low stomach acid. I started testing for this condition more often, and turned up more cases than I expected—not 20 percent of my patients, but a significant number. The amazing thing is, most physicians—even gastrointestinal specialists—rarely, if ever, test for hypochlorhydria (low stomach acid). In fact, physicians are so concerned with excess stomach acid that for many years the number one prescribed drug was one that inhibited the production of stomach acid.

The only way our immune system can communicate with us is through symptoms. I have come to regard symptoms as opportunities. Symptoms are the body's way of telling us it has needs that are not being met. After we figure out what those needs are, often we can meet them.

When I first saw Anne, she had several complaints—nothing dramatic, but enough problems that she knew she was sick. For years she had experienced headaches, muscle aches, and persistent fatigue. "Dr. Bock," she said sadly, "I feel like I'm in a mental fog all the time."

Anne's regular doctor used blood tests to rule out anemia or thyroid trouble, then told her she was probably under too much stress from taking care of her four teenagers and her sick mother. He recommended exercise—but Anne was so tired she couldn't even do the dinner dishes, let alone exercise.

Unfortunately for Anne, her symptoms did not point to any one particular diagnosis, so there was no "magic bullet" for her—no special pill or treatment her doctor could offer her. She had started to believe that for the rest of her life she would never feel quite like herself again.

When Anne and I reviewed her medical history, I learned that she had been repeatedly treated with antibiotics for recurrent sore throats. This immediately raised a red flag for me.

When antibiotics throw the intestinal flora out of balance, yeast overgrowth is common. Suspecting chronic candidiasis, I ordered certain blood tests for Anne that would help confirm this diagnosis.

Anne did indeed have a severe yeast overgrowth. For years she had been eating exactly the wrong foods for someone with a yeast problem: sugary baked goods, yeasted breads, and the occasional glass of beer or wine. After Anne overhauled her diet and started on nystatin (a prescription antiyeast medication), she felt dramatically better. Eventually she was able to proceed to a natural antiyeast preparation.

At her last office visit, Anne was delighted. "I can't believe how much better I feel! It makes me realize how sick I really was. When I think about it, I get angry that I wasted all those years feeling terrible—so I try not to think about it, and just celebrate being well again."

COMMONLY ASKED QUESTION NO. 2:

How come my previous doctor said there's no such thing as a chronic yeast problem?

Unfortunately, the diagnosis of candidiasis remains a clinical diagnosis—that is, a diagnosis based on the doctor's clinical judgment more than on laboratory tests. In the old days, clinical diagnoses were the art of medicine, but today we are so reliant upon lab tests (and so aware of malpractice lawsuits) that this art has become less fashionable.

The traditional medical establishment refuses to accept—for reasons unknown to me—the existence and importance of chronic candidiasis. Doctors recognize the normal presence of yeast in the gut, as well as severe, systemic yeast overgrowth in immunocompromised patients, but most are unable to accept the full spectrum of candida problems in between these clinical end points. Because people can tolerate varying amounts of candida in their gastrointestinal tract, there is no one definitive test to diagnose an excess of candida. I use several different tests, including blood work and stool samples, to confirm my clinical suspicion of chronic candidiasis.

Anne was under medical care for all those "wasted" years, but her doctors failed to help her because their minds were closed. I get extremely frustrated when I have to deal with doctors who refuse to venture outside the current medical paradigm. All medical progress comes from being willing to push the envelope and go beyond the accepted medical dogma. It will take many years for some of the therapies I use to become generally accepted, which means there are patients out there who are not receiving safe and effective treatments that I know would help them.

Schopenhauer once said, "All truth goes through three stages. First it is ridiculed, second it is violently opposed, third it is accepted as being self-evident." Examples of this resistance to change are everywhere. When Harvey Firestone first proposed the idea of a tire filled with air, he was laughed at. (He persisted in spite of this ridicule and went on to create an industry giant, Firestone Tires.) The Greek astronomer Eudoxus first determined that the earth was not the center of the solar system two thousand years before this fact became accepted. In medicine, it sometimes takes decades for effective cures to be recognized—and for ineffective treatments to be dropped.

In matters of healing, there is a great deal we know. We must also realize there are many things we don't know. But what keeps me up at night are the things of which we have not yet even dreamed—all that knowledge we're not even aware we're missing.

WHAT'S NEXT?

It is clear that conventional medical protocols are not the only valid approaches to healing. Most of us know or have heard about people who have been helped by healing therapies such as homeopathy and acupuncture. It is also clear that traditional medicine is slowly becoming more holistic. Even the venerable National Institutes of Health recently created a branch called the Office of Alternative Medicine to evaluate alternative therapies.

Ted Turner once said, "You don't want to go into the next war with the last war's weapons." Progressive medicine is what we will need to stay healthy in the future. It is also the approach we will need for illnesses that are difficult to diagnose and treat, such as immune-related disorders, allergies, Lyme disease, cardiovascular disease, and chronic fatigue immune dysfunction syndrome. The incidence of certain illnesses is skyrocketing in this generation. Clearly a new approach to health is needed.

As I mentioned earlier, we now know it is not just the germ (or virus, or parasite, or fungus) that makes us sick, but the germ set against the background of an immune system ravaged by the stresses and toxins of our present-day society. The immune system holds the ultimate key to health and well-being.

Researchers are currently investigating ways to harness the power and precision of a healthy immune system. Instead of focusing their efforts on directly destroying an antigen—for example, using chemotherapy to kill cancer cells—they are turning their attention to enhancing the ways in which the body successfully combats disease-causing organisms. Cancer vaccines, still under development, use this principle. The patient is injected with certain types of cancer-related materials that are recognized by the immune system, thereby provoking an immunological response that beats back all cancer cells in the body.

In HIV/AIDS research, attention is now being focused on how to use the immune system to fight AIDS.[1] There are people who test positive for HIV but who have not gotten sick, even after twelve or more years,[2] and there are people who have lived with AIDS for many years without succumbing to the disease. It's clear that some people have more immunological strength than others—and that we need to find out why.

Currently there is much speculation about the viruses of the future. Books like *The Hot Zone*, by Richard Preston, and *The Coming Plague*, by Laurie Garrett, are pretty scary, as are the killer virus movies. Every generation has had its life-threatening illnesses. We cannot predict what viruses or other immune system challenges will beset civilization in the years to come. What we can do to meet the illnesses of today and tomorrow is bolster the capacity of our immune system to defend our good health.

Nobody loves you more than your own immune system. When it is working correctly, it fights countless battles every day, large and small, to keep you healthy—whether you cooperate or not. Imagine how powerful your immune system could be if you provided it with all the nutrients it needs and took steps to protect it from the poisons and assaults of modern-day life.

As a society, we are no strangers to the concept of self-defense. We make all the safest choices we can about where to live, work, play, or travel, and with whom to do these things. No one would think you were being unreasonable if you walked briskly down a darkened street to discourage an unseen attacker, or installed an alarm system to guard your home from possible intruders, or bought insurance to protect your assets against unforeseen misfortune. On the other hand, many people would find you unreasonable (tiresome, even) if you refused a doughnut because of its fat and sugar content, or changed your restaurant table to get away from secondhand smoke—even though fat, sugar, and smoke are known health hazards.

Over the last ten years I have refined my Immune System Empowerment Program to the point where I know it works. When a new patient comes to see me, I know this program will be beneficial to him or her, especially in conjunction with whatever treatments the patient needs for any immediate health problems.

Some patients cannot expect to restore perfect health because they have tenacious conditions for which we at present have no cure. Other patients have an immune defect or missing immune factor that makes them susceptible to chronic illness. These patients cannot fully recover from diseases that other people are able to put behind them. For these patients, we keep searching for the next new development that might make the difference between sickness and health.

Some cases are very difficult to crack. Autism, depression, hyperactivity, and memory loss all can have organic causes. Sometimes finding just the right treatment or combination of treatments will enable a patient to function well in society.

We've had many, many heartwarming success stories over the years, but one of my favorites is that of little Mikey. Mikey was diagnosed as autistic at eighteen months of age. He was mute, unresponsive, and sealed off in his own world. Before coming to our health center he had received conventional pediatric care, including antibiotics for his recurrent ear infections and Benadryl for his allergies. Mikey's pediatrician had told his parents not to expect much—that this was simply the way Mikey would remain.

When we tested Mikey, we discovered that he had a yeast problem as a result of the antibiotics, plus many food and inhalant allergies, and chemical sensitivities as well. He was allergic to many substances in his diet, in his home, and especially in his day-care environment. While Mikey's mother quickly made the necessary changes in his lifestyle, we treated Mikey's yeast problem and started him on special allergy shots (more about these in Chapter 10, Immune System Super Boosters). Today, at age five, Mikey is interacting, smiling, and learning to talk. He even gives me a hug when he sees me. For a child who was previously diagnosed as autistic, this amounts to a monumental transformation. Everyone in the office loves to see Mikey because his emergence from his private world brings such joy.

The immune system is truly miraculous. Except in rare instances, people are born with all the immune system equipment they will ever need. We have what it takes to live a long and healthy life. What we have to do, then, is learn how to take care of our immune system so that it can take care of us. In the next chapter, we'll examine how the immune system strives to stay in balance, and what we can do to help or hinder this delicate equilibrium.

Because I combine traditional and alternative treatments for so many of my patients, it's hard for me to pick just one case history to illustrate progressive medicine in action. Most of the patients I treat have complex, interrelated medical problems that need to be teased apart and individually addressed with a comprehensive treatment program that synthesizes different modalities and approaches. In some of these situations (for example, when a patient has both Lyme disease and chronic candidiasis), the challenge is to treat each problem in a way that doesn't amplify the others.

In the case history that follows—and in the other in-depth case histories you'll find at the end of each chapter—I refer to treatments with which you won't be completely familiar until you finish reading this book. While you may want to reread these stories after you are more comfortable with some of the language, it's not essential that you fully understand the treatments at this point. What you will see in these case histories is men and women much like yourself who have been able to improve their health using the Immune System Empowerment Program and often certain Immune System Super Boosters (see Chapter 10) as well.

Many of my patients have Lyme disease, so this illness plays a role in a number of the case histories throughout this book. Not only am I located in an area endemic for Lyme, but I also have developed expertise in treating patients with this puzzling multisystem, multisymptom disease, so it is a significant part of my practice.

✑ CAROLYN'S STORY

Carolyn is a married mother of two who first came to see me when she was thirty-three years old. She had recently received several courses of antibiotics, including intravenous antibiotics, for Lyme disease. The trouble was that she was not feeling significantly better. She and her doctor had reached a dead end, but Carolyn knew she still was not well.

At the time of her initial evaluation, Carolyn was experiencing chills, joint aches, decreased appetite, and chronic fatigue, and just didn't feel like herself. Some days were worse than others, and her symptoms would go "up and down." Her physical examination was unremarkable, but her medical history was somewhat involved.

A little over a year before, Carolyn had moved from Manhattan to a suburb about forty miles from the city. Five days later she'd given birth to her second child. This was an intensely stressful time for her, with "too many things going on at once." By winter, Carolyn had developed joint pains and was suffering from recurrent infections, including sinusitis, pharyngitis, and conjunctivitis. She was also experiencing confusion, mood swings, emotional irritability, and insomnia. She had started to have bad nightmares, which would seem real to her, adding to her agitation and anxiety.

Carolyn had a history of food allergies when she was younger. She also had a history of ear infections dating from childhood, so she had taken frequent courses of antibiotics. She noted occasional vaginal yeast infections, especially just before her period or during stressful times, and she craved sweets and snacks during her periods. If she didn't eat or if meals were delayed, she would get shaky, light-headed, and cross.

Carolyn didn't recall any tick bite or rash, but her new home was in an area endemic for Lyme disease, and in fact everyone on her block either was being treated or at one time had been treated for Lyme. In April, a doctor had diagnosed Lyme disease and had prescribed a two-month course of Ceftin, an oral antibiotic. When she failed to improve, combination therapy (two antibiotics at once) was prescribed, but with no significant results. The next step was four weeks of intravenous doxycycline (another antibiotic), which didn't help her symptoms significantly, although she noted that her fingers were less numb and did not ache as much as when she was taking antibiotics.

Carolyn was switched to intravenous Rocephin (another antibiotic), but received this treatment only intermittently because she developed leukopenia (decreased white blood cell count). By August, this treatment had to be discontinued, and by October she was in my office.

So what was I to make of all this? It seemed to me that there was much more going on with Carolyn than a straightforward case of Lyme disease. I suspected underlying candidiasis (yeast overgrowth), allergies, reactive hypoglycemia (which could account for her dizziness when she was hungry), nutrient deficiencies, and possible hormonal imbalances, with this whole clinical picture complicated by Lyme. Difficult cases like this can be treated successfully with progressive medicine.

Carolyn's routine lab test results were normal, as were her Epstein-Barr virus profile and thyroid hormone levels. Her Lyme titer was negative, but her Lyme Western blot results were equivocal (three bands positive—the Centers for Disease Control considers five positive bands confirmation of Lyme), and one of three Lyme urine antigen tests was highly positive. These odd Lyme results indicate what a dynamic disease Lyme is, and how fallible lab results can be.

Carolyn's six-hour glucose tolerance test (used to measure blood sugar levels) was abnormal. At four hours, she had a blood sugar level of 50 milligrams/deciliter, associated with fatigue and an inability to concentrate. In addition, her immune profile was less than optimal, including a slightly decreased overall white blood cell count and decreased antibody levels. Blood testing revealed elevated candida antibodies, and intradermal skin testing was positive for several mild food and inhalant allergies.

At this point, I felt that Carolyn had immune deficiency, reactive hypoglycemia, allergic rhinosinusitis, chronic candidiasis, and probable Lyme disease. However, I did not believe that what she needed at the time was more antibiotics. I knew there were treatments we could use to boost her immune system and her level of health before trying antibiotics again, should that even be necessary. To get the maximal effect of antibiotics, it is sometimes helpful to rehabilitate the immune system first (if the situation is chronic rather than acute).

Carolyn's next steps included stress management counseling; nutritional counseling to help her implement a yeast-free, allergen-free, hypoglycemic Immune Empowering Diet; and various supplements, including a well-balanced, multivitamin/mineral supplement formulated especially for patients with joint pain, probiotics (such as acidophilus and lactobacillus), prebiotics (to support the probiotics), essential fatty acids, antioxidants, and ginseng (an immune system tonic). I also added the antifungal medication nystatin to this regimen (to combat candidiasis), and referred Carolyn for acupuncture. We discussed the fact that antibiotics might need to be restarted in the future after we got these other aspects of her health under control.

I started Carolyn on intravenous vitamin C for immune support, but she had an adverse reaction to her first treatment. It turned out that she had reacted to vitamins before, including prenatal vitamins, so we discontinued these treatments. Shortly after that, I started Carolyn on oxidative treatments, beginning with intravenous hydrogen peroxide. Carolyn noted much improvement with this therapy. Her sinuses cleared and she felt much better overall.

After a flu-like illness that winter, Carolyn felt her "Lyme symptoms" return, including pain and stiffness in her left hand, anxiety, nightmares, and frequent awakening at night. We started her on photo-oxidation therapy (a combination of intravenous hydrogen peroxide and ultraviolet radiation of the blood), which she tolerated well.

In June, we ran another Lyme titer, which was negative, and another Western blot test, which was definitively positive (five bands this time). It's possible that Carolyn's immune system, as it gained strength, was better able to respond appropriately to Lyme, resulting in a stronger positive result.

Photo-oxidation continued to help Carolyn immensely, but her symptoms—joint pain, bad dreams, etc.—still came back intermittently. She noted that they weren't nearly as bad as they had been, but still she did not feel completely like herself.

By now I was certain that Carolyn had chronic Lyme disease with arthralgias (the joint pains) and neuropsychiatric aspects (the mood swings, nightmares, etc.). We had tended to her overall well-being, so I felt it was time to return to antibiotic therapy. I started Carolyn on penicillin shots (a protocol that historically had been found to be effective for the neuro-psychiatric symptoms associated with late-stage syphilis), and she responded beautifully. I also added a low dose of Zoloft (an antidepressant) to ameliorate her mood swings, and natural progesterone for hormonal support.

At the insistence of her husband, who was concerned about Carolyn's symptoms and their persistence, Carolyn consulted an internist in New York City who did a complete standard workup and found *nothing wrong*. On the one hand, this was good news. Carolyn and her husband were happy that she didn't have any serious condition, like cancer, that had somehow escaped my detection. On the other hand, I find it a little scary that a patient with multiple abnormalities who was currently being treated for several conditions, including Lyme disease, could be told that nothing was wrong.

At her last visit, Carolyn was the healthiest and happiest I'd ever seen her. She had just thrown a large birthday party for one of her children—something she hadn't even been able to contemplate a year before—and she'd had energy to spare after it was over. It had taken her a year from her first visit to get to this point, and there had been some twists and turns on her road to recovery, but Carolyn now feels like herself again.

She has stopped the penicillin shots, is tapering off the nystatin, and no longer needs photo-oxidative treatments on a regular basis. To maintain her level of health, she takes supplements, keeps up with her acupuncture treatments, watches what she eats, and practices stress management techniques. She even has gone back to working out at the gym—a big deal for someone who felt as lousy as she formerly did. It is very rewarding for me to hear a patient say, as Carolyn recently did, "This is the best I've felt in a long time!"

Chapter 2

❧

THE IMMUNE SYSTEM KETTLE

The final appearance of disease, then, is a reflection of all the individual's past experiences, exposures and genetic predisposition.

—LEONARD A. SAGAN, M.D.
The Health of Nations[1]

I have a friend who refers to episodes of illness—the flu, an ear infection, strep throat—as "health terrorism." One minute you're fine; the next minute you're sick because a germ attacked you.

Many of my patients extend this point of view to larger health problems as well. They'll say, "I was perfectly healthy until I had that heart attack," or "Yesterday I was okay, but today you tell me I have cancer!"

I encourage my patients *not* to liken illness to a sudden event like falling off a cliff. Getting sick almost always involves a gradual descent, one we're not even aware of until symptoms appear. The initial changes that occur at the cellular level are undiscernible to us. When they advance to the tissue and organ level, we perceive them as symptoms. Once we feel terrible, we realize we have a problem.

In many ways we are engaged in a constant battle all our lives. Day in and day out our immune system protects us from innumerable threats to our health, from germs to damaged or mutated cells to toxins and carcinogens. Immune cells constantly seek out and destroy anything irregular within the body in daily skirmishes we can neither see nor feel. An overwhelmed immune system, however, is not able to mobilize as many troops as are needed to defend the body from a multitude of assaults. It starts to lose certain battles, symptoms appear, and we feel sick.

Whenever my patients get an unusual or unfamiliar symptom, they immediately think of cancer. It's a universal fear. That abdominal pain . . . is it cancer? This lump over here . . . is it cancer? Sometimes it is, but most often it is not. In his book *Beating Cancer with*

Nutrition, Patrick Quillin, Ph.D., notes that everyone gets cancer about *six times* in a seventy-year lifespan, yet only one in three people actually develops detectable cancer. This means the great majority of cancers are successfully handled internally by our immune system. "Think of these 20 trillion immune cells," says Quillin, "as both your Department of Defense and your waste disposal company."[2]

Neither good health nor illness just happens. How healthy you are depends upon a wide variety of factors that I'll explain in this book. The bottom line is that we have the power to strengthen our immune system by lessening its load and by supplying it with the support it needs, including adequate nutrients (proteins, vitamins, minerals, fatty acids), sunshine, fresh air, clean water, love, security, and peace of mind. By enabling our immune system to be strong, ready, and capable of fighting effectively at a subtle level, we may avoid having to fight a battle that much larger when illness is more easily recognizable.

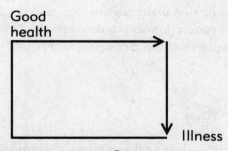

1. The "falling off a cliff" theory of illness is not a useful model. Disease usually develops over time.

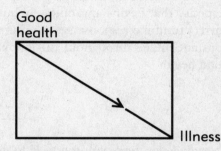

2. The descent into illness is apparent as more symptoms, or more severe symptoms, appear. Getting well again is an uphill climb.

IMMUNE SYSTEM BALANCE

Picture a tightrope walker on the high wire at the circus. As he carefully places one foot in front of the other, his arms are outstretched for balance. Each tiny movement to one side is counterbalanced by a movement to the other. Even when he pauses for a moment in the middle of the wire, seemingly motionless, his muscles are constantly reacting to keep him poised, thereby avoiding a plunge.

Like the tightrope walker, a healthy immune system is constantly doing a balancing act. As one of the most complex systems in the body, it must continually make intricate adaptations and adjustments to preserve many fine balances that are essential to our health. Even when all appears to be relatively quiet on the surface, on a cellular level the immune system is ceaselessly busy monitoring the balance maintained by cell membranes, adjusting the positive/negative charges of cells, maintaining the optimal acid/base environment, and stimulating and shutting off immune responses.

With all this activity, the immune system clearly is not in stasis (resting equilibrium). Instead, we say it is maintaining homeostasis (stability among opposing forces). Because of the dynamic nature of the immune system—and to avoid confusion over the term *stasis*—some people refer to immune system equilibrium as *homeodynamics*. Whichever term you prefer, the idea is that any one delicate balance can be thrown off, either by an excess or a deficit. Sometimes this leads to a cascade of events that trigger further imbalances. When the immune system becomes unbalanced, symptoms can develop.

One of the immune system's jobs is to protect us from foreign invaders. Due to the fact that we live in a world full of viruses, bacteria, fungi, and parasites, the immune system must be constantly vigilant in protecting us. A healthy immune system is able to react appropriately to foreign invaders—that is, to fight them, to neutralize them, and to return to its balanced state. An unbalanced immune system may not respond appropriately.

All incorrect immune responses can be attributed either to *overreaction* (for example, a response that begins appropriately but never shuts off) or *underreaction* (for example, the correct immune response never occurs). Immune overreaction and underreaction will be a constant theme throughout this book because proper immune system balance is vital for good health.

SELF/NOT-SELF

Friendly fire is the oxymoron used to describe gunfire or shelling that hits one's own soldiers in error. Obviously, this is a big mistake. When you're in the killing business, you need to spare your allies.

Similarly, the immune system needs to be able to correctly determine friend from foe, or "self" from "not-self." The scope and complexity of this task are staggering to contemplate. First of all, there are billions of cells within the body that need to be recognized and protected. In addition, there are thousands of substances (called *antigens*) that can provoke a detectable immune response. Some antigens are structurally very similar to "good" cells. Indeed, cellular mimicry is one of the ways in which viruses attempt to escape detection by the ever alert immune system.

That all-important line between self and not-self is not always sharp. *Exogenous* materials are those that enter the body from the outside. To complicate the immune system's job, some exogenous substances are friendly outsiders (for example, nutrients), while others are hostile (for example, viruses).

Endogenous materials are those that are normal inhabitants of the body or normal products of our own metabolism. Again, some are good (for example, tissue cells, or the beneficial bacteria that inhabit the intestines), while others are bad (for example, damaged or mutated cells).

The immune system maintains a *zone of tolerance* for beneficial cells, and most of the time, it does an astoundingly precise job of correctly determining what to tolerate and what to attack. However, sometimes the immune system gets confused. Problems with recognition can underlie both immune underreaction and immune overreaction. If the immune system fails to detect a threat, it will not initiate an appropriate response. This is how cancer cells escape immune surveillance and take hold in the body. Conversely, sometimes the immune system mistakes self cells as a threat and mounts an inappropriate defense. This is the mechanism that underlies autoimmune disorders.

	Internal threat	External threat
Immune overreaction	Overreaction to an internal threat = autoimmune problem	Overreaction to an external threat = allergic reaction
Immune underreaction	Underreaction to an internal threat = cancer	Underreaction to an external threat = infection

The rubric above is a helpful, albeit simplified, version of this concept. Realize that there is some overlap between quadrants—for example, a reaction to a food allergen (such as milk) can provoke an allergic-type reaction that ultimately involves self cells (such as those that line the joints), causing an autoimmune type of problem.

DEFENSE AND REPAIR

In addition to defending us against antigens, the immune system oversees the condition of our cells, tissues, and organs. Every minute of every day, the immune system is busy making repairs to cellular machinery. Some repairs correct the damage caused by the immune system's fight against antigens; other repairs are routine maintenance. Cells grow old and die. They also can be damaged, not only by infectious agents and toxic substances but also by the by-products of naturally occurring metabolic processes. Even when the threats to your health are minimal, your immune system is industriously taking damaged cells out of circulation, repairing cell membranes, cleaning up cellular debris, and helping usher waste products out of the body.

This constant activity takes place without our awareness. In fact, many repairs occur while we are sleeping. One theory holds that sleep is necessary to protect the brain against the cellular damage that occurs during our waking hours. Sleep deprivation actually has been linked to neuronal damage[3]—a powerful argument for getting enough rest!

A healthy immune system runs smoothly, dealing swiftly with intruders or impostors, repairing any damage from minor skirmishes, and scouting for trouble throughout the body.

However, when the immune system is overburdened and under constant attack, the body does not have the time and energy it needs to make repairs and build up its defenses. Imagine a castle that's under attack from four different directions. It's obviously easier to muster a sufficient defense in one location than in several places at once.

When the immune system is overburdened, cellular damage accumulates first, then tissues start to break down, and next organs begin to fail. Picture your kitchen. If you keep

The Illness Spiral

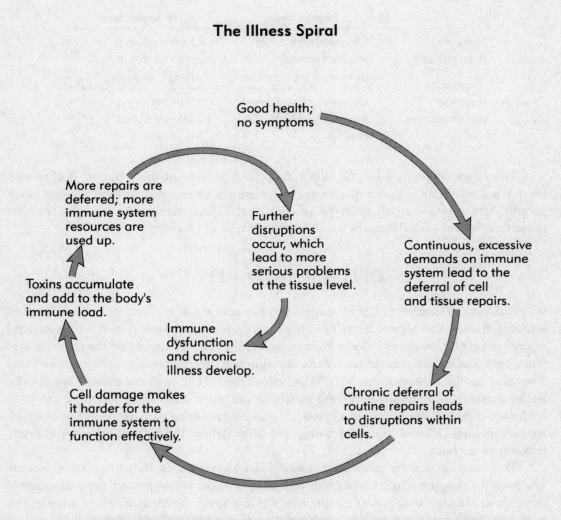

When the immune system is overburdened, it cannot take care of routine repair and cleanup work at the cellular level. This in turn can cause the immune system to function less effectively, and a vicious cycle begins.

cooking and cooking but have no time to do the dishes or take out the garbage, eventually an overwhelming amount of stinking debris will pile up.

The less energy your immune system is required to put into defense, the more it can put into cellular repair. On the other hand, if your immune system is constantly preoccupied with problems—and this can mean a single serious threat or a number of moderate stresses—deficits will build up. Eventually the deficits make it harder for the immune system to do its job. The less effectively it functions, the more problems develop, and the sicker you get. I call this chain of events the Illness Spiral. When the Illness Spiral proceeds unchecked, serious or chronic disorders can result.

In a comprehensive paper entitled "Immune Defense and Repair Systems in Biologic Medicine I,"[4] Russell Jaffe, M.D., Ph.D., an expert in immunology, details the kinds of problems we can expect to occur when the immune system is constantly stressed. They include the buildup of free radicals (and the damage they cause), abnormalities in mucosal permeability, the bioaccumulation of toxins, and disruptions in blood/tissue boundaries. I'll explain all of these problems later. For now, I just want to get you interested in reversing the Illness Spiral.

You have no doubt experienced the one-thing-leads-to-another syndrome, such as when you call a plumber for a routine repair and end up having to replace half your house. The immune system, too, is susceptible to chain reactions. Even a slight imbalance may eventually have huge ramifications. For example, when I first met my patient Stuart, he had been feeling lousy for so long that he couldn't remember when he had last felt well. He complained of achiness and fatigue and told me he was "too young to feel like an old man." He'd had to cut back on his activities, and his job performance was starting to slip. His wife was concerned and, because Stuart didn't seem to be taking any action, had actually made Stuart's appointment herself.

Stuart and his wife both had busy schedules and often ate on the run. I believe that Stuart's problems originally started with his poor diet. For many years he ate too much junk food, resulting in a chronic deficit of nutrients and antioxidants (antioxidants will be discussed in Chapter 4). Because his body did not have the resources it needed to keep up with routine repairs, oxidative damage started to accumulate. Eventually the lining of Stuart's gastrointestinal (GI) tract became irritated, and this in turn led to malabsorption problems. This meant that although Stuart continued to eat, his body was absorbing even fewer nutrients than before, which, as you can imagine, further contributed to his declining health. Eventually Stuart started to experience food allergies and other symptoms associated with chronic GI upset, including bloating and discomfort.

At this point we took firm steps to reverse Stuart's Illness Spiral, including a healthy diet, intravenous nutrients to bypass his ailing intestines and to promote the healing process, antioxidant supplements, and additional nutrients to support the cells of his digestive tract. In time Stuart found his way back to health again—and he has learned how to maintain his good health so successfully that I seldom see him anymore.

IMMUNE REGULATION

A healthy immune system regulates itself at appropriate levels. When an immune response is necessary, it springs into action. After the threat has been eliminated, the immune response shuts down. However, occasionally the immune system fails to regulate its responses appropriately, resulting in immune dysfunction.

An underactive immune system either fails to respond when it should or makes an inadequate response. A downregulated immune system is associated with chronic or recurrent infections, cancer, AIDS, and other types of immune deficiency.

An overactive immune system either fails to turn off an appropriate response or makes a hypersensitive response that really isn't necessary. An upregulated immune system is associated with allergies, autoimmune disorders, and a phenomenon known as immune dysregulation—another condition that is not acknowledged by most physicians.

With allergies, the immune system reacts to certain substances that are usually benign. Allergies are very individual, which is why one person may get hives from strawberries while another is sneezing from grass pollen (and another is not troubled by either).

With autoimmune disorders, the immune system reacts inappropriately to self cells. Persistent immune overreaction underlies illnesses like rheumatoid arthritis (in which the immune system attacks the joints) and multiple sclerosis (in which the immune system attacks the nerves).

Sometimes the immune system makes an appropriate response to an antigen—for example, a virus—but then when the fight should be terminated, the appropriate signals do not occur and the reaction persists. More and more antibodies are produced, even though they are no longer needed. It's as if the switch is turned on and the ability to turn the switch off is lost. My patients will say, "I got the flu (or hepatitis or mononucleosis or whatever) and never really felt well again after that." Immune dysregulation can actually cause flu-like symptoms because some of the substances produced by the immune system (which is furiously working overtime) are inflammatory.

When there is impaired host defense, the immune system needs to be strengthened and stimulated. When there is hyperreactivity, the immune system needs to be calmed down. And as if this weren't tricky enough, there are some situations in which the immune system is both down- and upregulated *at the same time.* For example, the Lyme bacterium can cause both immune suppression and autoimmune-type problems simultaneously.

When my patients have complex, chronic health problems involving immune dysfunction, we reverse the Illness Spiral one step at a time—like peeling off the layers of an onion. There is no one "magic bullet" that will eliminate all of the symptoms and problems that have developed over time. In my experience, the traditional one illness/one cure approach to restoring health in these complex, chronic cases is simplistic and shortsighted. This is why the Immune System Empowerment Program, as you will see, is a multilevel approach to strengthening and supporting the immune system so that the body's many delicate balances can be restored.

COMMONLY ASKED QUESTION NO. 3:

Just what is AIDS, anyway?

AIDS stands for *a*cquired *i*mmune *d*eficiency *s*yndrome—"acquired" meaning you aren't born with it, "immune deficiency" meaning an underactive immune system, and "syndrome" for the complex of symptoms that, taken together, present a clinical picture of AIDS. Without a functioning immune system, we are susceptible to a multitude of health problems that eventually are fatal. There is no known absolute cure for AIDS.

AIDS is thought to be caused by the human immunodeficiency virus (HIV), which affects helper T cells (which are explained in the next chapter). Many people believe that HIV is not the whole story, however. It's possible that HIV is lethal only in the presence of an immune system that is already overburdened. This could explain why some people who contract the AIDS virus die rapidly, while others live for many years without problematic symptoms.

ᕳᕲᕩ

DETOXIFICATION

When Antonio Benedi got the flu in February 1993, he took the pain reliever Tylenol Extra Strength in recommended doses. After taking the drug for several days, he slipped into a coma. At the hospital, it was discovered that he had sustained acute liver damage, and days later he received a liver transplant.

What happened? Although inconsistent reports appeared in the press, it appears that Mr. Benedi was accustomed to drinking wine at dinner. What do Tylenol and wine have in common? They are both processed in the body by the liver. Whether or not Mr. Benedi both drank wine and took Tylenol during his illness is not completely clear, but in any event, Mr. Benedi sued Johnson and Johnson, makers of Tylenol. His lawyers said that McNeil Consumer Products was aware as early as 1977 that people who consumed alcohol could suffer liver damage if they simultaneously took Tylenol, even in ordinary doses.[5] They said they had found evidence that sixteen people had died in this manner,[6] and argued that Tylenol lacked appropriate warnings on the package against drinking alcohol.

A federal jury awarded Mr. Benedi $8.8 million. Johnson and Johnson said the verdict would be appealed, and that Mr. Benedi's liver damage was caused by a preexisting viral infection.

Tylenol is made of acetaminophen, which is generally considered a safe drug. Not everyone who takes Tylenol and drinks wine is going to slip into a coma. However, Mr. Benedi's case interests me because it is clear that *something* overwhelmed his liver, and the liver is the organ primarily responsible for the biotransformation of toxins in the body. That is, the liver breaks toxins down into substances the body can eliminate.

Technically detoxification is not an immune system function. However, toxins greatly affect immunocompetence. Every day we are exposed to a multitude of *xenobiotics* (chemical compounds that are not-self). *Endotoxins* are internally arising and include harmful by-products produced by internal metabolic processes and toxins produced by bacteria in the gut. *Exotoxins* enter the body from outside and include drugs, microbes, chemicals, and pollutants in our air, water, and food.

A large part of the Immune System Empowerment Program is devoted to minimizing our exposure to toxins and to supporting the body's efforts to break down toxins and eliminate them via sweat, feces, urine, and exhaled air. When the normal detoxification pathways are overloaded or blocked, toxins can build up in the body, causing illness. And, as we've already seen, an accumulation of toxins makes the immune system function less effectively, which in turn leads to . . . you guessed it: a greater accumulation of toxins.

THE IMMUNE SYSTEM KETTLE

In his book *Spontaneous Healing,* Andrew Weil, M.D., compares the human body to a river.[7] You can keep dumping sludge and pollutants into a river and, to a certain extent, the river will be able to detoxify itself with its own healing mechanisms—for example, turbulence will oxygenate the water, sunlight will purify it, and plants will help remove contaminants. But if you keep burdening the river with toxins, eventually its flow patterns will change, the sunlight will no longer penetrate the murk, and the helpful plants will die. When its purification mechanisms are overwhelmed, the river loses its ability to heal itself.

However, if you stop polluting the river, eventually the levels of contaminants will drop to a level at which the natural healing mechanisms start to function again. If its burden is lessened, the river can be revived.

The body, too, has its own natural healing abilities with which it handles the stresses and strains of daily life. When these systems are overwhelmed, symptoms develop. When the burdens are lifted, health can be restored.

I often tell my patients to picture their immune system as a kettle. If you keep filling it with water, eventually it will overflow. The top of the kettle is your immune threshold. As your immune load builds up within the kettle, problems develop. When your immune load

The Immune System Kettle

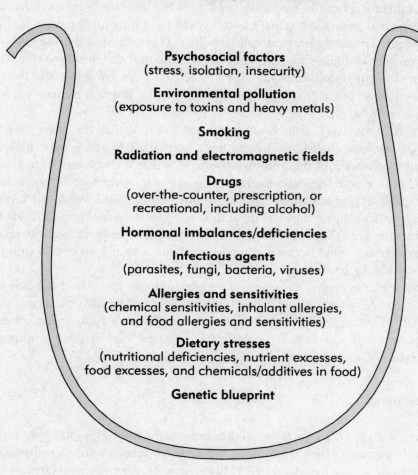

Psychosocial factors
(stress, isolation, insecurity)

Environmental pollution
(exposure to toxins and heavy metals)

Smoking

Radiation and electromagnetic fields

Drugs
(over-the-counter, prescription, or
recreational, including alcohol)

Hormonal imbalances/deficiencies

Infectious agents
(parasites, fungi, bacteria, viruses)

Allergies and sensitivities
(chemical sensitivities, inhalant allergies,
and food allergies and sensitivities)

Dietary stresses
(nutritional deficiencies, nutrient excesses,
food excesses, and chemicals/additives in food)

Genetic blueprint

Any one part of our immune system load can put us "over the top" of the kettle if our accumulated burden is high. On the other hand, if we keep our total immune system load low in the kettle, we are in a better position to accommodate an unexpected immune system challenge.

goes over the top, you get sick. Because the immune system is resilient, it can meet many challenges, but there is a limit to how many problems the immune system can handle all at once. The "straw that breaks the camel's back" could be a stressful situation, a virus, or a smoke-filled room, depending on your vulnerabilities. When stress is the last straw—which is common—people (including doctors) tend to overlook the other immune challenges that have contributed to the overall immune load and set the stage for going over the immune threshold. When these other challenges are eliminated, the immune system has a greater capacity for tolerating stress.

There are different layers in the Immune System Kettle, and all the layers are not of the same size. Your immune challenges depend upon your lifestyle and genetic makeup. The best part about the concept of the immune threshold is that it empowers us to consciously lower the level of our immune load. A certain amount of immune load is unavoidable, but all of us are capable of bringing down the level of our immune load within the kettle.

One of my patients has symptoms from food allergies only during pollen season when his inhalant allergies are at their worst. At other times of the year he can eat the same foods without any symptoms. Why? Because allergies are additive. When his overall immune load is lower in the kettle, he has fewer symptoms.

The same principle applies to groups of people. Suppose you attend a family reunion, and somebody shows up with a cold. Those members of your family who have a weakened immune system will have lowered resistance. Some might get a runny nose, others might even get pneumonia. If you have a relatively low immune load in your Immune System Kettle, you might not get sick at all.

Genetic Blueprint

The illustration shows all the layers of the Immune System Kettle sitting on top of your genes (genetic blueprint), which determine your personal predispositions and provide your underlying immune strength or weakness. This genetic blueprint is individual to you, and you have little control over it.

Biochemical individuality is absolutely fascinating to me. Each of us is biochemically unique, which explains why our reactions to both immune challenges and medical treatments are not completely predictable. If you were to expose a group of people to, say, a harmful pesticide, one person might develop sinusitis, another might get asthma, a third might get neuritis (inflammation of a nerve)—and the last person might show no symptoms at all.

Certain people have a stronger genetic immune constitution, which probably accounts for their innate resistance to certain infections or their ability to bounce back faster from illness than other people. These lucky individuals can tolerate a larger accumulation of immune system challenges, but they, too, have an immune threshold that can be surpassed.

Biochemical individuality also explains why some people are predisposed to certain illnesses. Your family history is extremely relevant to your health. Hereditary illnesses are passed directly from generation to generation and in some cases can be traced back hundreds of years. Family tendencies are a little more vague but account for higher-than-usual incidences of certain illnesses in certain families.

Not everyone has the same nutritional needs, either. Some individuals need more of a particular vitamin, mineral, or enzyme than most people. (This may be related, for example, to the sluggish functioning of a specific enzyme—something that is genetically determined.) Here's one example: People vary widely in their ability to maintain tissue levels of vitamin C. In one study, fifteen subjects were given 10 to 12 milligrams a day of vitamin C (a minimal amount) and observed for signs of vitamin C depletion. Within ten days, four people had drastic declines in leukocyte (white blood cell) ascorbic acid (vitamin C) concentration. At the other end of the spectrum, two people showed no significant drop after seventy days.[8]

Other individuals have inborn intolerances and need to avoid certain substances. For example, newborn babies are routinely tested for phenylketonuria (PKU), a disorder characterized by the inability to process the amino acid phenylalanine. If PKU babies ingest phenylalanine, phenyl ketones will build up in their bodies and cause brain damage. When PKU babies are not given phenylalanine, however, they grow up to be normal adults.

Some people have more sensitivities than others. I have patients with multiple chemical sensitivities who cannot shop in department stores, eat in restaurants, or wear synthetic clothes without having a reaction. These sensitivities may be due in part to genetic predisposition, nutritional deficiencies, chronic yeast infections, or chemical exposure (either long-term or sudden and overwhelming). In any event, people like this have to work harder at lowering their immune load to offset these biochemical sensitivities.

In the future, doctors will consider genetic predispositions more and more as tests improve. I do some biochemical testing, especially for tougher cases, but it's still expensive. Someday, when we are able to determine each individual's biochemical blueprint, people will be able to totally modify their environment (nutrients, enzymes, lifestyle choices, etc.) to match their unique genetic predispositions and needs. Biochemical individuality is discussed in greater depth in Chapter 4, Modern Life and Immune System Overload.

Dietary Stresses

The immune system is extremely sensitive to the body's state of nutrition. Every day the immune system produces billions of new cells, which busily communicate with one another by means of a vast array of biochemical messengers. The functioning of all these cells is profoundly affected by what we eat (and don't eat). The quality of our cellular machinery is only as good as the quality of the "building blocks" the body has to work with.

Chemicals and undesirable additives in food are discussed further in Chapter 4. Nutritional deficiencies, nutrient excesses, and food excesses are discussed in depth in Chapter 5, The Immune Empowering Diet. For now, here is a summary to show you why I am so passionate about nutrition.

Nutritional Deficiencies. Back in 1981, a landmark paper published in *The Journal of the American Medical Association* entitled "Single-Nutrient Effects on Immunologic Function" called attention to nutritionally induced immune problems due to deficits or excesses of many trace elements and single nutrients.[9] Doctors were already aware that generalized malnutrition caused impaired immunocompetence, but the effects of individual nutrients were not as well known. For example, volunteers with experimentally induced deficiency of vitamin B_6 (pyridoxine) showed a reduced antibody response to vaccines, and individuals deficient in vitamin A were observed to have a greater incidence of spontaneous infections. Many individual vitamins, minerals, trace elements, amino acids, and fatty acids were associated with immunologic changes in laboratory animals, pointing to the need for further testing on humans. Happily, we have been constantly adding to our knowledge about the link between nutrition and immunocompetence. The Immune System Empowerment Program includes diet and supplement recommendations to keep your immune system functioning at its optimal level.

Nutrient Excesses. Yes, there can be too much of a good thing. Nutrient excesses are usually the result of taking supplements (although it is possible to eat so many carrots that you develop yellowish skin from the excess beta-carotene!). Some vitamins—such as vitamins A and D, which are fat-soluble—have toxic effects when they are taken in large quantities. Also, because nutrients are used by the body in tandem, an excess of one can lead to a functional deficiency of another. For example, closely linked nutrients need to be balanced, so an excess of one doesn't induce a relative deficiency of the other. This is one of the dangers of self-supplementing, and why I've included guidelines for safe levels of supplements in the Immune System Empowerment Program.

Food Excesses. Modern food excesses—such as overconsumption of caffeine, saturated fats, and refined carbohydrates—are definitely harmful to the immune system. Here's just one example: sugar. America has a giant sweet tooth. We consume 134 pounds of sugar per person per year (about a pound every three days!).[10] Sugar consumption dramatically inhibits immune function. Studies have shown that sugar has an immediate effect on the white blood cells in the bloodstream, reducing their ability to engulf bacteria. Consuming 24 teaspoons of sugar (the amount in, for example, two cans of soda) causes a 92 percent decrease in white blood cell efficiency—an effect that lasts for up to five hours.[11] (By contrast, eating a starch like rice has no effect on immune cells.) It is also worth noting that certain kinds of tumors rely on sugar for their predominant source of energy. When you figure that most people indulge in more than one food excess, you can see how as a nation we are undermining our immunocompetence. Most physicians, by the way, are not going to protect you from sugar. When my father was hospitalized with severe pneumonia, his hospital diet—when he was able to eat again—included pudding, Italian ices, coffee with sugar, frozen yogurt, and other sweetened liquids at a time when he needed optimal nutrition, not a lot of sugar.

Chemicals and Additives in Food. Hormones, antibodies, pesticides, and herbicides all find their way into our food due to the way animals are raised and crops are grown. In addition, processed, packaged foods contain many additives, including colorants, preservatives, and artificial flavorings. Again, let me pick just one example for now: aspartame. A memorandum from the U.S. Department of Health and Human Services reveals that since 1980 the Food and Drug Administration (FDA) has received over seven thousand complaints of adverse reactions to aspartame alone. Over ninety different symptoms were reported, including headaches, seizures, difficulty breathing, and mood changes.[12] At a recent American College for the Advancement of Medicine conference, one doctor devoted his entire lecture to the hazards of aspartame. According to one study, aspartame consumption in the United States as of 1991 was 17 pounds per person,[13] so we clearly are not going out of our way to avoid troublesome additives.

The basic American diet is not doing our immune system any favors. Survey results published in 1995 show that of 23,699 American adults contacted during a random telephone survey, only about one in five reported that they'd eaten the recommended five or more servings of fruits and vegetables a day,[14] even though a diet high in fruits and vegetables is associated with a reduced risk of heart disease and cancer.

Another earlier survey showed that *not one* of the 21,500 Americans contacted had consumed 100 percent of the government's recommended daily allowances (RDAs) for calcium, iron, and vitamins A, B_1, B_2, B_6, B_{12}, and C.[15] I find this especially distressing because I believe the RDAs are too low in the first place. Developed as minimum amounts necessary to prevent deficiency diseases in mass populations, the RDAs do not allow for individual biochemical needs and do not take into account the fact that by the time deficiency diseases appear, many of the body's major systems have broken down. Most people probably need much higher amounts than the RDA of at least one of these nutrients, and probably several of them.

Eating right is one of the simplest, most effective, and most worthwhile steps we can take to strengthen our immune system, which is why I've included guidelines for the Immune Empowering Diet in the Immune System Empowerment Program.

Allergies and Sensitivities

I've touched on allergies and sensitivities briefly already. We are susceptible to food allergies and sensitivities (reactions to substances we ingest), inhalant allergies (reactions to particles we breathe in, such as dust, dust mites, mold, pollen, and animal dander), and chemical sensitivities (reactions to chemicals, such as gas fumes, perfume, etc.). Signs and symptoms of allergies and sensitivities can be highly obvious, or subtle and difficult to detect. The best way to deal with an allergy or sensitivity is to avoid whatever it is that gives you trouble. For many ubiquitous allergens, that may be very difficult, so it becomes even more imperative to adopt a program that will strengthen your immune system and lower your immune load as much as possible. Minimizing exposure to problematic substances is discussed in Chapter 4, Modern Life and Immune System Overload.

Infectious Agents

These include viruses, bacteria, fungi (yeast), and parasites. An associated immune burden is the toxic by-products of these infectious agents. Some people take rather extreme precautions against contamination, such as the microbiologist who has been known to douse toilet seats with alcohol and set them on fire to sterilize them. Obviously, this is highly unusual behavior, but there are many more practical precautions you can take, which will be discussed in Chapter 4.

Hormonal Imbalances and Deficiencies

Hormones are released into the bloodstream by various organs and glands and can affect virtually every cell in the body, so hormone imbalances and deficiencies can cause significant problems. We are finding that hormones play a role in many more disorders than was previously believed. A doctor is needed to diagnose and correct hormonal imbalances; hormone therapy is discussed in Chapter 10, Immune System Super Boosters.

Drugs

Drugs of all types—over-the-counter, recreational (including alcohol), and prescription—can contribute to our immune load. Some can have minor side effects, some can cause organ strain, some can cause death. The fact that a medication is available over the counter (without a prescription) does not mean it is harmless. Being prescribed by a physician doesn't make a medication harmless, either. Drugs are discussed further in Chapter 4.

It worries me that conventional medicine tends to overlook the body's natural healing abilities, and even to override them. In one study of breast cancer patients, there was a 71.6 percent postoperative reduction in natural killer cell function. With chemotherapy around the time of surgery, natural killer cell function dropped 95.7 percent. These statistics led the researchers to conclude that conventional treatment for breast cancer significantly impairs the natural immune system and may place women at an increased risk of metastases.[16]

COMMONLY ASKED QUESTION NO. 4:

What is meant by iatrogenic?

Conventional medicine can make you well, but it also truly can make you sick. Each year an estimated 300,000 Americans die from complications due to drugs or surgery.[17] Iatrogenic, or doctor-caused, problems also include thousands of nonfatal complications.

We are still dealing with the long-term ramifications of diethylstilbestrol (DES), which was prescribed for pregnant women to avoid miscarriage and ended up causing congenital abnormalities in their babies. There are many prescriptions I would rather write only as a last resort, including those for synthetic estrogens and immune-suppressing steroids. I prefer to prescribe effective, safer alternatives such as natural estrogens and progesterone or high doses of anti-inflammatory immunoactive nutrients.

I am not advocating throwing conventional medicine out the window. I do think we all need to be aware that there are steps we can take to support the immune system either before or while using traditional medical approaches. Yet for years when I advised my cancer patients to take certain immune system boosters such as vitamin C and beta-carotene with their chemotherapy (although not immediately before, during, or immediately after), oncologists told them these nutrients would protect the cancer and make treatment less effective. This myth finally has been exposed. In truth, these nutrients selectively protect the body's normal cells, thereby potentiating the killing of the tumor cells.

Radiation and Electromagnetic Fields

Radiation takes many forms. We are exposed to high-energy radiation from sun rays, radiation therapy, X rays, and certain diagnostic medical tests. It is well known that this type of radiation can cause cellular damage, and that its effects are cumulative. Examples of low-energy radiation include microwaves, transmissions from radio and television stations, and electromagnetic fields generated by computer monitors and electric blankets. The health consequences of low-frequency radiation are less clear, but this type of energy may also be problematic. Minimizing unnecessary exposure to all forms of radiation is discussed in Chapter 4.

Smoking

You don't need me to tell you that smoking is unhealthy, and that it introduces poisons into the body and causes cancer. I tell my patients it is frequently the single worst immune insult that they can do to themselves, especially over the long term. You might not be aware, however, of the remainder of the long list of side effects associated with smoking (and secondhand smoke), which I'll tell you about in Chapter 4. Here all you need to know is that every day over a thousand American smokers die from their addiction—roughly the equivalent of three fully loaded jumbo jets crashing each and every day of the year.[18]

Environmental Pollution

Poisons that have been released into the environment include industrial smoke and other industrial wastes, pesticides, herbicides, and chemical fertilizers. These toxins contaminate our food, water, and air, not to mention our offices, workplaces, homes, lawns, and gardens. In 1940, the birth of the petrochemical era, 1 billion pounds of petrochemicals were manufactured that had never existed before. By the late 1980s, this figure had risen to over 500 billion pounds.[19] Where do you think all these chemicals are going?

Heavy metals that find their way into the body include lead, mercury, cadmium, arsenic, nickel, and aluminum. Heavy metals can inhibit immune function by competing (often preferentially) with other minerals on the cellular level. When a heavy metal binds with an enzyme, the enzyme can no longer do its job.

Pollution affects every system of the body. Petrochemicals can cause a wide variety of illnesses, including cancer and neurological problems. Avoiding exposure to toxins will be covered in Chapter 4.

Psychosocial Factors

Stress, loneliness, isolation, depression, and anxiety suppress the immune system. It is well documented that feelings of hopelessness, helplessness, and insecurity contribute to poor health. The ability of the immune system to function effectively is profoundly influenced by our thoughts, feelings, and emotions, which are translated by the body into chemicals that have measurable, observable effects. The study of the mind/body connection, called *psychoneuroimmunology*, is discussed in Chapter 8, Stress Management Techniques.

We are a stressed-out nation. The Institute of Stress reported that in 1994, up to 90 percent of all visits to primary care physicians were stress related.[20] Family, financial, and work-related stresses contribute to all kinds of modern maladies, including back pain, insomnia, substance abuse, and headaches.

I always advocate reducing stress as much as possible, but as a doctor I also see many people who are temporarily in very distressing situations. Stress frequently becomes a very large part of the Immune System Kettle and very often it moves us over our immune threshold and into an overtly symptomatic state. Some of my patients have already been told by other health care practitioners that their symptoms are caused by stress. However, we find that when they lower their total immune load, they can tolerate a fairly large amount of stress without physical symptoms.

There's more good news, as well: joy, love, and contentment bolster the immune system. In his book *Anatomy of an Illness*, Norman Cousins describes how he cured himself of a potentially fatal disease with a positive attitude and lots of laughter. I am not suggesting that putting on a false happy face is curative. I do believe, however, that nurturing our emotional selves nurtures our physical selves, and that having fun and enjoying life, as well as loving oneself and sharing love, all contribute to immune health.

CELLULAR SELF-DEFENSE

I don't want you to come away from this chapter feeling overwhelmed. Instead, I hope I've persuaded you to embark on the Immune System Empowerment Program. There is a great deal we can do to help our immune system help us, including eating well, taking supplements, minimizing our exposure to troublesome substances, and taking advantage of natural treatments and therapies that will bring our immune system back into balance. By providing our immune system with what it needs and protecting it from what it doesn't, we can greatly improve our powers of cellular self-defense.

ᏆᏔᎯ   *JOHN'S STORY*

Life is change. Our internal landscape is never the same from minute to minute. The body has an almost magical ability to transform what it *has* into what it *needs*. For example, we metabolize food to release energy, transduce thoughts and sensations into biochemical messengers, and transform toxins into less harmful waste products.

The human body is always active, even when it is at rest. Day in and day out, cells are being constructed and torn apart, tissues are being built up and torn down, and myriad substances are synthesized and secreted. Newly invading microorganisms are being detected and destroyed, even as old enemies are recognized and challenged.

When the immune system is overburdened, it cannot adequately participate in all of the body's processes of defense and repair, and our health declines. My patient John is a good example of a very sick individual whose Immune System Kettle was simply overflowing. One by one we worked on reducing the layers in his kettle until he reached the point where his immune system could rebalance. For John, the one diagnosis/one treatment medical model was totally inadequate.

At the time of his first visit to my office, John was fifty-one years old. He'd been feeling unwell for five years, and recently his symptoms had been worsening. He had numbness and tingling in his hands and feet, muscle weakness, cold feet, persistent fatigue, and stiffness in all his joints. He also had chronic gut problems, including gastritis and diverticulosis, and he was highly stressed and anxious about his health. John also was depressed, although he made an effort to joke with me and my staff. His wife indicated that sometimes John's pain and despair were so great that he would weep in private. It was not immediately clear to me whether his depression was physiological in origin—part of his illness—or whether it was purely psychological.

I asked John about his medical history and found that he had received some kind of insect bite—he wasn't sure what it was—five years before, and that his symptoms had started shortly after that. His health had been steadily worsening, starting with a stiff neck, headaches, and joint pains, and progressing to difficulty concentrating, some problems with balance, episodes of blurry vision, feeling woozy, and vertigo.

John had consulted numerous medical doctors and had been through many diagnostic tests, including an MRI of his head and a CT scan of his sinuses. All his test results were negative except for some that indicated immune irregularities (he tested positive for anticardiolipin antibody and antinuclear antibody, both signs of autoimmune problems). John's previous doctors had ruled out lupus, but no one had been able to tell him what was wrong with him. Each new symptom scared him, and he was worried that he was trapped in a downward spiral with no apparent end.

I learned from John that he had just been informed by his previous doctor that his Lyme titer test was positive. Lyme definitely could have been causing many of John's symptoms, including the immune dysfunction, but after three weeks of amoxicillin he did not feel significantly better. However, when he was off the antibiotics, he felt worse. When another Lyme titer came back positive, we moved on to combination therapy (two oral antibiotics at once), but John developed a lot of gastrointestinal upset, so we discontinued this approach.

We ran further Lyme tests on John, and his titer again came back positive. Even though only four bands of his Western blot test came back positive (not the five bands that the Centers for Disease Control considers indisputable evidence), I felt confident that John had chronic Lyme disease.

I started John on intravenous antibiotics, but he made a very slow clinical response and also developed a "drug rash." I switched him to a different intravenous antibiotic. After eleven weeks, he showed noticeable overall improvement (by his estimate, he felt 50 percent better), but still he had persistent fatigue, achiness, stiffness, and coldness. It now seemed clear to me that he had other problems as well as Lyme disease that were preventing him from recovering fully.

John's body temperature was subnormal, and some of his other symptoms were consistent with an underactive thyroid, so I placed him on a small amount of natural dessicated thyroid. This was helpful, but still he felt unwell.

The more I talked with John, the more I felt that it was essential that he receive some stress management counseling. John was very pleasant and likable, and not the kind of person to take out his problems on others, but privately he was constantly worried and agitated about his health. John consulted the stress management specialist in our office and began to use relaxation techniques daily, but he still was having a great deal of trouble accepting his illness and the limitations that being sick placed upon him. He wanted to go back in time and be able to do everything just as he used to, and he did not want to accept the fact that he was ill. Because he could not bring himself to accept his illness, his ongoing health problems did not get any easier to bear.

Ultimately, John was hospitalized for depression and mental confusion. In the hospital he was started on Effexor, an antidepressant, which was definitely helpful. He stopped obsessing over his every symptom and finally recognized the impact of his emotional upsets on his well-being. He left the hospital less depressed . . . but still not healthy.

The Lyme antibody blood tests that John received in the hospital came back negative. At this point we also ran a Lyme urine antigen test (this is used to detect actual fragments of Lyme spirochetes in the urine, as opposed to antibodies in the blood). The results were negative, so, in light of his negative test results and clinical situation, I felt he no longer had an active Lyme infection. However, he was still experiencing pressure in his head and ears, facial pain, burning eyes, a chronic sore throat, muscle aches, joint pains, some dizzy spells, and weakness and fatigue, especially after exertion. Symptoms like these are debilitating for the patient and frustrating for the doctor, for they do not point to any one disorder that can be easily corrected.

Suspecting that John had chronic candidiasis, I started him on the prescription antifungal medication Diflucan. We also did an allergy workup on John and discovered he had multiple food and inhalant allergies, so we instituted changes in his diet as well as environmental changes in his home. I also started John on enzyme-potentiated desensitization (EPD) immunotherapy for food and inhalant allergies.

John was actually relieved to learn that Lyme had accounted for only some of his symptoms, and that there were treatments that would help the rest. As he got control of his allergies, he was able to see a definite correlation between his health (particularly his sinus troubles) and his diet and environment.

To help John's immune system rebalance itself, and to help kill off any residual fungi, bacteria, or viruses in his body, I started him on photo-oxidative therapy. This was extremely helpful, especially with his chronic aches and pains.

To treat John's ongoing gastrointestinal troubles, I recommended nutritional supplements (including high doses of glutamine) and the prescription medication Prilosec. He also undertook a three-week liver detoxification program, which was also very beneficial. Eventually John's gastrointestinal health was so much improved that he was able to discontinue the Prilosec.

John's psychotherapy and stress management techniques were helpful with the mind/body component of his illness. To help him get to sleep at night, I recommended tryptophan capsules. (You may remember that this amino acid was in the news because a tainted batch from a Japanese supplier, sold through health food stores, made some people very sick. At that time, all tryptophan was taken off the market, but today it is available by prescription from specialized compounding pharmacies.) We started to see John come out of himself, with less depression and more motivation. He started feeling better and better for longer periods of time.

At his last visit, John noted that he is "doing more and suffering less." He feels more in control of his health and his life now that he understands what is happening to him. His energy bank account is still depleted and any overexertion exhausts him, but now he recovers more quickly. He also has become more accepting of his limitations. John is still a worrier, but his anxiety has lessened, and the Effexor continues to be helpful. Every day he takes his thyroid medication, a special multivitamin/mineral that is beneficial for people with joint pain, antioxidant supplements, glutamine (for gastrointestinal support), and oral magnesium (to help his circulation and his muscle spasms). He will continue with EPD every two months (at least for the near future) and with the photo-oxidation treatments every three to four weeks as needed.

John's case involved the complicated interplay among many different immune system challenges. Level by level, we were able to reduce the burden in his Immune System Kettle to the point where his downward spiral of worsening symptoms was reversed, and his health most noticeably improved.

Chapter 3

⌒∾⌒

IMMUNOLOGY 101

Our rapidly expanding technology has brought us trips to the
moon, powerful notebook computers, laser surgery and
satellite communications. But in spite of our accomplishments,
we cannot make a baby, or an apple, or even a feather. Life is
far more complex than many people are willing to admit.

—PATRICK QUILLIN
Beating Cancer with Nutrition[1]

The immune system is like the last frontier, even though it lies within ourselves. Every day researchers make new discoveries that contribute to our knowledge of how the immune system operates, yet each breakthrough only deepens the mystery. The immune system is so responsive and so adaptable that the more we learn about it, the more complex it becomes.

Sometimes I ask my patients to think of an immune response as a symphony. Each instrument plays a vital part at its own appropriate time, working in concert (pun intended) with myriad other instruments, all within a great concert hall. If you were to isolate the contribution of the bassoon, or the piccolo, or the double bass, you would learn something of the music, but you would not appreciate the depth and breadth of the fully orchestrated piece.

And so it goes with the immune system. We have isolated different types of immune cells and have even learned how to synthesize biochemical messengers in the laboratory, but we cannot orchestrate a full immune response. Not yet, anyway.

There are times, too, when the immune system's performance is flawed. Imagine a concert in which something goes wrong— the cymbals crash at the wrong moment, or the trumpet blast lasts too long, or the musicians get up and leave one by one. When the immune system misfires, or overreacts, or underreacts, doctors try to compensate for the error until harmony is restored.

Or suppose the concert hall itself is at fault. During the recent renovations of Carnegie Hall in New York, the stage was improperly constructed, which in turn affected the sound of all the instruments. If the foundation of your health is undermined—for example, poorly nourished—the quality of your immune responsiveness will suffer. When the stage upon which your immune responses are conducted—your cellular integrity—is compromised, then the symphony of your response will be affected as well. This seems like common sense, but it is not so obvious to the typical physician, and therefore seldom mentioned to patients.

Happily, we do know a great deal about immunology. I've included the basics in this chapter because I'd like you to have a working knowledge of how the immune system operates before you start your Immune System Empowerment Program in Part II. I think you'll find that the program makes more sense when you understand what processes you are strengthening. Also, after you've read this chapter, you'll understand more of what I'm talking about when I refer to the various components of the immune system and the different problems that can occur. For example, you may want to try some visualization techniques later on. Your understanding of how the immune system operates will help you visualize your cells doing what they need to do.

I realize this may not be the easiest chapter for everyone, so I've tried to make it as user-friendly as possible. If you're finding it hard to get through, take a break, or read the chapter twice—but please do read it.

THE POWER TO HEAL

A healthy immune system is more effective than any drug. It can defeat deadly bacteria, conquer cancer, and even hold the AIDS virus at bay.

Several best-selling books already have been written about those miraculous reversals of disease people call "spontaneous remissions," "remarkable recoveries," or "healing mysteries." Physicians tend not to like these stories on the grounds that they are unscientific and their results are not reproducible. I think we doctors are bothered by these stories for a deeper reason as well. When you're supposed to be healing people, it's difficult to accept that very, very sick patients sometimes fully recover without any help from a doctor whatsoever.

Do these stories touch a vein of insecurity in the doctor, making him or her feel less necessary? Or do they just go against what we doctors were taught in our training: that there is a natural progression of "incurable" illness, and that the inevitable outcome is death? Who knows?

I've thought a lot about what *incurable* really means. It doesn't mean no cure exists. It simply means we don't know what the cure is. Sometimes when you're open to alternative approaches, the incurable becomes curable.

Paradoxically, I've found that many doctors would rather believe in spontaneous healing than in the effectiveness of alternative therapies. Sometimes extremely sick patients come to me who have been seen by traditional medical doctors and told there is nothing more that can be done for them. In some cases, this means living with a debilitating condition. In other cases, this means dying. However, after we utilize some alternative treatments, these patients often progress beautifully. When they return to their original doctor, they are told they had a spontaneous remission.

One of my patients, a young woman in her thirties, had been diagnosed with an unusual and severe type of cancer. She had seen expert oncologists in New York City and had been told her case was hopeless. Few things are more lethal than being told by a doctor that you are going to die. When Audrey consulted me, I recommended that she utilize some alternative therapies, including lots of nutrient support and intensive mind/body work. I knew the spiritual work would be important not only to give Audrey hope, but also to allow her to access the power of her own immune system. She took these approaches very seriously, and for her they were effective. Eventually she went into complete remission. Ten years later, Audrey is counseling cancer patients and teaching them how to use visualization techniques.

That's the great news. The disturbing part is that when Audrey returned to her oncologists, they could see she was well—but rather than acknowledge that alternative therapies had succeeded where they had failed, they backtracked and questioned her original diagnosis. It disturbs me that they did not even ask her what she'd done. What a learning opportunity they missed, and what a lack of appreciation they showed for the power and potential of alternative medicine.

I think remarkable recoveries are tantalizing evidence of the largely untapped power of the immune system. We don't know how these recoveries occur, and we can't will them to happen, but as time moves on we are learning more and more about how to allow a patient's immune system to make previously unheard-of responses.

As we now turn our attention to immune processes, I hope you'll keep in mind that our continuum of knowledge about the immune system stretches from the laboratory-tested and scientifically verifiable to the inexplicable and perhaps even miraculous. Like the smell of lilacs outside, or the thought of a friend in another country, the essential mystery of the immune system is always with us.

FIRST, SOME DEFINITIONS

If you were very tired, and if you knew you absolutely had to wake up at four o'clock in the morning to make a plane, you might set two or even three alarm clocks. If you ignored the first, perhaps the second would do the job. If you slept through the second, the third would surely get you up.

The immune system, too, has backup systems and even overlapping systems to protect your health. The processes involved in an immune response are so interdependent that it is difficult to tease them apart. However, by examining the different aspects of an immune response, we can see where problems develop and how intervention might be helpful.

Nonspecific Immunity

The body's first line of defense is called *nonspecific* or *innate* immunity. There are several maneuvers the body can use against antigens that don't require any specialized information about the antigen's exact molecular structure. All-purpose immune responses of this nature include:

Phagocytosis. *Phagocytes* are cells that eat other cells (including microorganisms such as viruses and bacteria) as well as cellular debris (including old or dead cells). This process is called *phagocytosis*. Like fraternity boys at a beer party, phagocytes are not fussy about brands. Once they recognize an antigen, they'll eat it. Some immune cells need to be told what to do, but phagocytes don't necessarily need any biochemical messengers to be activated. Other immune cells have specific receptors that recognize particular antigens. Phagocytes don't have these receptors, so their effectiveness is wide-ranging. In addition to consuming microorganisms, phagocytes can also release substances called *pyrogens* that cause fever. Some phagocytes circulate in the blood; others reside in tissue.

The Reticulo-endothelial System. This system is made up of tissue-based cells (located in the liver, spleen, and elsewhere) that help to filter and remove debris from the blood, including antibody-coated cells (i.e., immune complexes). The cells of the reticuloendothelial system line the so-called sinusoids of those tissues, which are like small pools of circulating blood. In this way they are constantly exposed to cellular elements and substances in the blood, and thus can perform their valuable function.

Inflammation. When tissue is invaded by a microorganism, or is injured, an inflammatory response kicks in right away. The affected area sends out biochemical distress signals that attract phagocytes. Blood vessels widen and become more permeable, allowing more substances and cells that augment the immune response to flood the tissue. Inflammation is characterized by redness, swelling, and pain.

Complement Proteins. The *complement system* comprises about twenty enzymatic proteins (C1, C2, C3, etc.) that activate each other in serial fashion and circulate in the blood to augment an immune response. The complement cascade is triggered by the surface of an invading organism. Complement enzymes can attack antigens and digest pieces of their cell membrane, causing them to rupture and die. They also attract phagocytes to an area of inflammation and increase the efficiency with which the phagocytes destroy invaders. Somehow complement proteins make foreign invaders more "tasty" for the phagocytes (a process called *opsonization*).

Other Soluble Factors. The immune system is not "hard-wired" like the nervous system, which has interconnected nerve fibers all over the body. Immune cells travel around in body fluids. How do you get a message to a cell that is moving around? With a cellular phone—in this case, a soluble biochemical messenger. The immune system produces many of these substances. Some involve local phone calls between neighboring cells, while others mediate long-distance communications.

Natural Killer Cells. Natural killer cells, also called NK cells, are *cytotoxic* (cell-killing). NK cells scout for infected or malignant cells and destroy them through direct contact. NK cells also can secrete biochemical messengers, which means they probably have an immunoregulatory function. Like phagocytes, NK cells react to antigens without being told what to do by other immune cells. NK cells are not involved with immunologic memory. For them, each antigen is a new challenge.

Specific Immunity

If the body's nonspecific immune responses fail to eliminate an antigen, the next alarm clock goes off. *Specific* immunity—which is also called *acquired* or *adaptive* immunity—is an immune response tailor-made for a particular antigen. Cells are manufactured for the express purpose of destroying a specific microorganism. This is accomplished on two fronts:

- *Cell-mediated immunity* involves activities that immune cells engage in directly. For example, certain immune cells lock onto other cells that are under attack and destroy them. Cell-mediated immunity is an important response against organisms that hide within cells (including many viruses, many fungi, some bacteria, and some parasites).
- *Humoral immunity* depends upon *antibodies* that circulate in body fluids. Antibodies are soluble substances—actually, immune proteins (also called *immunoglobulins*)—that are specifically created to attack a particular antigen. Humoral immunity is an important response against organisms that are present in body fluids (including many bacteria, some viruses, some fungi, and some parasites).

Specific immunity is based on recognition. It requires specialized knowledge about an antigen and takes time to develop.

Long-Term Immunity

Lasting immunity depends upon the long-term survival of memory cells that are sensitized during an immune response. Immunity can be conferred only against a very specific organism. After the body has completed a specialized defense against an infectious agent, it carries a grudge for as long as memory cells live to remember the invader.

COMMONLY ASKED QUESTION NO. 5:

How do vaccinations work?

During *passive immunization,* antibodies are taken from the blood of a person (or animal) who has already been exposed to a particular illness and are injected into someone else. Passive immunity provides short-term protection. If you step on a nail and haven't had a tetanus vaccine, you would receive not only a regular tetanus vaccination but also tetanus immune globulin, which would work immediately to neutralize the bacteria. (The same holds true if you once had a tetanus vaccine, but failed to get a booster shot within the recommended period of time. In this case, your immunity against tetanus may have fallen below protective levels.)

During *active immunization,* the person to be protected is injected with a killed or altered version of an antigen. The immune system's defense against the modified microorganism generates memory cells. If the real antigen ever enters the bloodstream, the memory cells can quickly mediate a specific immune response.

THE BIG PICTURE

The immune system fights its battles on the organ, tissue, and cellular levels. The primary organs of the immune system are the bone marrow and the thymus gland. Immune cells originate in the bone marrow. Some of them go on to be educated or processed in the thymus (which is located behind the sternum). We believe others are further educated by the bone marrow. (More about this in a moment.)

The Lymphatic System

Immune responses are made possible by your *lymphatic system.* Just as the circulatory system includes veins and arteries that carry blood throughout the body, the lymphatic system includes a network of vessels that collect *lymph* from all over the body. Lymph is a milky fluid that consists of water, protein, and immune cells; it is the lifeblood of the immune system. Unlike the circulatory system, which is powered by a beating heart, the lymphatic system depends upon muscle movement and exertion to move lymph through the lymphatic vessels. (Another good reason to exercise!)

Lymph accumulates in the intercellular spaces of body tissues. It is collected by the lymph vessels and transported to *lymph nodes,* small masses of specialized tissue that house certain kinds of immune cells and filter out antigens before draining lymph into the bloodstream. Lymph nodes also help in the production of antibodies. Any time you've experienced "swollen glands," your lymph nodes have been working overtime.

In addition to the lymph nodes, the tonsils, spleen, and Peyer's patches (located in the wall of the small intestine) all contain lymphoid tissue.

The Mucosal Immune System

The *mucosal immune system* comprises our skin and the mucous membranes that line our respiratory tract, gastrointestinal tract, and urogenital tract. These are the body surfaces that come into contact with particles from the outside world and provide protection against invading organisms.

On the outside of us, skin is an impenetrable barrier against infectious agents. On the inside of us, mucous membranes prevent antigens from gaining access to our bloodstream or inner tissues. This type of protection is sometimes referred to as *mechanical immunity.*

The mucosal immune system has several tricks at its disposal. Oil glands in the skin secrete chemicals that are highly toxic to many bacteria. Mucus on the mucous membranes contains substances that can kill bacteria. So do tears in the eyes, saliva in the mouth, and acid in the stomach. Hairs inside the nose filter out dust particles and harmful organisms. (This is why you don't want to be within range of a germ-laden sneeze.) Tiny hairs called *cilia* that line the respiratory tract sweep microbes up and out. (This is why you don't want to be exposed to an antigen-laden cough.)

The gastrointestinal tract has to handle extensive amounts of antigens, which probably explains why it contains almost 50 percent of the body's immune mass.[2] (It has been said that the entire surface area of the GI tract would cover a tennis court.) The gut mucosal system contains all kinds of immune cells, including B cells, T cells, monocytes, macrophages, and plasma cells. It contains more neutrophils and macrophages than all other organs combined.[3] Now let's clarify what all these cells do.

THE IMMUNE SYSTEM UNDER A MICROSCOPE

As I've already said, the immune system is constantly active as it battles bacteria, viruses, parasites, and fungi and clears the body of infected or damaged cells. When you think of the thousands of antigens and the multitude of cellular defects and mutations that can lead to abnormal cells, you see that the immune system's job is highly complex and neverending. There's a cellular team at work to make it happen, and each of the players brings a particular strength or talent to the process. By combining the efforts of many different specialized kinds of cells, the immune system successfully *recognizes* an antigen, *reacts* appropriately to it, and *remembers* how to destroy it should it ever show up again.

The Derivation of White Blood Cells

The body uses white (transparent) blood cells to orchestrate an immune response. White blood cells are bigger than red blood cells, but fewer in number.

Bone marrow produces basic *stem cells* that develop along two different cell lines: *myeloid* stem cells and *lymphoid* stem cells.

• Myeloid stem cells further differentiate into *platelets* (the smallest type of blood cell, important in the formation of blood clots), *red blood cells* (oxygen-carrying cells), *granulocytes* (phagocytic white blood cells that actually can be seen to contain granules), and *monocytes* (other phagocytic white blood cells).

• Lymphoid stem cells further differentiate into *T cell lymphocytes* (which are educated in the thymus) and *B cell lymphocytes* (which we believe are educated in the bone marrow— their place of birth). T cells and B cells work together to coordinate an immune response.

More About the Granulocytes

Granulocytes provide nonspecific protection against microorganisms, mostly by means of phagocytosis. There are three types of granulocytes:

• *Neutrophils* are stored in the bone marrow and are released into the bloodstream as needed. They are like foot soldiers—numerous but lightly armed. Neutrophils are an important part of the inflammatory response. They isolate and ingest bacteria, but because they can't excrete the by-products, they have a limited capacity and die relatively quickly. Dead neutrophils are found in pus. Neutrophils normally make up approximately 56 to 65 percent of circulating white blood cells.

• *Eosinophils,* which are relatively few in number, have a role in allergic reactions and parasitic conditions. Eosinophils make up approximately 1 to 3 percent of circulating white blood cells.

• *Basophils,* which are even scarcer than eosinophils, are responsible for early inflammatory changes. When basophils migrate to the affected tissues during an inflammatory response, they are called *mast cells.* Mast cells generate chemical messengers such as *histamines* that attract other immune cells to the site of the inflammation and help create an escalating immune reaction. (*Antihistamines* modify the severity of an allergic reaction by blocking the release of these inflammation-causing histamines.) Basophils make up approximately less than 1 percent of circulating white blood cells.

The Derivation of Cells

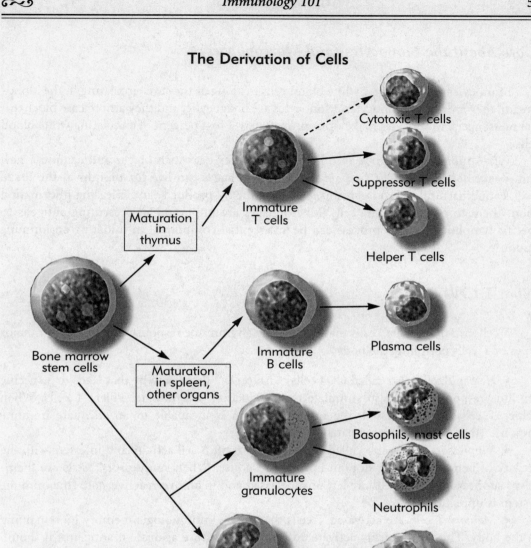

Immune cells are derived from stem cells, but they mature in different ways. The derivation of NK cells (not pictured) is not known for certain at this time, but the majority opinion is that they are derived from cytotoxic T cells. The minority hypothesis is that they derive from a non-T cell substance.

Illustration by Gary Carlson

More About the Monocytes (and Macrophages)

Monocytes are the largest white blood cells. As long as they are circulating in the bloodstream, they are called monocytes. Monocytes are phagocytic, and they also release biochemical messengers. Monocytes make up approximately 2 to 4 percent of circulating white blood cells.

When monocytes migrate into body tissues, they get much bigger and acquire a new name: *macrophage* (literally "large eater"). Macrophages can live for months at the tissue level, eating harmful microorganisms, excreting the by-products, and releasing information about them to other immune cells. Macrophages are important in presenting antigens to specific lymphocytes. This process can be an essential component in initiating an immune response.

What T Cells Do

T cells are the "smart" cells that orchestrate an immune response. There are four major types of T cells patrolling the body:

• *Helper T cells* (also called CD4 cells) turn on the B cell activity that leads to a specific immune response. They also stimulate the production of cytotoxic (killer) T cells. When helper T cells are suppressed, the immune system is incapable of an adequate immune response (that is, it is downregulated).

• *Suppressor T cells* (also called CD8 cells) turn off B cell activity and interfere with the activity of helper T cells to stop an immune response. When suppressor T cells are themselves suppressed, the B cells are left unsupervised and in an overreactive state (the immune system is upregulated).

• *Memory T cells* are activated T cells that create immunologic memory by remaining in the body. They will quickly activate an immune response against an antigen if it should reappear.

• *Cytotoxic (killer) T cells* (another type of CD8 cells) are T cells that kill infected or cancerous cells. Unlike NK cells, cytotoxic T cells have different surface receptors so they recognize specific antigen targets.

As you can see, T cells are vital because they influence the activities of other immune cells. They do this by releasing biochemical messengers to which other cells respond. Actually, the first three subsets of T cells are involved in the regulation of the immune response, and are appropriately called *regulatory T cells.* The cytotoxic T cells are directly involved in cell killing, and are therefore referred to as *effector cells.*

What B Cells Do

B cells tend to cluster near lymph nodes. Because they have surface receptors that react with antigens, they don't need help to be activated. However, B cells generally need help from T cells to mature.

Different B cells have different antigen receptors. When a particular strain of B cell has detected an antigen, it starts to multiply and, with encouragement from helper T cells, the newly proliferated B cells turn into *plasma cells*. Plasma cells are B cells that produce antibodies. Plasma cells are the end of the developmental line for B cells; they do not further differentiate.

Some B cells remain in the body as memory cells. If the antigen dares to show its face in town again, these memory cells will rapidly produce antibodies against it. This is why we get certain illnesses (such as measles and mumps) only once. (We can get a hundred colds, but that's because there are so many different cold-causing viruses. You catch the *same* cold only once.) The response time of memory cells is much quicker than the initial reaction that created them.

Antigens are interested in surviving, so they have devised a way of getting around antibodies: they mutate. A virus that has mutated will require a brand new immune response and the manufacture of new and improved antibodies to combat it. Bacteria, too, can show up in so many different antigenic variations that an infection to one version will not confer immunity to another. (This explains why you can get Lyme disease, for example, more than once.)

The scope and speed of the immune system's activities are staggering. In the time it takes you to read this page, your immune system produces about 10 million new lymphocytes and trillions of new antibody molecules.[4]

More About Antibodies

Antibodies have a characteristic Y shape that is perfectly suited to the job they do. The top of the Y is the antigen-binding site. This part of the antibody molecule is variable—that is, it can be adapted to fit different antigens. (Actually, one arm of the Y includes a variable region, and the other arm includes a hypervariable region.)

The bottom part of the Y is constant. This part of the antibody molecule interacts with receptors on other immune cells. Let's look at an example. Each mast cell has receptors on its surface that lock onto the base of an antibody molecule. This leaves the top part of the Y open and ready to latch on to the antigen for which it was made. When the antibody latches on to the antigen, this causes the mast cell to release its inflammatory/allergic mediators (including histamine, kinins, and slow-reacting substance of anaphylaxis, or SRS-A).

Antibody Structure

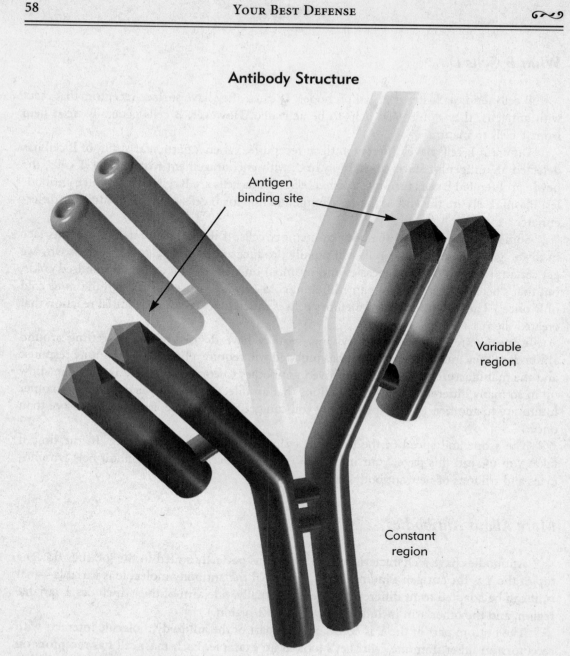

Antigen
binding site

Variable
region

Constant
region

Antibodies have a characteristic Y shape. The top part of the Y can adapt to different antigens, while the bottom part stays constant. This illustration shows two antibodies, with different antigen binding sites.

Illustration by Gary Carlson

Some antibodies adhere to the surface of B cells, while others are sent off to circulate throughout the body. When the top part of a circulating antibody grabs an antigen, the resulting combo-organism is called an *antigen/antibody complex* or *immune complex*. This complex is then either eaten by phagocytes or filtered out of the blood by means of the reticuloendothelial system. Occasionally—for example, when phagocytes are overwhelmed by autoimmune disease—these complexes are deposited in the tissues. This can cause inflammation wherever the complexes accumulate.

Antibodies can also attack antigens directly. Some rip open an antigen's cell membranes, while others cover up an antigen's toxic site. Antibodies also can activate the complement system as well as mediate some cytotoxic reactions.

At any given time, the body has 10 million antibody shapes carried on the surfaces of B cells, ready to do battle with antigens.[5] Only a few of these 10 million antibodies will recognize the shape of a particular antigen, and the fit may not be exact. What happens next is extraordinary. The select B cells with the closest fit undergo mutations to improve the shape of the antibodies on their surface so that they better lock on to the antigen. Subsequent new and improved antibodies will fit the antigen precisely.

Scientists believe that "swollen glands" (enlarged lymph nodes) occur when the immune system makes a frantic burst of B-cell-mutation activity. Only one cell feature mutates: the shape of the antibody on the cell's surface. However, the B cells mutate at a rate that is 10 million times faster than the normal mutation rate for cells. Of the antibody variations that are created, some may fit worse, but others will fit the antigen better. Those that don't fit die off. Those that successfully bind tightly with the antigen move out of the lymph node into the bloodstream and release millions of copies.

There are five main classes of antibodies. Each class is used for a different purpose within the body, so an elevated level of one class of antibody in the blood has certain implications.

- *Immunoglobulin G (IgG)* is the most common type of antibody. IgG antibodies pursue antigens. They are produced later in an immune response, so their presence is a sign of an ongoing or established infection. There are four subclasses of IgG: IgG1, IgG2, IgG3, and IgG4. If one subclass of IgG is deficient, this can create clinical problems, even if the other subclasses are present in normal amounts. In one study of adults with IgG deficiency, the response to hepatitis B or tetanus boosters was blunted even when IgG1 and IgG2 were normal.[6]
- *Immunoglobulin A (IgA)* antibodies protect mucous membranes and are present in saliva, tears, and other secretions. IgA in the blood is called serum IgA. The inside of the gastrointestinal tract is lined with secretory IgA. Few doctors (or patients) appreciate how important this first line of defense is. A lack of adequate secretory IgA is the most common immune deficiency in humans.
- *Immunoglobulin M (IgM)* antibodies also pursue antigens, but their presence is a sign

of a recent infection. IgM is the first antibody that is mobilized following an attack by a new pathogen. It takes a few weeks for IgM levels to peak.

• *Immunoglobulin E (IgE)* antibodies are involved in allergic responses. There are many different types of IgE molecules. The presence of elevated levels of these antibodies in the blood can be an indication of classic IgE-mediated allergies. (Hay fever, eczema, and asthma are all symptoms of classic IgE-mediated allergic reactions.) Another, albeit infrequent, cause of very elevated levels of IgE in the blood is parasites.

• *Immunoglobulin D (IgD)* antibodies are the rarest. We aren't sure what they're for, and we don't routinely test for IgD levels.

It is now possible to generate in the laboratory pure forms of antibodies that are effective against specific antigens. These immunoglobulins, called *monoclonal antibodies,* are produced by means of a process that fuses a normal lymphocyte with a tumor cell. The resulting hybrid cell proliferates like the parent tumor cell, but produces the same antibodies as the parent lymphocyte.

This process is known as *hybridoma technology.* If you want to produce antibodies, you start with a parent B cell. If you want to produce a biochemical messenger secreted by a

COMMONLY ASKED QUESTION NO. 6:

How do antibiotics work?

An antibiotic (literally, "against life") is effective only against bacteria. If you have viral pharyngitis, it may look and feel like strep throat, but an antibiotic won't help. On the other hand, if you have strep throat (caused by the streptococcus bacterium), an antibiotic can help.

Antibiotics buy time while your immune system rallies. Some antibiotics are bacteriocidal, meaning they kill bacteria outright; others are bacteriostatic, meaning they prevent the bacteria from growing or multiplying. Antibiotics do not harm normal cells, and each antibiotic is effective only against specific types of bacteria. Even if you're on antibiotics, your immune system still has to mop up and filter out the debris caused by an infection.

Bacteria believe in survival of the fittest. Short-term use of antibiotics can kill off the less resistant bacteria while leaving the tougher ones intact. If they are allowed to multiply, you'll have a tougher infection to beat. This is why your doctor will insist that you take an antibiotic for the entire recommended time.

T cell, you can use the same process but start with a parent T cell. *Recombinant DNA* technology also permits the production of large amounts of pure proteins. In this process, human genes are placed within bacteria or yeast cells that secrete the desired protein. Both antibodies and biochemical messengers created in this way have been used in clinical trials to treat certain diseases. Because they affect the course of an immune response, they are called *biological response modifiers.* (Biological response modifiers will be discussed in more detail in Chapter 10, Immune System Super Boosters.)

PUTTING IT ALL TOGETHER

Let's suppose a virus enters your body. A macrophage discovers the invader and processes it, then presents the processed antigen to a helper T cell. The helper T cell binds to the macrophage, causing the macrophage to release a biochemical messenger that stimulates other resting T cells. In addition, the helper T cell, now fully activated, releases a different biochemical messenger that stimulates B cells to initiate their part of the immune response.

Some viruses are easier to beat than others. It may take time for your B cells to produce a really effective antibody in large enough amounts to defeat the invader. In the meantime, you may develop symptoms. Your aches and pains and fever are in part the result of your immune system's efforts to conquer the virus.

B cells are like well-trained infantrymen: they'll keep going until somebody tells them not to. After the B cells mount their defense and the virus is controlled, suppressor T cells need to order the B cells to cease and desist. Then your immune system can return to its previous homeostasis, and you feel well again.

Obviously, there are plenty of opportunities for error during this complicated process. Things can and do go wrong during an immune response, just as they can and do go wrong during any event that involves careful coordination, whether it's a performance by a full symphony orchestra or by a string quartet.

BIOCHEMICAL MESSENGERS

The body is constantly sending messages by means of its language of chemicals. The nervous system sends messages via *neurotransmitters;* the endocrine system sends its intercellular messages via *hormones;* and the immune system sends its messages via *cytokines.*

Neurotransmitters, hormones, and cytokines are like people talking in interwoven dialects. Different systems eavesdrop on one another's conversations, so it's difficult to keep a secret within one system. Receptors for neurotransmitters can be found on immune cells, and receptors for cytokines can be found on certain nerve cells. This explains why cytokines produced by the immune system can have neurological effects. It also explains why acupuncture, by enhancing the production of endorphins (natural painkillers), can have immunomodulatory effects. (I'll talk about this in more depth when I discuss the mind/body connection in Chapter 8, Stress Management Techniques.)

The biochemical messengers produced by lymphocytes are called *lymphokines*. Those produced by monocytes are called *monokines*. All cytokines are proteins. Immune cells have "lock and key" receptors that recognize the molecular shapes of these messengers. A particular combination of molecules sends a certain message. Cytokines can act locally (at the point of release) or at a distance, depending where the receptor cells are located.

The discovery of an antigen within the body is like a murder in a small town. Lots of cellular discussion ensues, and the biochemical phone lines are humming as the immune system upregulates, confronts the antigen, and downregulates.

The earliest detected cytokines were named after the effects they caused (for example, T cell growth factor). Eventually, however, researchers discovered that the same biochemical messenger could have different effects, and different biochemical messengers could have related effects. Now new agents are all named *interleukins* to avoid this confusion. As of this writing scientists have identified over thirty interleukins and they're still counting.

Because of technological advances, purified interleukins can now be synthesized in the lab. This has resulted in a tremendous increase in our knowledge about each of these molecules.

Many different biochemical messengers are involved in the communication between cells and in regulating an immune response. Here is a list of some of them:

• The *interferons,* or IFNs, were first identified in 1957. Different types of interferon (alpha, beta, and gamma) are released by different types of immune cells. Interferons can promote antiviral activity (by making uninfected cells resistant to a virus), augment NK cell activity (by stimulating NK cells to kill virally infected cells or tumor cells), and induce fever. Interferons are produced in the early stage of an infection and are the body's first line of defense against many viruses. Instead of directly inactivating viruses, interferon acts against viruses indirectly. The Food and Drug Administration has approved the use of interferons in the treatment of certain diseases such as Type C viral hepatitis and hairy-cell leukemia, and new antiviral, antitumor, and immunoregulatory indications are under study.

• *Colony-stimulating factors,* or CSFs, form a group of cytokines that are important for cell growth and differentiation. These molecules are released by different types of immune cells and fall into three classes roughly based on which types of cells (i.e., neutrophils, eosinophils, and macrophages) are being proliferated. Because they promote the proliferation of these three kinds of cells, CSFs have an important role in regulating their concentrations in the circulation. Interleukin-3 (see below) is a type of CSF. Some CSFs have been produced in the laboratory and approved for treatment.

• *Tumor necrosis factor,* or TNF, is released primarily by activated macrophages. It is cytotoxic to some tumor cells, stimulates the production of lymphokines, and also causes systemic responses such as fever. Blood samples from cancer patients contain materials that inhibit the activity of TNF. (These blocking factors are not found in the blood of patients who don't have cancer.)[7] Synthesized TNF is available.

• *Transfer factor* is a lymphocyte extract taken from a healthy donor and injected into a sick patient. Transfer factor is like an immune "soup" that contains many cytokines capable of stimulating an immune response in the recipient. Under the influence of transfer factor, the recipient's lymphocytes rapidly reproduce, mature, and get to work. This treatment has been used to treat particularly stubborn viruses, including HIV.

For the benefit of curious readers, descriptions of some of the interleukins follow. Clinical use of interleukins is still in the experimental phase, but they are being researched for use in treating specific illnesses.

• *Interleukin-1,* or IL-1, is released primarily by activated macrophages and was initially known as lymphocyte-activating factor (LAF). IL-1 stimulates resting T cells, stimulates the production of other lymphokines that upregulate the immune system, and causes systemic responses such as fever.

• *Interleukin-2,* or IL-2, is released primarily by helper T cells and was initially known as T cell growth factor (TCGF). IL-2 is a potent immunomodulator because it is involved in the proliferation of T cells. IL-2 also induces synthesis of other lymphokines and activates cytotoxic lymphocytes. IL-2 acts by binding with IL-2 receptors on immune cells. Receptors for IL-2 appear on T cells shortly after they are activated. Laboratory-produced IL-2 is currently approved for certain rather experimental treatments.

• *Interleukin-3,* or IL-3, is produced primarily by activated T cells. IL-3 supports the growth of stem cells in bone marrow as well as the growth of mast cells in tissue. IL-3 is known as a multi-CSF because it supports the growth of multiple types of cells. IL-3, too, has been produced in the laboratory.

• *Interleukin-4,* or IL-4, is released by activated T cells, and was initially known as B cell growth factor (BCGF) because it stimulates the production of activated B cells. However, IL-4 also stimulates the proliferation of resting T cells and mast cells and enhances the capabilities of cytotoxic T cells. Laboratory experiments with mice indicate that IL-4 has an effect on the production of certain antibodies (IgG and IgE). Other studies with mice have shown that deliberately lowering IL-4 levels inhibits IgE response.[8] Perhaps IL-4 will therefore be helpful for patients with allergies. Laboratory-produced IL-4 is currently in early phase clinical trials.

• *Interleukin-5,* or IL-5, has colony-stimulating effects on eosinophils, augments killer T cell activity, and increases the expression of IgA antibody.

• *Interleukin-6,* or IL-6, is released by activated T cells and other immune cells, and was initially known as B cell differentiation factor (BCDF). IL-6 induces the differentiation of activated B cells into antibody-secreting plasma cells. It also has an important regulatory role in the growth of myeloid cells. IL-6 and IL-3 work synergistically.

It's easy to see why cytokines are so exciting. They are powerful immunomodulators with a proven ability to influence basic immune system mechanisms. In the future, cytokines will undoubtedly play a larger role in the treatment of many immune-related disorders.

Remember those helper T cells? There are two major subsets of helper T cells, known as TH-1 and TH-2, which produce different lymphokines. TH-1 and TH-2 have distinctly different functions. TH-1 cells produce lymphokines that boost cellular immunity, which is important in an immune response to infection (due to a virus, bacterium, fungus, or protozoa). TH-2 cells play a more significant role in humoral immunity, such as an allergic reaction or an antibody-mediated response to a parasite. A TH-2-mediated response is not always sufficient to clear an infection. Also, in certain circumstances, TH-2 cells can cause the production of autoantibodies, which can be destructive to self cells. Because TH-1 cells are more protective, current research is focused on how to promote the production of TH-1 cells (or selectively inhibit the production of TH-2 cells, causing a relative increase in the TH-1 cell population).

Ironically, increasing levels of cytokines during an immune response can actually make us feel sick. Cytokines can amplify and perpetuate tissue inflammation. IL-2 can cause all the symptoms that we usually associate with the flu, including body aches and general malaise. This means an appropriate immune response to an infection can cause symptoms that look just like the infection itself! Or, if cytokines are not correctly regulated by the immune system, they can be overproduced, and the inappropriate levels of cytokines in the body can produce symptoms. This situation is one of the possible explanations for chronic fatigue immune dysfunction syndrome (CFIDS).

HOW DOES THE IMMUNE SYSTEM RECOGNIZE SELF/NOT-SELF?

We've all had the experience of seeing someone unexpectedly and doing a double take. Is that my neighbor talking to the school principal—or isn't it? Is that my old college roommate waiting for the bus—or isn't it? The difference between human faces can be subtle, and so can the difference between human cells.

All cells of the body have proteins on their surface. One genetic region of chromosome 6, called the *major histocompatibility complex,* or MHC, is responsible for tagging cells by coding these proteins. In humans, the MHC is called the *human leukocyte antigen* system, or HLA. The surface proteins in question are sometimes called *histocompatibility antigens.* These proteins enable the immune system to recognize self cells.

We inherit half of our genes from each parent, so each of us has a unique protein code on the surface of our body cells. Cells without the proper identification are taken in for questioning, so to speak. Virally infected cells that display self proteins sound an alarm and set off an immune system reaction. This understanding of the immune system response is so important, and the implications are so far-reaching, that Peter C. Doherty and Rolf M. Zinkernagel received the 1996 Nobel prize for physiology or medicine for their early work in this area.

The MHC genes are responsible for encoding three classes of molecules. Class I molecules are the proteins found on most nucleated cells and play an important role in recognition processes. Class II molecules are largely limited to cells that present antigens to helper T cells. Class III molecules are soluble proteins released into the blood, including complement enzymes (the proteins that circulate in the blood to augment an immune response). The more we find out about the immune system, the more we realize how much genetic factors influence how an individual responds to an immune challenge. As I've already mentioned (and will talk about again), genetic predispositions can play a critical role in the development of disease. The more we learn about our inborn predispositions, the more we will recognize how to modify our environment (both internal and external) to promote the health of our immune system.

Matching cell surface proteins as closely as possible is important for medical procedures such as bone marrow transplants and tissue transplants. You've undoubtedly heard of "tissue typing," and of searches for appropriate bone marrow donors. A successful transplant depends upon being able to "blindfold" the immune system so it believes the transplanted tissue is self and does not reject it. This in turn depends upon finding tissue that matches the patient's as closely as possible, and also upon giving the patient immunosuppressive drugs to help stave off an immune response.

Recognition Problems

In the previous chapter, I mentioned how crucial it is that the immune system correctly distinguish between self and not-self. Recognition problems can create immune system havoc. Imagine if you mistook a burglar for your uncle Charlie and welcomed him into your home—or if you mistook your uncle Charlie for a burglar and hit him with a baseball bat.

When the immune system fails to detect a threat, an antigen can take hold in the body. If internally arising cancer cells go undetected, you'll end up with cancer. Cancer indicates a downregulated immune system. Pregnancy and cancer are the only two biologic conditions in which foreign tissue is tolerated by the immune system.[9]

Cancer cells often escape immune surveillance. Researchers have had trouble proving the existence of any surface antigens that are unique to tumor cells and not seen on normal cells.[10] It seems that some cancer cells hide behind normal surface antigens.

At the other end of the spectrum is the hypersensitive, or upregulated, immune system. A touchy immune system will set off an allergic response to substances from outside the body that normally are not troublesome (for example, dust that is inhaled or food that is ingested). The mechanism of an allergic reaction is not in itself abnormal, but it is a misplaced immune response—a misfiring, not a malfunction.

Antigenic Mimicry

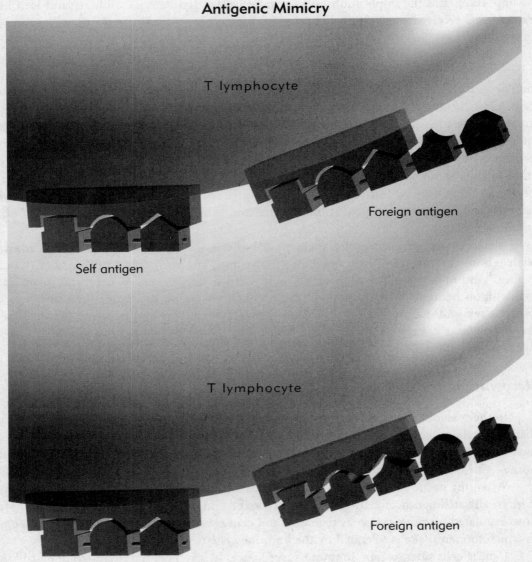

Antigenic mimicry refers to the resemblance between a self protein and an antigen protein. Sometimes certain subunits are not actually identical, but they look very similar (bottom). In other cases, the same sequence occurs within a self protein and a foreign protein. In either situation, a cross-reaction may occur when the immune system mistakes self for not-self.

Illustration by Gary Carlson

Another puzzling form of immune upregulation is autoimmune disorders, which occur when the immune system misidentifies the body's own proteins as antigens and fires up a disease response. The antibodies the body produces against itself are called, not surprisingly, *autoantibodies*. With autoimmune diseases, the body is at war with itself. An autoimmune reaction is persistent, unrestrained, and self-destructive. The resulting inflammation has different names, depending upon where it is located. (When you hear *-itis*, as in colitis or neuritis, that's an indication that some form of inflammation is present.) Examples of autoimmune disorders include multiple sclerosis (in which the sheaths surrounding the nerves are affected), rheumatoid arthritis (joints), myasthenia gravis (muscle cell receptors), Hashimoto's thyroiditis (thyroid), Crohn's disease (colon), diabetes mellitus (pancreas), systemic lupus erythematosus (connective tissue), and scleroderma (skin and internal tissues).

Why would the body mistake self for not-self? Basically, it's an honest mistake. Both antigens are made up of the same building blocks: proteins, carbohydrates, nucleic acids, and lipids. Cell receptors on the reactive immune cells don't lock on to the full chain of building blocks; the process of recognition requires only a small piece of the antigen known as an *epitope* (rhymes with *rope*). This epitope may closely resemble or even match a self antigen. Some pathogens deliberately make selflike antigens as a means of disguise, a process known as *antigenic mimicry*.

Autoimmune disorders can develop when a disruption of the immune system allows B cells to escape suppression. If suppressor T cells are themselves suppressed, or if for some reason suppressor T cells fail to turn off an immune response after the correct amount of antibodies have been produced, there is a loss of feedback regulatory control and an excess of rampaging B cells on the loose, producing excessive antibodies.

Sometimes the body becomes sensitized to its own tissues as a result of illness (or treatment for illness). For example, suppose an infectious agent looks molecularly similar to your own tissue. In the process of making an appropriate immune response to the antigen, your immune system may cross-react inappropriately with your own cells. This dynamic is believed to underlie rheumatic fever, an inflammation of the heart, joints, and nervous system, which can follow strep throat but is not actually caused by streptococcal bacteria. Your immune system makes antibodies to the strep bacteria, and then these antibodies mistakenly react with your heart or joint cells.

This dynamic may also underlie multiple sclerosis (MS), a disease in which immune cells attack the myelin sheath that protects the nerves in the brain and spinal cord. Researchers have discovered that T cells from MS victims react strongly with several infectious organisms, including the herpes simplex virus (which causes cold sores) and the Epstein-Barr virus (which causes mononucleosis).[11] When an autoimmune disorder follows closely on the heels of an infection, it can be difficult to tell where the infection ends and immune upregulation begins. This situation is not uncommon in the later stages of Lyme disease and can contribute to the perplexing nature of this illness.

Abnormal production of cytokines can lead to chaotic immunoregulation, which may result in the production of autoantibodies. Continuous production of cytokines from activated immune cells can lead to chronic inflammation (either localized or systemic). Researchers have determined that abnormal production of IL-6 is frequently associated with autoimmune diseases.

Autoimmune cross-reactivity can also be triggered by foods. For example, research indicates that the protein in cow's milk (bovine serum albumin) closely resembles a molecule on the surface of certain pancreatic cells. This resemblance can set off an autoimmune attack against insulin-producing pancreatic cells that results in insulin-dependent diabetes. In one Australian study, it was found that children who were given baby formula based on cow's milk in the first three months of life were 52 percent more likely to develop insulin-dependent diabetes than children who were not given the cow's milk formula.[12]

Researchers recently determined that psoriasis is a T-cell-initiated disease and used this knowledge to create a treatment. First it was discovered that activated killer T cells were present in psoriasis lesions. Then it was found that the T cells were releasing IL-6, which was making the skin cells overgrow. Both the inflammation and skin cell death of psoriasis were linked to T cells.

Next researchers tried selectively killing the killer T cells. This was possible because killer T cells have IL-2 receptors on their surface. They can be killed off with a drug that hooks diphtheria toxin to IL-2. When the T cells take up the IL-2, they are killed.

After patients received intravenous treatment with this drug, all the pathological changes that define psoriasis were reversed.[13] This treatment is still experimental and expensive, it could have unforeseen side effects, and it's possible that its effects are only temporary. Still, this is more exciting evidence that future treatments for disease will involve manipulating the immune system.

BLOOD/TISSUE BOUNDARIES

It's a little surprising, but the immune system does not have access to every nook and cranny in the body. Certain areas, called *immunologically privileged sites,* are shielded from the immune components of blood and lymph. All of the cells of the body need to receive fresh oxygen and nutrients and need to have their waste products taken away, but this can be accomplished without exposing body tissues to immune cells. (If you're wondering whether or not infectious agents can "hide" in these immunologically privileged sites, the answer is yes, they can.)

Each cell of the body has its own integrity. A cell's membrane keeps the correct substances in and incorrect substances out. Each cell maintains its own cellular environment, preserving its optimal inner levels of potassium, magnesium, calcium, salt, etc. This is accomplished through the work of different cellular pumps that act as gatekeepers (more about this on page 83).

As I mentioned in Chapter 2, a slowdown in the rate of routine repairs can lead to an accumulation of cellular wear and tear. If the appropriate repairs aren't made, changes occur in the material surrounding the cells (the *extracellular scaffolding*). Eventually the barriers that normally separate organs from blood cells and immune cells become compromised. Vessels become abnormally permeable. With an increase in blood/tissue permeability, immune cells and substances start to go where they've never been before.

At first this process can stimulate repair. However, if further deficits build up, inappropriate accessibility increases, and the immune system may react to the cells of this new, uncharted territory. This sets the stage for autoimmune disorders.

MEASURING IMMUNE SYSTEM HEALTH

You will get a sense of the condition of your immune system when you complete the Immune System Profile in the next chapter. As a physician, however, I have diagnostic tests at my disposal that I can use to evaluate specific aspects of my patients' immune system health.

Tests present *part* of the picture of overall health. Some people who feel sick will have normal general test results. Others who feel fine will have results that indicate biochemical abnormalities that will eventually cause problems. The optimal approach is to "catch" a disorder while there is time to reverse the changes—and the earlier in the process, the better.

Almost all doctors use general tests like the complete blood cell count (CBC), which is used to check the number of red blood cells as well as the number and types of white blood cells, and a chem screen, which is used to measure liver function, kidney function, serum blood sugar levels, serum cholesterol levels, serum electrolytes, etc. (I'll discuss tests more in Chapter 12, Getting the Right Diagnosis.)

If the results of these tests are within normal ranges, many physicians tell a patient he or she is healthy, despite the patient's symptoms, which point to the contrary. If the doctor doesn't look further for causes of illness, or ask the right questions, he won't find the answers. Many times I find underlying causes missed by previous doctors because I am willing to be a medical detective and I know where to look for the fingerprints of the perpetrator. I am willing to follow subtle clues into waters that are not routinely navigated by conventional physicians. These clues are often missed by doctors who attempt to fit a patient's history into a diagnostic box.

To determine the condition of your immune system, I could take a sample of your blood and count the number of different kinds of immune cells. The ratio between the number of helper T cells and suppressor T cells is important. A normal cubic centimeter of human blood contains over six hundred helper T cells (but this number depends upon the total white blood cell count and the percentage of lymphocytes). Too few helper T cells could indicate an immune system imbalance. HIV infects helper T cells, so the progression of AIDS is measured with a T cell count that specifically looks at the ratio between CD4 (helper) T cells and CD8 (suppressor) T cells. Too few helper cells will yield a low ratio of helper/suppressor cells. On the other hand, too few suppressor cells—which occurs in upregulated disorders like autoimmune diseases, chronic fatigue immune dysfunction syndrome, and late-stage Lyme disease—will yield an elevated ratio of helper/suppressor cells.

It's sometimes helpful to add specific antibodies to a blood sample. The antibodies bind with the kind of cell you wish to target, making it easier to do a differential count of specific types of lymphocytes (like the CD4/CD8 ratio just mentioned). The general CBC will reveal the overall level of lymphocytes, but this immune profile test will indicate the status of different types. An increase in certain types of immune cells could indicate that the body is responding to an infection. A decrease could signal immunosuppression.

It's also possible to measure the immunoglobulins present in a blood sample or saliva sample. Elevated or decreased levels of different immunoglobulins have different implications. Lower levels of secretory IgA in saliva correlate with decreased immune function—and are associated with higher amounts of stress. (When the stress is decreased, the levels of secretory IgA can increase.) As I've mentioned, an elevated level of IgE in blood can indicate the presence of allergies and, less frequently, parasites. Elevated IgM indicates an early-stage infection, while elevated IgG indicates an older or more established infection. As I mentioned earlier, testing for IgG subclasses (IgG1, IgG2, IgG3, IgG4) can reveal a deficiency of a particular immunoglobulin even though *total* IgG levels are normal. Certain patients with recurrent respiratory infections can have IgG subclass deficiencies. Again, to find answers, you need to know where to look—or at least be willing to look. I can't tell you how many patients (including children) I've seen who have been plagued with recurrent respiratory infections who have never had any kind of workup (either allergic or immune) and whose only treatment has been antibiotic after antibiotic.

Skin tests measure how quickly and how markedly your immune system reacts to an antigen. In the tuberculosis (TB) tine test, inactivated tuberculosis bacteria are injected beneath the skin. A positive reaction indicates you've been exposed to TB and your body has mounted an immune defense. A similar principle applies to allergy testing. A minute amount of a substance is introduced into your skin by a pinprick or, preferably, under the skin *(intradermally)*, as is done in our office. A positive response indicates a sensitivity. These responses differ in that a positive TB wheal is a delayed reaction, whereas a classic allergic response occurs within minutes.

Another way to look at general immune responsiveness is to take a blood sample and mix it in a test tube with an antigen or immune system stimulant. A strong reaction indicates greater immune responsiveness. This test has been used to measure the response of the immune system to grief, which is known to suppress the immune system (more about this in Chapter 8, Stress Management Techniques).

Another test tube procedure is used to measure the activity of NK cells. The key here is not number, but function. Low NK cell function is associated with chronic fatigue syndrome and can be seen with nutritional deficiencies. It's also a risk factor for developing malignancies.

In measuring immune system health, each of these tests represents just part of the picture. It's possible to have a low T cell count, or an elevated IgE level, or a high antibody titer, and to feel completely healthy. It's important to view these kinds of tests not as harbingers of doom, but as tools your doctor can use to decide on the best treatment for you.

IMMUNOLOGICAL UNIQUENESS

What do your last three colds have in common?

You!

It is important to recognize that you are the common denominator of your own mishaps, immune and otherwise. I do not in any way say this to place blame or to make you feel guilty. However, accepting this fact gives you the opportunity for positive change. How to do this? That's what this book is about!

Each individual has a unique genetic makeup that determines everything from hair and eye color to nutrient needs, predisposition to certain illnesses, and yes, immunological responses. However, genes are not destiny. We can devise strategies to help us express those genetic predispositions that are healthy and downplay those that aren't.

People sometimes refer to the kind of medicine I learned in medical school as "modern medicine." I prefer to call it traditional medicine. In traditional medicine, the emphasis is on identifying a condition or classifying a complex of symptoms into a diagnostic box and then applying a standard protocol—usually drugs or surgery. This approach does not take biochemical individuality into account. To me it's just common sense that interventions need to be tailored to meet individual differences between patients.

Recently I spoke at a national conference that included medical speakers at the tops of their fields. Several of the lectures on infectious diseases included slide after slide about drugs and their side effects, and I actually started to get bored. Now, I am a doctor who loves learning and going to conferences, and I am constantly seeking leads that will help me help my patients in their pursuit of wellness, so it isn't really in my nature to be bored. However, all this emphasis solely on drugs just misses the point. There was no discussion about the patient's total clinical picture, which could include allergies and sensitivities, individual nutritional requirements, covert infections, environmental exposures, or even life stresses. Our persistent attempts to fight disease only with new and improved drugs—without harnessing the power of the patient's immune system—seem like going into a war with pop guns.

Truly modern medicine—progressive medicine—is based upon an appreciation of the body's own healing mechanisms and an understanding of the biochemical uniqueness of each one of us. The Immune System Empowerment Program takes these principles and puts them into practice.

ᏄᏉ *MELANIE'S STORY*

Traditional medicine often relies on destructive therapies (for example, antibiotics to kill bacteria, or chemotherapy to kill cancer cells) and the suppression of symptoms. Progressive medicine relies upon preventive therapies as much as possible (for example, antioxidants to prevent free radical damage and optimal nutrition to support immune function) and aims to reverse, not just mask, symptoms.

After enduring the ravages of traditional cancer treatment, Melanie finally said "enough" to her oncologist and came to my office for help. She knew her chances of a full recovery from her type of cancer were not good, but she did not want to spend her last months weakened by destructive cancer treatments of uncertain benefit. Instead, she sought constructive therapies that would enhance her quality of life and perhaps allow her to live longer as well.

Melanie's medical history was harrowing. A formerly healthy nonsmoker, she developed a persistent cough in her twenties that was accompanied by shortness of breath when she exerted herself. Sometimes Melanie would cough up blood. Repeated courses of antibiotics did not help. Inhaled medications cleared up the blood, but her cough persisted. Eventually a chest X ray, CT scan, and bronchoscopy yielded the diagnosis nobody wants to hear: small cell lung cancer. By the time it was detected, the cancer had spread to Melanie's liver.

We will never know why Melanie developed cancer, particularly so young, but she did have some family history of cancer, she had been exposed to secondhand smoke all her life at home and at work, and she lived just blocks from a chemical-tank-cleaning company. An extremely sweet person, Melanie also has the classic nonconfrontational "cancer personality" that often accompanies immune system underreactivity.

Surgery was not an option for Melanie's type of cancer, so she received six months of chemotherapy, after which her cancer went into partial remission. She needed blood transfusions to correct her red blood cell count, but she was happy to have improved.

Several months later, Melanie was hospitalized for a bone marrow transplant. (Bone marrow transplants are usually performed while the patient's cancer is not active.) In this procedure, the patient's immune system is destroyed in order to allow the transplanted bone marrow of a healthy donor (or, in some cases, the patient's own bone marrow that has been treated) to take hold. When the operation is a success, the new marrow reconstructs the patient's immune system and eliminates the cancer.

Three months later, a CT scan of Melanie's lungs and liver revealed no cancer. Soon Melanie was healthy enough to go back to work—a mixed blessing, actually, because her secretarial job was very stressful.

Melanie's next CT scan, scarcely two months after she had resumed working, revealed a recurrence of her cancer in her lungs and liver. A lung biopsy confirmed this diagnosis. At this point, Melanie's situation was not good. She had a virulent type of cancer that had recurred after aggressive treatment; she did not care for her oncologist (whom she regarded as cold and uncaring); and the only therapeutic option she'd been offered was more chemo-therapy, which her oncologist admitted had a low chance of successfully treating her cancer. Melanie refused this therapy and, on the recommendation of one of her friends, came to see me.

I first evaluated Melanie in May. We talked about what she hoped to accomplish with her cancer treatment, and about the importance of the mind/body connection in illness. I tried to get as complete a picture of Melanie as I could, knowing that I was treating not just renegade cancer cells but an entire human being.

Melanie's immune boosting regimen ultimately included:

- An Immune Empowering Diet (Melanie had admitted that she would "eat anything," so it was important for her to concentrate on eating more nutritious food)
- Many different supplements (to correct her nutrient deficiencies and support her im-mune system), including a high-dose multivitamin/mineral with antioxidant-rich algae, high-dose vitamin C powder, high doses of essential fatty acids, high doses of vitamins E and A, high doses of CoQ10, and plenty of bioflavonoids
- Probiotics (such as acidophilus and bifidus), prebiotics (food to support the probiot-ics), and enzymes (for gastrointestinal support)
- Chinese herbs (including astragalus) and mushroom preparations
- Bovine cartilage (which is believed to have anticancer properties)
- Psychotherapy (to help her deal with her feelings)
- Healing visualizations

I also started Melanie on intravenous vitamin C three times a week and placed her on a liver detoxification regimen (including special nutrients) to support her ailing liver. Eventu-ally I switched her to what we call our "tri-ox" treatments, which include intravenous chela-tion, vitamin C, and hydrogen peroxide.

Three weeks after starting on this new immune-empowering regimen, Melanie felt bet-ter and brighter and looked wonderful. She had a smile on her face, her color was better, and my staff was thrilled to see her so full of life. Her quality of life was improved, and she felt she had more control over her health. Her mother, who came to me for her own health concerns after seeing Melanie's dramatic turnaround, gave me the most heartfelt thanks for giving her daughter her life back, even knowing that the severity and aggressive nature of Melanie's cancer would most likely make this time, however long it might be, a precious gift.

A follow-up visit with her oncologist confirmed that Melanie's general state of well-being was very good. On examination, her lungs were clear, her heartbeat was regular, and she had no edema (swelling). Her most recent CT scan, however, showed progressive cancer in all sites. The diagnosis: asymptomatic progressive cancer. The options: continuing with her Immune Empowering Program as long as she remained well, or starting systemic chemotherapy. Melanie again opted not to pursue chemotherapy, and, given her excellent quality of life, her oncologist supported her decision at that time, noting that her cancer was behaving in a "very unusual" way. Despite her sobering CT scan results, Melanie is actually feeling better.

I wish I could say that Melanie was cured of her cancer, but this is not always possible. Sometimes what patients and I are able to achieve together is improvement of their overall health so that they stay as comfortable and as energetic as possible for as long as possible. Paradoxically, some of my sickest patients are also my healthiest. Despite the fact that their immune system can't indefinitely fight off a chronic disease, by devoting themselves to a comprehensive immune-empowering program, they are able to live the life they have remaining productively and, even more important, lovingly and joyfully.

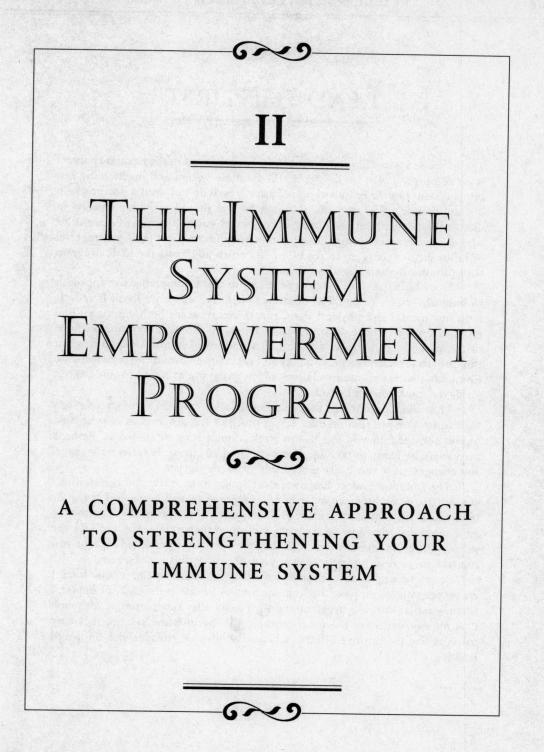

II

THE IMMUNE SYSTEM EMPOWERMENT PROGRAM

A COMPREHENSIVE APPROACH TO STRENGTHENING YOUR IMMUNE SYSTEM

READ THIS FIRST

The Immune System Empowerment Program presented in the next six chapters is an all-purpose plan for bolstering the immune system and maintaining immune system health. People who are basically well do not need a doctor's help in implementing this program, although no one should make big changes in diet or lifestyle without consulting his or her physician. People who are ill or who are under extreme stress can use this program to boost their general level of health before going on to read Part III, which augments the basic program with Immune System Super Boosters.

There is no question that it is necessary to take a comprehensive approach to immune system health. The immune system is "where we live." It reflects both our mental and physical state, and therefore needs both emotional and physical support. Please do your best to follow all the basic recommendations of the program. If you eat a perfect diet and avoid harmful substances but skip the stress management, you may still experience immune system overload. Combining all the recommendations of the program, at least to some degree, yields the most powerful effect.

That said, I need to add that you should follow only the recommendations with which you are comfortable. Try as much of the program as is acceptable to you and see how you feel in two weeks, four weeks, or six weeks. Perhaps then you'll be ready to take another step. Gradual change is easier to manage, and changes made slowly are more likely to be permanent.

The Immune System Empowerment Program is gentle and compassionate, not harsh or judgmental. It is not supposed to make you feel guilty or inadequate; it's supposed to make you feel better. Some people have further to go than others; some people are more motivated than others. You can take the steps of the program in sequence, as they are necessarily presented here, or you can take them all at once. Proceed at your own pace; this is not a race.

It can take up to three months for changes to occur at the cellular level. I encourage you to complete the Immune System Profile at the end of Chapter 4 when you first start the program and then again after three months. Although it is impossible to see the inner workings of the immune system, it is easy to recognize the positive effects of beneficial lifestyle changes and improved health.

Chapter 4

❧

MODERN LIFE AND
IMMUNE SYSTEM OVERLOAD

Avoid the avoidable, and seek safer alternatives.
—SAMUEL EPSTEIN, M.D.

Sitting across from me was a distressed little triangle of people: Nick and Sandy with their daughter, Lauren. Only a few months before, Nick and Sandy had proudly dropped off Lauren at Brown University. Now it was February, and Lauren was on the verge of dropping out.

"Dr. Bock," Lauren said softly, "I'm exhausted all the time. My skin is breaking out, my head aches, and I've got some kind of permanent cold. But the worst part is, I can't think straight anymore. I honestly can't study. I try, but I'm not remembering things. I can't keep up." Lauren looked like she might cry.

Nick and Sandy were eager to assure me that Lauren had always been vivacious and industrious. She'd had many interests and friends in high school, and had not only worked part time in a deli but had also volunteered at a local shelter.

The Lauren I now saw across my desk looked a little scared and a lot tired. All three looked at me expectantly. What was Lauren's problem?

THE IMMUNE THRESHOLD

Back in Chapter 2 we took a look at the contents of the Immune System Kettle. Every day our immune system has to deal with a multitude of challenges, some of which occur naturally within us (for example, toxins that are released by bacteria in the gut, or cells that are damaged during metabolic processes) and some of which are imposed on the body from outside (by viruses, bacteria, pollution, radiation, and poor food choices, among other

77

things). These burdens add up until one last stress puts us over the top of our Immune System Kettle and we get sick.

Although stress is frequently the most visible immune challenge and the one that tends to top off our Immune System Kettle, it is in fact just one of many possible immune challenges. What we call "stress-related disorders" usually are not, in fact, solely due to stress. They're due to stress added on to multiple other immune challenges, of which many physicians are not even aware. Without recognizing the other immune challenges, doctors tend to attribute a patient's entire constellation of symptoms to stress alone. Although stress may indeed be the largest immune challenge we have, and although it definitely needs to be handled, lowering the contents of our Immune System Kettle by attending to our other immune challenges can help us tolerate stress without going over our threshold and developing symptoms.

I see patients every day whose immune systems have been ravaged by a typical modern lifestyle. Lauren's case was not at all unusual. Lauren wasn't doing anything "wrong," but the cumulative effect of her new college lifestyle had exceeded her immune system's coping mechanisms.

Lauren was stressed out, and her family doctor had already suggested that she drop some courses or even take a semester off. But Lauren had successfully handled stressful situations before, and she wanted to stay at school. So we began to look at the whole picture.

Lauren revealed that it was pretty much impossible to sleep in her dorm. Sometimes she would opt to take a nap during dinnertime, when the dorm was usually quiet. Then she'd grab a snack later. Lauren wasn't a big partyer, but she and her friends tended to stay out late socializing. Lauren's room was partially below ground, so her view out the window was at ankle level. Smoking was not permitted on her floor, and although Lauren's roommate smoked, she would go elsewhere with her cigarettes. Lauren had selected all challenging courses, and she found some of her fellow students academically intimidating.

So Lauren ate poorly, slept poorly, and was under constant pressure. I suspected that her "permanent cold" was in fact an allergic reaction to mold in her basement-level room. Her fuzzy thinking could also be due to this allergy. In my experience, mold is one of the allergens that can be associated with cognitive problems (as well as dizziness, headaches, and sinus pressure).

Lauren tested positive for allergy to mold. I recommended that she move into another dorm as soon as possible and told her to avoid moldy areas like indoor swimming pools, damp basements, and old houses with water damage. We could not make Lauren's mold allergy disappear, but I was certain that modifying her environment and lowering her total immune burden would bring her some relief. Before Lauren returned to college, I gave her some intravenous vitamin C to boost her immune system and prescribed various nutritional supplements for her to take on an ongoing basis. I also discussed some basic stress management techniques with her.

With a letter of medical necessity from me, Lauren was able to switch dorm rooms. She was conscientious about taking her supplements and about eating as healthfully as she could, which in her case involved staying away not only from sweets but also from fermented or mold-related foods such as mushrooms, aged cheeses, and beer. She still couldn't get much sleep, but she did cut back on the late-night socializing. With all of these changes, in about two weeks her head (and skin) cleared. When she started feeling better, Lauren felt more like exercising, which in turn helped her stress level. Lauren reversed her downhill slide, stayed in college, and ultimately did quite well.

In this chapter, you will learn how to recognize immunotoxicants (substances that poison your immune system) and minimize your exposure to them. Once you know what's dangerous, you can make informed decisions about living healthfully in an increasingly toxic world.

The Immune System Threshold

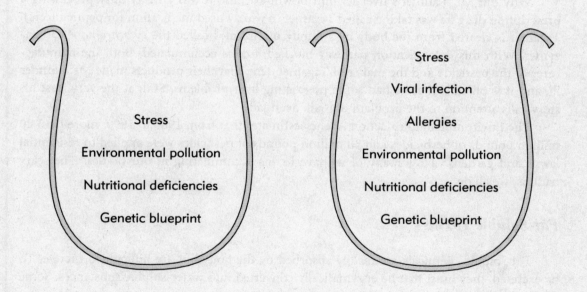

Stress

Environmental pollution

Nutritional deficiencies

Genetic blueprint

Stress

Viral infection

Allergies

Environmental pollution

Nutritional deficiencies

Genetic blueprint

Stress is just one layer in our Immune System Kettle. Lowering our overall immune load helps us handle stress without getting sick.

THE BIOACCUMULATION OF TOXINS

According to *The Wall Street Journal*,[1] Thomas Latimer was a successful, vigorous, athletic man . . . until he mowed the lawn.

Mr. Latimer spent an hour or so cutting the grass and cleaning up the clippings. Soon he felt dizzy and nauseated, and he developed a terrible headache. Ten days later, he was still sick, and his symptoms were worsening. Five months later, he developed testicular cancer. Years later he still had seizures, difficulty walking, and several other health problems.

Doctors determined that Mr. Latimer was poisoned by a pesticide used to treat his yard. The toxin was absorbed through his skin and inhaled into his lungs. Normally the body flushes out a moderate amount of organophosphate in a day or two, but Mr. Latimer's liver was unable to metabolize the poison, which consequently accumulated in his body and attacked his nervous system.

Why did Mr. Latimer's liver let him down? Because it was already busy processing a prescription drug he was taking called Tagamet (a widely used medication for peptic ulcers). Tagamet is cleared from the body by a family of enzymes called the *cytochrome P-450* enzymes. With this detoxification pathway blocked, toxins accumulated. Both the manufacturer of the pesticide and the maker of Tagamet deny that their products made Mr. Latimer ill, and it is possible that he had some preexisting liver problems. Still, at the very least his story calls attention to the problem of toxic overload.

The Environmental Protection Agency estimates that from 1980 to 1990, more than 20 million pounds of herbicides and 30 million pounds of pesticides were applied to residential lawns and gardens.[2] How many of us have toxins accumulating in our bodies? The scary truth is, we all do.

Fat-Soluble Toxins

Fat-soluble chemicals are readily absorbed by the body but are difficult to excrete. To be excreted, they must first be enzymatically converted into water-soluble substances. Some of them can't be converted at all.

Fat-soluble chemicals tend to accumulate in fatty tissues, including cell membranes. The 1990 National Human Adipose Tissue Survey by a department of the Environmental Protection Agency found that 100 percent of the people tested had styrene (used in the manufacture of plastics) and xylene (a solvent found in gasoline and paints) in their fat. In addition, 96 percent tested positive for benzene (found in gasoline and other compounds) and 91 percent for toluene (another solvent).[3] And this is only a partial list!

In her address at the 1993 Hazardous Waste Conference, Ellen K. Silbergeld, Ph.D., sounded an alarm about the body burdens of dioxin, DDT (a pesticide that was banned in 1972), and PCBs that were discovered by the Human Adipose Tissue Survey, noting that "these levels may now be in a range that raises concern about health endpoints such as neurologic, neuroendocrine and immunologic effects."[4] The increasing incidence of many common diseases and disabilities—including low birthweight, neurodegenerative diseases of aging, and asthma—may be related to environmental factors.

One reason that so many people are walking toxic dumps is that we humans are at the top of the food chain. When a chicken, for example, eats treated feed, toxins accumulate in the chicken's body. When we eat the chicken, we get a concentrated dose of bioaccumulated toxins.

Toxins that enter the body from outside are called *exotoxins*. We are constantly exposed to industrial wastes, herbicides, pesticides, and heavy metals in our food, air, and water (more about this later). We also ingest medications, hormones, food additives, and other substances that can have a damaging effect on our cellular machinery. What we think of as a typical day—doing our regular job and eating our usual foods—imposes toxic burdens on our immune system that didn't even exist fifty years ago.

Toxins produced internally are called *endotoxins*. Some are natural by-products of our digestive flora, and some are by-products of illness. While the body generally has mechanisms to cope with endotoxins, a sudden or chronic overproduction of them can overburden the immune system.

Detoxification Pathways

Detoxification actually means several different things. The body naturally detoxifies itself by excreting waste products through sweat, urine, feces, and exhaled air. We can hasten these processes with detoxification treatments like saunas and enemas.

Years ago, I used to avoid being too involved with colon cleansing because some of its advocates take an extreme position, and some of their protocols (such as frequent colonic irrigations and coffee enemas) were viewed as a little weird. We now know, however, that gastrointestinal health is crucial to overall good health, and that GI imbalances can cause problems that affect the entire body. There is an important place in the Immune System Empowerment Program for cleansing and rejuvenating the GI tract (see Chapter 9).

Toxins need to be broken down into products the body is able to excrete. As we learned from Mr. Latimer's example, if these toxins are not broken down successfully, they will simply accumulate in the body.

The organ primarily responsible for detoxifying the body is the liver. In the liver, two detoxification processes occur that restructure undesirable chemicals. Some toxins pass only through Phase I (an oxidation reaction—more about oxidation in a moment). Others go through only Phase II (a conjugation reaction, which adds a molecule). Others go through both steps: in Phase I, they are broken down into intermediate products, and in Phase II, these intermediate products are conjugated into water-soluble end products that the body can excrete.

Sometimes these phases get out of sync. If Phase I proceeds very quickly, a buildup of intermediate products will occur, even though Phase II is proceeding at a normal rate. If Phase II moves too slowly, this, too, causes a buildup of intermediate products, even though Phase I is proceeding normally.

Phase I intermediates can be highly reactive and are often more toxic than the parent (original) compound. If these intermediates are produced in significant amounts, or if they hang around awhile before being further broken down, they can cause cell and tissue damage.

People vary widely in their inborn capacity for liver detoxification. Some people just can't detoxify as others do. (My colleague Jeffrey Bland, Ph.D., an expert on nutritional medicine and liver detoxification, calls these individuals "metabolic yellow canaries," after the canaries used in mines to detect lethal fumes miners could not smell.)

Even if you have been blessed with a strong liver, it is possible for your detoxification pathways to be overwhelmed, either by a slow and steady exposure to toxins or by a sudden massive influx. The liver also can fall behind if it does not have at its disposal the nutrients it needs to transform incoming toxins into exiting waste products.

Once the liver starts to function less effectively, the problem builds upon itself. Toxins build up, and the liver falls further and further behind, creating a biochemical bottleneck. Other detoxification pathways are overburdened, and the accumulated toxins can cause symptoms ranging from aches and pains to neurological abnormalities. (Research on Parkinson's disease, for example, shows that patients with this illness tend to have less efficient detoxification pathways and may be unusually vulnerable to environmental chemicals.)

The Immune System Empowerment Program helps to break this vicious cycle. By lessening your exposure to immunotoxicants and by taking in adequate nutrients, you can help ensure that your body's detoxification processes are keeping up with the demands placed upon them.

OXIDATION

The chemical process called *oxidation* is essential to life as we know it. During oxidation, oxygen combines with another substance to release energy. Oxidation causes fires to burn, metal to rust, and vegetation to decay. When oxygen is combined with gasoline in the engine of your car, the resulting combustion provides the energy that allows you to drive around 2,000 pounds of steel and glass.

We need to keep breathing in order to take in oxygen, which is used by the body to "burn" carbohydrates and fats to produce energy for our cells. Each and every cell of the body needs a constant supply of energy if it is to stay alive and function properly.

Without oxygen, the human body cannot generate energy. You may have noticed feeling tired in a low-oxygen environment such as a smoke-filled room or airplane cabin. If their oxygen supply is cut off, brain cells start to die within minutes.

Within each cell are *mitochondria,* little engines that use oxygen to break down molecules to create energy. In a step-by-step enzymatic process, energy is converted into cellular ATP (adenosine triphosphate) stores that are like tiny batteries. (This process is covered in depth in Chapter 11.) ATP is the fuel we use to move and think. On a cellular level, ATP provides cellular pumps with the energy they need to maintain the correct balances of potassium, magnesium, calcium, sodium, and other substances. Because there is more potassium and magnesium within a cell, and more calcium and sodium outside it, each cell needs a constant supply of energy to resist the natural movement toward equilibration of minerals. It's a dizzying concept to realize that even when we rest and sleep, energy is constantly being expended to maintain cellular integrity and proper electrochemical balances and charges.

No reaction burns 100 percent clean, so oxidation produces by-products. Just as burning wood in the fireplace creates soot, so, too, cellular oxidation produces by-products: carbon dioxide and water (which are harmless) and also highly reactive molecules called *free radicals* (which can be harmful). Free radicals are not the protesting hippies of the sixties, but, rather, active and potentially dangerous molecular marauders.

Free Radical Damage

Free radicals are unstable because they have an unpaired electron. Electrons are generally paired, and in fact prefer to have company. Free radicals try to achieve stability by grabbing another electron wherever they can find one—if necessary, by tearing up a nearby stable molecule. This creates a new free radical, and the resulting chain reaction can cause structural changes and cell damage in a string of molecules. When I discuss this with patients, I liken it to a fireplace throwing off hot sparks that are able to ignite a fire some distance away.

So, ironically, oxidation—a process that is essential to life—stresses the body. Over many years, free radical damage accumulates, which is why free radicals have a lot to do with the aging process. The disease progeria (which is very rare), characterized by extremely rapid aging, is associated with a genetically caused inability to counteract oxidative stress. Children who develop early-onset progeria start to age at around four years and die by puberty. You may have seen a picture of a ten-year-old child with progeria who looks ninety. Without protection from free radical damage, the health of progeria sufferers degenerates quickly.

Our cell membranes are particularly vulnerable to free radical attacks. Because the cumulative surface area of all cell membranes in the body is so vast, and because cell membranes play an active role in so many processes, free radical damage to cell membranes is something we need to take seriously. When free radicals attack cell membranes, they can cause a rupture and the cell may leak, or bacteria and viruses may enter. If the free radical breaks off the cell's identifying proteins, the cell's identity is destroyed. By fusing together membrane fats and proteins, free radicals can alter the structure of the cell membrane and cause it to become brittle. Just as flexibility helps us adapt to life's challenges, flexible cell membranes are important for molecular life processes. For example, a red blood cell needs to be able to squeeze into a tiny capillary to oxygenate tissue—a feat it can achieve only if it is malleable.

The chromosomes inside cells are also vulnerable to free radical damage. When free radicals attack chromosomes, they can rewrite or destroy genetic information. This can cause mutations on the cellular level and can trigger the transformation of a healthy cell into a cancerous one. If this damage goes uncorrected, all succeeding generations of cells will be defective. So, yes, there is a direct and observable link between free radicals and cancer.

Free radicals can undermine health on many fronts. Free radical stress contributes to degenerative problems, from wrinkled skin to heart disease, stroke, emphysema, and eye problems (including macular degeneration and cataracts). Recent research shows that oxidative stress is associated with neurological problems, including Alzheimer's disease. The list is long—and it is getting longer.

The free radicals that are manufactured within the body during oxidation are called *oxygen free radicals* (free radicals derived from molecular oxygen). There are other kinds of free radicals as well. Air pollution, radiation, toxic wastes, food additives, and pesticide residues all contribute to our free radical burden. So do infectious agents, surgery, stress, smoking, drugs, alcohol, and certain fatty acids. As free radical damage builds up, we become more and more susceptible to disease. Happily, there is a solution.

Reduction and Antioxidants

Free radicals are not, in and of themselves, "bad." Phagocytes use free radicals to destroy the antigens (including viruses and bacteria) they digest, so free radicals are actually helpful in fighting infections. The liver produces free radicals as it breaks down toxins. As always, it's a question of balance. Large numbers of scavenging free radicals are unhealthy unless the body is able to swiftly quench them.

Antioxidants take free radicals out of circulation. Remember that fire throwing off hot sparks? Antioxidants are like a screen in front of a fireplace. They prevent damage by changing free radicals into harmless compounds. They do this by adding back that missing electron, a process known as *reduction*. Antioxidants give away electrons to free radicals before harm occurs.

Confused? You're not alone. Just remember that oxidation and reduction are two sides of the same coin. In fact, together they are sometimes referred to as *redox*. Oxidation is defined as the loss of an electron (don't confuse this with oxygenation, which is providing oxygen where it is needed). Reduction is defined as adding an electron. In the process of giving up an electron to stabilize a free radical, an antioxidant is itself oxidized. This changes the chemical composition of the substance so that it can no longer function as an antioxidant—unless it is regenerated by another antioxidant. This is another reason why we need a constant fresh supply of antioxidants!

Again, we're back to the importance of good nutrition and its effects on the cellular level. When you eat plenty of fresh fruits and vegetables, you take in natural antioxidants like beta-carotene and vitamin E (both of which are fat-soluble and help protect the fatty membranes of cells) and vitamin C (which is water-soluble and helps protect cells from inside).

Antioxidants work synergistically—that is, taken together they are more effective than when used alone. This is one reason why studies that use only one antioxidant do not show the same efficacy as studies using several. In their book *Living with the AIDS Virus,* Drs. Parris Kidd and Wolfgang Huber refer to the vitamins, minerals, and enzymes that have antioxidant effects as an "antioxidant tapestry."[5] Together, antioxidants help regulate oxidation/reduction reactions and help maintain homeostasis within the body. Antioxidants also need various cofactors—minerals, vitamins, and amino acids—to do their job effectively, so it's important to take in a wide range of nutrients, not just vitamin C pills

Bruce Ames, Ph.D., a professor of molecular and cellular biology at the University of California, has taken the controversial and well-publicized position that the amount of man-made toxins to which we are exposed is insignificant compared to the amount of toxins that are naturally present in our food. Dr. Ames feels it is a waste of time to worry about things like pesticide residues and air pollution. This point of view flies in the face of what we now know about the soaring rates of cancer, asthma, autoimmune disorders, and other modern health problems. However, Dr. Ames and I do agree on the importance of antioxidants. He has stated, "If you don't get enough antioxidants, it is the equivalent of irradiating yourself."[6] Eating antioxidant-rich fruits and vegetables has finally become a universally accepted rule of good health.

That important balance between oxidants and antioxidants can be disrupted from either direction: the scales can be tipped by an overabundance of oxidizing agents on the one side, or by a scarcity of antioxidants on the other. Some people have a genetic predisposition to decreased activity of antioxidant enzymes, so they don't produce reducing agents as efficiently as they should. The effectiveness of antioxidant enzymes can also be reduced by the presence of lead and other environmental toxins. The only sure way to boost your reserves of antioxidants is to eat a good diet (see Chapter 5, The Immune Empowering Diet) and to take supplements (see Chapter 6, Immune System Boosters).

Now let's review the contents of the Immune System Kettle to see how we can lessen our total immune load.

YOUR GENETIC BLUEPRINT

As you observed back in Chapter 2, in the bottom of the Immune System Kettle lies your genetic blueprint. Your lifestyle choices and environmental exposures are all layered on top of your individual, innate predispositions.

In the 1950s, Dr. Roger J. Williams proposed the idea that individual differences in nutrient requirements could influence health and disease. In his groundbreaking book, *Biochemical Individuality,* Williams proposed that normal people can vary in their nutrient requirements by ten times or more. That is, while I might need 25 milligrams of a certain nutrient each day to stay healthy, you might need 250 milligrams of the same substance. (We now know that serious inborn metabolic errors can lead to the rare case in which someone needs a thousand times the average amount of a particular nutrient, but my focus here is on what can be considered normal.)

Here's one example. If you've had a baby lately (or known someone who has), you are probably aware that prenatal multivitamins contain higher levels of folic acid than everyday multivitamins. This is because certain women run a higher risk of delivering babies with neural tube defects (for example, spina bifida) if they don't take extra folic acid while they are pregnant. So experts recommend that *all* women increase their doses of folic acid during pregnancy. This won't hurt the women who don't need it, but for those who do, it will help prevent devastating birth defects.

Several large studies concluded that folic acid is protective against neural tube defects, but researchers only recently found a specific gene that explains why. This gene is encoded to produce an enzyme that uses folic acid in the metabolism of the amino acid homocysteine. The aberrant version of the gene produces a variant of the enzyme that is unusually inefficient—that is, it requires more folic acid to do its job. (Interestingly, adults with this aberrant gene are more likely to develop heart disease, which is associated with elevated homocysteine levels—something that can be measured with a simple blood test.)[7] The bottom line is that because of genetic variations, some people need much more folic acid than others.

Until that time when we can reliably and affordably ascertain each individual's precise nutrient requirements, I feel it is important to take in sufficient amounts of nontoxic nutritional supplements that will cover the probability that each of us has an increased need for one or more nutrients. Roger Williams proposed that if an individual's genetically determined nutrient needs are not met, this might lead to what he called "genetotrophic" disease (genetic disease of nourishment). It figures that a functional deficiency on the cellular level will eventually have repercussions in the tissues and ultimately in the organs. We have since learned that genetotrophic diseases do indeed exist.

Understanding Genetic Predispositions

Biochemical individuality can be observed in our different needs for vitamins, minerals, enzymes, and amino acids. People also detoxify substances differently, respond to medications differently, and have different hormonal patterns. Perhaps this knowledge will make us more compassionate toward people whose sensitivities are not like ours. (Don't be too quick to judge someone who says she suffers from terrible premenstrual symptoms, or someone who claims cold medications knock him out. You may not have these problems, but others truly do.)

Within the nucleus of each cell are chromosomes that carry genetic information. Each chromosome contains several thousand genes, and each gene is responsible for one small aspect of body chemistry. All the cells of any one person (except egg or sperm cells) carry exactly the same chromosomes. This is because each of us starts out as a single fertilized egg, and with each cell division the original chromosomal material is faithfully reproduced.

Each of us receives genes from our father and from our mother. This makes us each genetically unique (except for identical twins, who derive from the same fertilized egg). Our genetic makeup determines our gender, hair and eye color, height, and other obvious characteristics, as well as other aspects of our individuality that may be considerably more subtle or even invisible, such as the way in which our enzymes function or the serotonin levels in our brains.

Each gene can be printed out as a sequence of four letters (A, C, G, and T) that stand for the four chemical compounds (adenine, guanine, thymine, and cytosine) that make up DNA (deoxyribonucleic acid, the double helix within our chromosomes that carries genetic

---

GENETIC ABNORMALITIES

. . . A C C G T A A C . . .
. . . A C C G T T A C . . .

Genetic information is encoded in DNA, which is made up of four different chemical compounds (nucleotides) represented by the letters A, G, T, and C. The enormous number of variations made possible by this sequencing enable different cell functions to be encoded in the chromosomes. In this tiny segment of a gene, a "misspelled" nucleotide has changed the genetic message.

information). If you were to print out the sequence for one gene, it could be a hundred pages long.

Genetic mutations are like spelling mistakes in the code. Some occur spontaneously, while others are inherited. If you have one "misspelled" version of a gene, you may be a carrier for a certain genetic disorder—that is, you can pass the disorder on to your offspring without actually having any symptoms yourself. If you have two sets of the "misspelled" gene, you may develop a full-blown genetic disorder. Some disorders are more complicated and can be traced to "misspelled" versions of more than one gene.

Genetic abnormalities run the gamut from increased nutrient needs to fatal disorders. The key concept here is that *when we are aware of our genetic predispositions, we can work to offset them.* We can't change our genes, but we can certainly modify our diet and behavior. Sometimes simple changes in our environment are enough to keep a genetically influenced disorder from expressing itself.

Remember those people who don't produce reducing agents as efficiently as others? These individuals can experience greater oxidative stress, which in turn can be associated with asthma. However, if they recognize that they have an increased need for antioxidants, and if they are aware that they are at increased risk for asthma, they can increase their intake of antioxidants and avoid asthma triggers—and possibly outsmart their genetic predisposition. The same principle applies to other genetically influenced diseases, including cancer.

I have a friend with two beautiful children—a son and a daughter. His son has a rare kidney disorder that affects only males. Little is known about this disease except that it is inherited and that it causes kidney degeneration. There is no cure. However, it is believed that a low-protein diet will place less strain on the kidneys and postpone the onset of disease. While researchers look for a cure, my friend and his wife give their son carrot sandwiches and "veggie subs" to take to school and remain optimistic. By carefully monitoring his diet from birth, they may successfully delay the expression of this disease until a cure is found.

The Human Genome Project

The National Center for Human Genome Research in Bethesda, Maryland, is in the midst of what is called the Human Genome Project: the staggeringly complex task of mapping all of the body's 80,000 genes. According to Francis Collins, M.D., director of the project, if you were to print out the entire genome of a human being, it would fill twenty-three sets—not volumes, but sets—of the *Encyclopaedia Britannica*. To locate a single gene, you'd have to first find the right volume and then the right page.[8]

So far geneticists have located the genes that cause cystic fibrosis, Lou Gehrig's disease, and Huntington's disease, plus a gene linked to breast cancer. Researchers suspect there are genetic links to other forms of cancer, as well as to problems like heart disease, diabetes, and high blood pressure. Recently the field of genetics has even invaded the controversial territory of personality traits, sexual orientation, and mental health (for example, schizophrenia and manic depression).[9] As hard as it is to locate the one gene responsible for a single-gene disorder, it is even harder to find the several genes that may in combination cause other disorders.

In the future, we will be able to identify each individual's genetic predispositions and nutrient needs. This will allow us to practice the medicine of the individual, rather than the medicine of the masses. By understanding our own biochemically unique needs, we will be able to provide our cells with just the correct amounts of the right nutrients—and thereby prevent genetotrophic diseases from ever expressing themselves.

DIETARY STRESSES

It is only common sense that what people eat influences their health for better or for worse, and yet I doubt you have ever received nutritional advice from your doctor.

Jeffrey Bland, the expert on nutritional medicine I mentioned earlier, is used to physicians' being unaware of his work and its importance.

"Doctor," Jeff will say, "do you practice nutritional medicine?"

"Certainly not," most doctors will reply. "Nutrition is for nutritionists."

"Do your patients eat?" Jeff will then ask.

"Of course!" the doctor will answer. So in fact doctors do need to be aware of their patients' nutrition. Even surgeons, who probably don't view nutrition as relevant to their practice, could improve their surgical results by making sure their patients are optimally nourished. When I heard that a well-known New York City plastic surgeon now recommends nutritional and homeopathic supplements to hasten the recovery of his face-lift patients, I knew it wouldn't be long before nutritional intervention would become a fairly standard part of many different types of medical practices.

The next two chapters will discuss how to avoid nutritional deficiencies, nutrient excesses, and food excesses with the Immune Empowering Diet and Immune System Boosters. For now, I just want to mention the chemicals that find their way into our food and therefore into our bodies.

According to one source, the average American consumes about *6 pounds* of synthetic chemicals each year.[10] I divide these chemicals into three categories:

• First, there are chemicals that are deliberately used in growing, shipping, and selling food. This category includes antibiotics and hormones in poultry, meat, and milk; pesticides and herbicides in crops and in animal feed; ripening agents; and other treatments and coatings that prevent premature spoilage and make food better able to withstand being shipped thousands of miles. Consumers have no way of knowing which of these residues are on or in their food, or how much.

• The second category includes chemicals that are added to processed foods to make them palatable and to increase their shelf life. This includes preservatives, coloring agents and dyes, flavorings and flavor enhancers, conditioners, emulsifiers, stabilizers, sugar substitutes (remember aspartame, back on page 39), and other additives. While these additives are permitted by the Food and Drug Administration, some are so problematic for so many people that they must by law be specifically listed on package labels.

• Finally, there are substances that no one could possibly want to add to our food, but which are present nonetheless. This category includes dirt and other contaminants (rodent droppings, bug bits, fungi, etc.) and chemicals that are inextricably part of our food chain because of global pollution (for example, mercury and PCBs in fish).

A sourcebook entitled *Alternative Medicine: The Definitive Guide* lists the top ten food additives to avoid as aspartame (a chemical sweetener); brominated vegetable oil (used in many soft drinks); BHA and BHT (common preservatives); Citrus Red Dye No. 2 (used to color the skins of oranges); monosodium glutamate (a flavor enhancer); nitrites (preservatives often used in meats); saccharin (another artificial sweetener); sulfur dioxide, sodium bisulfite, and sulfites (more preservatives); tertiary butyhydroquinone (a preservative used in packaging); and Yellow Dye No. 6 (which has been banned in Norway and Sweden).[11]

Most of the substances mentioned above cannot be washed off, and the vitamins and nutrients lost during the refrigerating, freezing, canning, boxing, dehydrating, and packaging of processed foods cannot be replaced. Yet because commercially prepared foods are what everybody eats, we have as a culture lost track of the fact that a chicken nugget, a "creme-filled donut," a can of soda, and a bowl of frosted cereal are all in fact highly artificial, chemical-laced food substitutes.

We all know that it's better to buy organic foods and to prepare healthful meals from scratch. I think what keeps attracting us to processed foods is the convenience. Unless you're in the habit of buying your vegetables and soaking your beans and cooking your grains ahead of time, it's a heck of a lot easier just to get fast food for dinner.

One of my patients now looks back at her family's fast-food past with horror. Emily's son, Patrick, had many allergic reactions as a baby, and in particular he always reacted to antibiotics. Patrick often would break out in hives all over, especially when his pediatrician put him on an antibiotic for an ear infection. Eventually his chart in the office was so covered with "do not prescribe" stickers that Emily felt forced to seek alternatives and came to us.

When I first heard Patrick's medical history, I immediately considered the possibility of an underlying chronic yeast problem in addition to allergies. (Multiple courses of antibiotics can predispose someone to developing chronic candidiasis, which can provoke or worsen allergies and sensitivities.) We were able to determine that Patrick was not allergic to all these antibiotics, as it first seemed, but rather to the red dyes used in them and in many other liquid pediatric preparations. These same red dyes are also present in lollipops and other candy, Popsicles, fruit drinks, gelatin desserts, and more, including some antibiotics and even in a pink children's allergy medication (unbelievable as that might seem).

Once Emily started noticing how many chemicals her family was eating, she made some sweeping and unpopular changes in their eating habits. Now the family eats fresh, organic food as much as possible and as little processed food as possible. Emily is the first to admit that they owe this lifestyle change to Patrick's allergy—and that without his medical history, they would probably still be eating sugar-coated cereals.

ALLERGIES AND SENSITIVITIES

As Patrick's story illustrates, allergies and sensitivities are adverse reactions to substances that are usually tolerated by most people. A classic allergic reaction is IgE-mediated. The IgE mechanism is a response that all allergists will agree is a truly allergic reaction. For example, if you have a classic allergic reaction to peanuts, you will have an increased production of IgE immunoglobulin (specific to peanuts) that will be detectable in your blood. To complicate the picture, however, some allergic reactions are IgG-mediated or cell-mediated, and a sensitivity is mediated by other mechanisms altogether that are not classically immunologic.

Only approximately one third of food allergies are IgE-mediated. Traditional allergists refer to any reaction to foods other than an IgE-mediated reaction as a food "intolerance." However, an intolerance—for example, lactose intolerance—is nonimmunologically mediated. Because reactions that are IgG- or cell-mediated don't fit the mold of a classic allergic reaction, they can be overlooked by many doctors.

Classic IgE-mediated allergies are called *atopic* and usually involve a family history of allergy plus some combination of rhinitis (runny and/or stuffy nose), hay fever, eczema, asthma, and hives. Individual patients can have variable immune responses—that is, you might produce both IgG and IgE antibodies to one allergen, but only IgG or IgE against others. The non-IgE-mediated reactions *(nonatopic)* can cause myriad symptoms, including gastrointestinal upset and difficulties with concentration (as seen with attention deficit disorder), and can also play a part in autoimmune illnesses as well as many other problems.

Some allergies and sensitivities are obvious, some aren't. Some are immediate (such as IgE-mediated reactions), some are delayed (such as IgG- and cell-mediated reactions). A study of asthmatics published in the *Lancet* found that the delayed, IgG-mediated reaction takes from two to four hours to kick in and lasts from six to ten hours.[12] In his medical textbook *Basics of Food Allergy,* J. C. Breneman, M.D., describes delayed-type allergic reactions as late as three to four days after exposure.[13] Delayed allergies are the least obvious and most undiagnosed. One reason for this is that they are not IgE-mediated.

We do a lot of allergy testing at our health centers because we find that many people are walking around with significant allergies of which they are completely unaware. They don't feel well, but they also don't connect their symptoms to allergies or sensitivities.

One of my more stressed-out patients, a successful litigator and father of three, was experiencing episodes of what he called being "out of it." Sometimes he'd have headaches or just feel exhausted. It got to the point where Gary would be unable to finish dictating a letter or focus on what was happening in the courtroom. Although he had lots of sinus infections and went through repeated courses of antibiotics, his family doctor found no other problems and his CBC blood test results were normal.

Suspecting allergies, I ordered additional tests and found that Gary had hidden allergies to wheat and yeast. After he made changes in his diet (eliminating all wheat- and yeast-containing foods, as well as mold-related foods like aged cheese and mushrooms), he felt like a new man. The difference in his performance was night and day. "Dr. Bock," he said at his next office visit, "my wife makes this great homemade bread, and I was eating slabs and slabs of it, and I really thought it was healthy, you know? I *hated* cutting that out of my diet. But I feel so much better now, I could never go back to eating that way again. I figure one man's meat is another man's poison, right?"

The best way to deal with allergies and sensitivities is to minimize your exposure to anything that is problematic for you. This will immediately lower your immune load. Some allergies can be treated with medications or immunotherapy such as conventional allergy shots, neutralization, or enzyme-potentiated desensitization (more about these in a moment).

Signs and Symptoms

Someone who is having a pronounced allergic reaction may be coughing and sneezing, with a runny nose and red, itchy eyes. Or he may be covered with hives that disappear from one area only to reappear in another. Some people—including adults—experience behavioral changes, either becoming depressed and lethargic or angry and uncooperative. If an allergic reaction is grave, it can lead to anaphylaxis (swelling, shock, and death).

Chronic allergies show up a little differently. Signs and symptoms can be localized or systemic, and can include:

- Puffy or red-rimmed eyes, dark circles under the eyes
- Sinus infections; runny nose, the "allergic salute" (constantly rubbing the nose)
- Ear infections; red, burning earlobes
- Swollen tonsils
- Coughing, sneezing, wheezing, asthma
- Edema (swelling)
- Eczema, rashes, canker sores
- Headaches, migraines
- Dizziness, light-headedness, vertigo
- Gastrointestinal problems, including bloating, burping, gas, heartburn, ulcers, "nervous stomach," diarrhea or constipation, nausea, vomiting
- Excessive perspiration, sweatiness

- Excessive salivation, drooling (babies), spitting while talking
- Muscle aches, joint stiffness
- Burning sensations, numbness and tingling
- Twitchy legs, leg cramps
- Aggressive behavior, tantrums, irritability, depression, anxiety, racing pulse
- Sleep problems, insomnia, bed-wetting
- Lethargy, fatigue
- Cognitive problems, difficulty concentrating or thinking clearly, "brain fog," forgetfulness
- Changes in speech

I'm no longer surprised by what my patients tell me about their allergic reactions. Food allergies, in particular, can mimic almost any disease. If a patient tells me she has noticed that eggs always make her dizzy, well, who am I to say she's wrong? Why would I not believe this information? Allergic reactions are systemic and can affect all areas of the body, including the brain. Why is it that most allergists want to confine allergic reactions mainly to the skin, nose, and lungs?

There is a mysterious aspect to allergies, in that we know they are influenced by thought and emotions. Distress can trigger or worsen an asthma attack, and someone who is allergic to roses can have an allergic reaction to a plastic rose. Even more confusing is the report that a patient with a multiple personality disorder exhibits allergies only in one personality.

People who don't have allergies are quick to conclude that this means allergies are all in the head and that allergy sufferers are slightly hysterical. I think these detractors would revise their position if they could see a three-month-old baby with an allergic reaction to milk-based formula, as I have.

There is an emotional element to all illness, and it is clear that the mind/body connection plays an important role in allergic reactions. However, as we've seen, symptomatic illness is a result not only of the most obvious emotional or psychological stress, but also of each individual's cumulative immune burden. To effectively treat illness, we need to deal with both its emotional and physical aspects, attending to all the different levels in the Immune System Kettle. I believe my job as a physician is not to judge, but to do everything I can to help those people who, for whatever reasons, have multiple sensitivities.

Allergies and Immune Load

Allergies are closely related to each individual's immune threshold. If you are fighting an infection, you may suddenly discover that you can't eat peaches or let your neighbor's cat sit on your lap. Or, because allergies are additive, if you have an allergy to ragweed, you may react to eggs only during ragweed season.

Allergies tend to run in families, which suggests that a predisposition to allergies is inherited. Your family history is useful information. For example, if you know your parents were troubled by asthma, you may be able to adopt preventive strategies to minimize potential asthma problems.

Inhalant Allergies

Inhalant allergies are allergies to particles we breathe in. Many people are allergic to dust, dust mites (little microscopic critters that live in bedding and carpets), mold, pollen (such as ragweed), and animal dander. People who are allergic to latex may be troubled by urban air, which is full of rubber tire particles. It's also common for people to react to inhaled chemical smells or perfumes, but this is considered a chemical sensitivity and will be discussed separately.

Inhalant allergies can be seasonal. Ragweed allergies kick up in late summer, mold allergies tend to be worse in the fall, and dust allergies can be worse in the winter when we spend more time indoors with closed windows.

ᏸ᠊ᨠ

COMMONLY ASKED QUESTION NO. 7:

Why am I allergic all of a sudden?

Signs and symptoms of food allergy can develop at any age. Infants can develop food allergies to allergens in breast milk or formula. However, not all disorders are present from birth. It can take time for problems to develop or for predispositions to be expressed. Some of my patients developed food allergies as adults, which on closer examination is not as puzzling as it seems.

Food allergies are often a consequence of abnormal permeability of the lining of the gastrointestinal tract. When the intestine is abnormally permeable, larger-than-appropriate molecules of food may be absorbed into the bloodstream, where they are perceived by the immune system as foreign invaders. Permeability, in turn, can be affected by many things, including changes in GI flora, low levels of secretory IgA in the lining of the GI tract, and nutrient and enzyme deficiencies. Food allergies also may be a consequence of low stomach acid (hypochlorhydria), which causes inadequate digestion of proteins, resulting in the subsequent absorption of larger molecules of food.

Allergies are closely related to overall immune load. Previously unapparent inhalant allergies may not rear their (sneezing, wheezing) head until your Immune System Kettle is full of additional immune challenges.

ᏸ᠊ᨠ

Food Allergies

Basically anybody can be allergic to any food (whether it's wholesome or not!). Food allergies are more common than most people think. Dr. Breneman, the expert on food allergy I mentioned earlier, refers to food allergies as "the plague of our times," noting that 95 percent of food allergies are undiagnosed.[14]

An article in *The Journal of the American Medical Association* lists the most common food triggers as eggs, milk, tree nuts, peanuts, whitefish, and crustacea (shrimp, lobsters, etc.).[15] To this list I would add chocolate, wheat, corn, soy, and oranges.

Fixed food allergies are usually predictable and immediate. This type of allergy is less common and accounts for 5 to 15 percent of allergic reactions. Fixed food allergies are seldom outgrown. Anaphylactoid allergic reactions are an extreme example of fixed food allergies. For example, someone who is highly allergic to shrimp will experience throat swelling and associated symptoms each and every time he eats shrimp. In the most severe cases, an individual can react to just the smell of the offending food. One physician had an anaphylactic reaction to a batch of nut-free cookies that were baked especially for him—by a friend who used a spatula from a previous batch of cookies that contained nuts. One of my young patients who is allergic to peanuts got hives on his face when his grandfather kissed him on both cheeks after eating salted peanuts on an airplane.

Variable food allergies are less predictable and are affected by the amount of food that is eaten, how often, other foods that are consumed in combination, how the food is prepared, and the presence of other immune challenges. These allergies are usually manageable and may even be "outgrown." By this I mean that if you avoid the offending food long enough, and then reintroduce it at infrequent intervals (at most every four to seven days), you can avoid adverse reactions to that particular food. I frequently hear from patients that they have outgrown food allergies, but in reality what happened is that the allergy is just expressing itself differently (e.g., wheat, which used to cause colic and gastrointestinal problems, is now causing eczema and fatigue).

Many symptoms of food allergies—for example, hives, nasal congestion, eczema, and wheezing—are classic IgE-mediated reactions. However, food allergies can also cause GI symptoms that are not IgE-mediated, including nausea, vomiting, constipation, and diarrhea.

Diagnosing and Treating Allergies

There are three traditional ways to test for classic allergies:

1. **Skin tests.** In conventional testing, allergy extracts (diluted preparations of allergens) are placed on pinpricks on the skin or slightly beneath the skin's surface (intradermally). A positive reaction creates a red, raised wheal. Skin tests are used to detect classic IgE-mediated

allergies and will not pick up reactions that are mediated in other ways. I never use pinprick skin tests for food allergies, as I have found intradermal testing to be more accurate. Also, the process of intradermal testing helps to determine the treatment dose (see below).

2. Blood work. RAST (radioallergosorbent tests) and ELISA (enzyme-linked immuno-sorbent assays) will detect the presence of serum IgE antibodies to specific antigens (for example, foods, inhalants, insect venom, and certain drugs). Blood tests are useful for patients who are extremely sensitive and who should not be exposed to allergy extracts because of the risk of anaphylaxis. They are also useful for children because they avoid the need for multiple intradermal skin tests.

3. The elimination diet. An inexpensive way to test for allergies is to follow a severely restricted allergen-free diet (usually lamb, rice, water, and possibly a few other foods) for one to two weeks, and then to reintroduce foods one at a time and watch for any reactions. (Timing is important. If you wait longer than two weeks, you may have become tolerant.) The good news about the elimination diet is that it presents clear clinical evidence. A positive reaction to a food challenge is more meaningful than the results of any blood test, positive or negative. The bad news is that the diet is not easy to follow, and you have to be 100 percent strict. Even a tiny bit of the wrong food at the wrong time can skew the results. Also, the process of reintroducing foods is time-consuming, because you can do only one food challenge at a time. The elimination diet can be done under strict medical supervision or, in less troublesome cases, at home. This approach is not helpful for people who have severe, acute food allergies, but in most cases these individuals have learned the hard way what foods will set off an anaphylactic reaction.

If traditional skin tests and blood work fail to reveal any IgE-mediated allergies, many traditional allergists will tell you that you don't have allergies. This may be untrue. Broader-minded physicians recognize that other methods are needed to diagnose allergies that are IgG-mediated or cell-mediated. A delayed-onset reaction to cow's milk is common, with symptoms that include asthma and eczema occurring from hours to days after ingestion. This type of sensitivity to milk is not IgE-mediated, but can be diagnosed by detecting raised serum levels of IgG antibodies to milk proteins.[16]

The IgG serum antibody test is used to measure the amount of serum IgG antibodies to specific food antigens. Another useful, though expensive, tool is the ELISA/ACT test, which is able to detect the presence of both cell-mediated and antibody-mediated food allergies. This test can be useful for diagnosing allergies that have been extremely difficult to pin down. The originator of this test, Russell Jaffe (an expert on immunology whom I mentioned earlier), is on the forefront of clinical immunology and immunological diagnostic testing. His groundbreaking research and publications have helped to educate physicians about the importance of hidden food allergies, which in turn has allowed countless patients to obtain diagnostic and treatment information that wasn't available before.

Diagnosing and treating allergies has become a large part of my practice. Over the years

I have evaluated several different approaches, and I've found methods that are extremely successful and that bring great relief to many people.

Some of the patients who come to my office already know they have allergies, but the vast majority do not. Sometimes the diagnosis is easy—for example, allergic rhinitis is very common and easy to spot, and anaphylactoid food allergies are unmistakable. Covert (hidden) allergies, on the other hand, are more difficult to detect. The symptoms of allergies are so vast and so vague, particularly the symptoms of non-IgE-mediated allergies, that I first take a careful medical history to see if there is any connection between a patient's complaints and a particular season, food, location, or activity. Hidden allergies are always a possibility in the back of my mind.

Any time I see a new patient with an autoimmune disorder, I test for food allergies because of the phenomenon of cross-reactivity (an allergic reaction to a food can contribute to an autoimmune reaction). When we are able to determine a food allergy and alleviate it, the patient's autoimmune symptoms sometimes lessen. Traditional physicians do not endorse this approach, but I have seen the beneficial results time and again in my own patients.

When the clinical evidence suggests the possibility of allergies, I may first simply test for the more common allergens (for example, wheat, corn, milk, and yeast). If these test results are positive, we often proceed further.

To test for food allergies, I use intradermal testing with progressively weaker dilutions of food allergens. We start with a dilution that is likely to produce a positive response, which is a skin wheal of a certain diameter, and keep testing weaker dilutions until no positive response is observed. Also associated with a positive response can be other allergic symptoms such as a stuffy nose, headache, or fatigue; as testing is continued, these symptoms may be alleviated by a neutralizing dose (see below). Intradermal testing generally is not appropriate for people who have severe food allergies (except possibly in centers providing close monitoring and sophisticated technical support, should an anaphylactic reaction occur), but it is quite safe for most other food allergies. This method is time-consuming because only one food is tested at a time, but the test results are in my experience among the most accurate (there is no one foolproof method for diagnosing food allergies) and they also give us a good sense of exactly how allergic the patient is.

Some physicians provoke an allergic response by placing drops of antigen solution under the patient's tongue (sublingually) and watching for signs or symptoms. At a certain dilution, the patient's symptoms (such as headache, irritability, or difficulty concentrating) will be provoked; at another dilution, his or her symptoms will be neutralized. The neutralizing dose becomes the patient's immunotherapy. He or she takes the drops on a regular basis to prevent symptoms. This neutralizing dose is effective, but often needs adjusting.

This method is called *provocation/neutralization,* or P/N. The principle behind P/N is that an allergen that provokes a reaction when given at one dose will actually cancel out the same reaction when given at a different dose. This principle is akin to that of homeopathy, in which minute quantities of certain substances are used to correct symptoms they would actually cause if they were taken in larger quantities. Both P/N and homeopathy work because of the harmonic nature of an immune response. (Harmonic recognition is not always immune-mediated, as we will see in the discussion of energetic medicine in Chapter 10.)

Consider the sine curve intersecting a horizontal plane (see below). It looks like a sea monster cruising along the surface of the ocean. The horizontal plane (the surface of the ocean) is the state of immune system equilibrium. The sine curve (the sea monster) moves along both above and below this plane, intersecting it at several points. The part of the sine curve above the horizontal plane represents immune overreactivity, and the part below represents immune underreactivity.

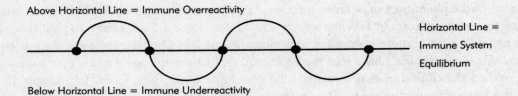

The purpose of P/N testing is to find exactly the dose of an allergen that stimulates a response at the level of immune system equilibrium. Note that there are multiple points on the curve that represent this equilibrium. A dose either higher or lower than the neutralizing dose will provoke symptoms. When this neutralizing dose is administered, you can eliminate allergic symptoms. Over time, you can desensitize the patient and his or her reactivity.

Although P/N is not accepted by traditional allergists and their societies, it is utilized and promoted by members of the American Academy of Environmental Medicine and the American Society of Otolaryngologists. I believe that P/N is valuable, but I prefer to observe and measure the actual skin wheals that are caused by intradermal testing, in addition to noting provoked symptoms. Also, I've found other methods that help control allergic symptoms very successfully.

For suspected inhalant allergies, I use intradermal testing, but in this situation I start with a very weak dilution of allergen extract and work up toward a stronger one. This method, called *serial dilution titration (SDT),* is very safe (with inhalant allergies you must be careful not to provoke an asthma attack) and uses panels of related antigens—a pollen panel, a mold panel, a dust panel, etc. An allergic patient may have no reaction (no skin wheal) to a weak dilution, a moderate reaction (medium-sized wheal) to one of the moderate dilutions, and a pronounced reaction (larger-sized wheal) to a stronger dilution. The dilution in the middle is the most important, for it becomes the basis of the patient's treatment—strong enough to stimulate the immune system, but not strong enough to provoke a serious reaction.

Intradermal testing for inhalant allergies is, like the intradermal tests for food allergies, very time-consuming, but the results often enable me to take a shortcut in the patient's treatment. Instead of commencing allergy shots (see page 100) at the lowest level and adding slightly larger doses of allergen over a period of many months, often we can begin at a higher level and get results in only a month or two. Also, because serial dilution testing is much more dose-specific for individual patients than conventional allergy testing, we can create immunotherapy shots that patients can administer safely and effectively at home, which is more convenient and cost-effective for them than repeated office visits.

Sometimes allergies can be cured, especially if the underlying causes are attended to. In other situations, they can be successfully managed. The best way to manage allergies is to avoid allergens (an example of "less is more"), but this is difficult to do with ubiquitous allergens like dust, or common foods such as wheat and corn.

Because most food allergies are variable, you may not be stuck with a moderate food allergy for life. To manage food allergies, you can try limiting your intake of your problem food. You may be able to tolerate it in moderation. If this doesn't work, you may need to eliminate the problem food from your diet altogether for a period of time. After two to six months, depending upon your sensitivity to the allergen, it is often possible to reintroduce a food on a rotating basis, meaning you eat a certain food (and, often, foods in the same family) every four days or less often, but not more frequently. A rotation diet allows people with allergies to remain within a zone of immune tolerance in which they tolerate a food and do not react to it.

Children who do not eat foods to which they are allergic sometimes outgrow their allergies after a year or two. However, reintroducing foods can be tricky. If they resume eating a problem food in large amounts or very frequently, they may develop symptoms again. This time, however, they may have new and different symptoms. If soy caused eczema before, it now may cause chronic fatigue or confusion. The connection between the old allergy and these new symptoms is often missed.

Be aware, also, that it is possible for inhalant allergies and food allergies to provoke each other. For people who have mold allergies, exposure to a moldy, mildewy environment can cause symptoms. Eating mold-related foods can also cause a reaction, either alone or in combination with the symptoms of inhalant allergies. Again, allergies are additive.

Although traditional allergists do not give shots for food allergies, I have found that enzyme-potentiated desensitization (EPD), a form of immunotherapy that was pioneered in England by Dr. Len McEwen, is very effective in treating food allergies and other sensitivities. This technique uses an injection that combines extremely small doses of allergens (the "allergen mix") with the enzyme beta-glucuronidase, which is present in all parts of the human body. When beta-glucuronidase combines with the allergen mix, it potentiates the immune system response. I feel EPD offers an exciting advance in the field of immunology, and therefore it is discussed separately in Chapter 10, Immune System Super Boosters.

If you have inhalant allergies, cleaning up your environment may bring you substantial relief. Here are some examples of what we call environmental controls:

- Use an air filter in winter; run the air conditioner and/or dehumidifier in summer. (Make sure your air conditioner is not growing mold.)
- Buy dust covers for your mattress and box springs.
- Wash your bedding often in hot water, and dry it in the dryer (clotheslines expose bedding to dust and pollen).
- Get rid of any heavy drapes, upholstered furniture, and dust collectors like stuffed animals, bookcases, and silk flowers.
- Remove carpets and have wood floors instead.
- Fix any leaks and seal any cracks; water damage promotes mold growth.
- Vacuum as often as possible (excellent "allergy" vacuum cleaners are available that filter any dust from the air exiting the machine), and damp mop whenever possible.
- Keep pets out of your bedroom (most people refuse to part with their pets).

The traditional medical treatments for inhalant allergies are medications and allergy shots. Medications are used to relieve the signs and symptoms of allergies, but they do not change the mechanisms that cause the allergic reaction in the first place. There are a number of commonly used drugs.

- Steroids (cream, liquid, tablets, or inhaled) are used to combat inflammation. Steroids also suppress the immune system, and by doing so, stop allergic responses.
- Antihistamines (liquid or tablets) work quickly to block the effects of histamines released during an allergic reaction. (Histamines dilate blood vessels, causing swelling, and irritate nerve endings, causing itching.)
- Bronchodilators (liquid, tablets, or inhaled) rapidly open up the air passages in the lungs, allowing air to move in and mucus to move out.
- Cromolyn sodium (capsules, drops, or inhaled) blocks the release of histamine. This drug is used preventively over several weeks or longer.
- Decongestants can decrease swelling and congestion in nasal passages and provide symptomatic relief for allergic rhinitis.

Conventional allergy shots may be safe and effective for most inhalant allergies, but they are not effective for food allergies. Patients who receive allergy shots are injected with tiny amounts of the substances to which they are allergic. The dose is increased very slowly over time. Generally they receive shots on a regular basis until their body builds up a tolerance to the allergens. When the ever-increasing doses are carefully kept below a concentration that will stimulate an adverse reaction, the body is desensitized into accepting a higher and higher level of a particular antigen. When the patient becomes symptom-free, the number of shots can be reduced until eventually they are stopped. Unfortunately, this form of immunotherapy can take eighteen months or longer to have an effect.

In addition to EPD injections and allergy shots based on SDT, I also use nutrients, homeopathic remedies, and herbal preparations to combat allergies. I use high doses of vitamin C, specifically a buffered vitamin C that can be more helpful in allergic situations (and, at times, intravenous vitamin C); bioflavonoids such as quercetin and pycnogenol; vitamin B_6; pantothenic acid; certain Chinese herbs, including glycerrhizin; borage oil, which is a source of gamma-linolenic acid (an essential fatty acid); and adrenal and thymus extracts. (All of these supplements are discussed separately in later chapters.) I use a system of homeopathic remedies called Heel or Heel/BHI remedies that are not classic homeopathy, in that they are combination remedies, but which I find helpful. Euphorbium is a homeopathic spray used for nasal and sinus symptoms.

Chemical Sensitivities

Many people find it difficult to believe that someone could have an adverse reaction to the smell of bleach, or nail polish, or ink, or gasoline. Many doctors find it difficult to accept that a patient could have an acute sensitivity to the smell of a plastic shower curtain—or to dry-cleaned clothes or car exhaust—that cannot be verified by a standard medical test. Chemical sensitivities, environmental illness, and clinical ecology are still considered by some to be on the fringe of respectable medicine. This attitude is lessening over time as people gain a greater understanding of them.

I once had a patient who was *panallergic*—allergic to practically everything. Her severe chemical sensitivities made her so sick that I admitted her to the local hospital. A physician from a nearby practice who was covering my hospital rounds one weekend made comments about this patient that were far from compassionate. He thought, of course, that she was completely crazy.

As it turned out, this patient's sensitivities were so disabling that she had to be transferred to an environmental unit in Dallas, Texas, where she underwent extensive immune testing. Multiple specialists were involved in her case. When she had surgery for an abdominal problem, it was discovered that she had severe lymphadenopathy and multiple organ involvement from her allergies. The surgeons were actually able to take biopsies that gave physical evidence of her heightened allergic state.

This patient was treated for lengthy periods with intravenous therapy and had to live in a structured environment free of any types of allergens. Her life as she had known it was basically over. She was probably one of the sickest patients the experts in Dallas had ever seen, and yet my colleague had completely discounted her symptoms.

Modern life means being besieged by chemicals in our air, food, and water. (Environmental pollution is discussed further on page 112.) Inside our homes and offices we are exposed to a multitude of synthetic substances and their vapors. Everything seems to be scented, from fabric softeners, soaps, candles, colognes, and room deodorizers to cosmetics.

Other chemical odors are released by:

Aerosol sprays	Mothballs, moth crystals
Arts and crafts supplies	Newsprint
Bleach, scouring powders	Oven cleaner
Carpet, carpet adhesive	Paint, paint remover
Cleansers, detergents	Permanent marker pens
Disinfectants	Plastic
Dry-cleaned clothes	Plywood, fiberboard
Floor polish or wax	Polyurethane, varnish
Gas appliances	Radon
Glue, rubber cement	Tobacco smoke
Insecticides, pesticides	Turpentine

Outdoors we are exposed to myriad other chemical smells, including those from:

Asphalt	Herbicides, lawn sprays
Chemical spills	Insecticides
Exhaust (diesel, bus, auto)	Paints, sealants
Factories	Refineries

Signs and symptoms of chemical sensitivity include everything on the list on page 92. However, the most common are fatigue, headache, dizziness, nausea, irritability, burning sensations, muscle aches, neuropsychiatric problems, and hypersensitivity to odors. Obviously, these symptoms can be caused by a wide variety of conditions, but if they are consistently linked to chemical exposure, they may indicate a sensitivity. Many people do not recognize the connection or realize that chemical sensitivities are even a possibility. Your symptoms will depend upon your genetic blueprint, your nutritional state, your overall immune load, the amount of chemical exposure you receive, and the duration of the exposure.

Interestingly, the body will sometimes become less reactive over time to a certain chemical exposure. For example, someone who starts working at a dry-cleaning establishment might have runny eyes. If she persists, however, this symptom might eventually subside, a phenomenon known as *adaptation*. Instead, more serious symptoms might develop, such as chronic fatigue, difficulty concentrating, or lung problems. The sensitivity doesn't go away, but the symptoms change.

It's easier to check for the presence of chemicals in the body than it is to diagnose a particular sensitivity. Various tests involving blood, urine, hair, breast milk, or fat can confirm that you have been exposed to certain chemicals. Fat-soluble chemicals can remain in the body for many years and can be released from fat years later (for example, during fasting or weight loss). For this reason, you may develop symptoms some time after your exposure.

It is possible to check for chemical sensitivities by using extracts or provocation/neutralization procedures. If a patient tells me he consistently and repeatedly gets a rash, runny nose, or headache from a specific kind of chemical exposure, that to me is good clinical evidence of a chemical sensitivity. However, sometimes a patient is unaware that certain symptoms are related to chemical exposure until we discover this through a careful, detailed review of his or her medical history.

As with all allergies, avoidance is key. Stay away from any chemicals that trouble you. One of my patients runs to close her windows every time her neighbor has the lawn sprayed (unfortunately, she can't stop him from spraying). We ask nurses and patients alike not to wear perfume or scented lotions at our health centers in consideration of those people who have chemical sensitivities. You may need to make expensive alterations at home, such as replacing wall-to-wall carpet with hardwood floors and replacing oil- or gas-burning appliances. At the very least, try to make your bedroom an allergen-free safe haven.

To help your body detoxify chemicals, get plenty of nutrients to support the breakdown process and drink lots of water to help flush the by-products out of your system. Sometimes it is helpful to boost liver function with a liver detoxification program. (These nutrients and liver detoxification are discussed separately in Chapter 9.) Exercise and massage therapy both increase circulation and help remove toxins from tissues. Saunas are detoxifying, but with some precautions: you need to be in a well-ventilated space, and you need to scrub down afterwards. For more serious cases of exposure, intravenous vitamin C (see Chapter 10) is a mild chelator (it binds with chemicals) and also is helpful in decreasing chemical sensitivities, especially when glutathione and glycerrhizin (derived from the licorice herb) are added. Oxidative therapies (see Chapter 11) help metabolize toxins, enhance oxidative metabolism, and help improve tissue and cellular oxygenation.

INFECTIOUS AGENTS

On the microbial level, it's a busy world out there. We are surrounded by viruses, bacteria, fungi, and parasites that would love to make us their permanent residence. All are common, and all can contribute to immune overload.

Viruses

Viruses range from relatively benign (for example, a cold virus) to lethal (HIV). The virulence of a virus depends not only on the organism but also on the state of your immune system. Some viruses, once acquired, remain in the body indefinitely. A classic example is the Epstein-Barr virus, which causes mononucleosis. We now know that Epstein-Barr can be kept in check by a healthy immune system, but can be reactivated, either acutely or chronically, when the immune system is stressed. It was formerly believed that Epstein-Barr caused chronic fatigue immune dysfunction syndrome, but we now believe that the reemergence of Epstein-Barr symptoms as well as evidence of reactivation revealed by blood testing is a consequence, not a cause, of CFIDS.

Bacteria

Bacteria also range from the garden variety to the virulent. Antibiotics have knocked out some of the weaker strains; some of the stronger strains have become antibiotic-resistant. Not only are bacteria becoming tougher to beat, but also our immune system is increasingly stressed. Some bacterial infections are insidious. The Lyme spirochete can cause symptoms that subside without treatment but reoccur in a more problematic form months or years later. Other examples of chronic bacterial infections include sinusitis (bacteria hidden deep in the sinuses, where they are hard to reach, behaving almost like an occult abscess) and dysbiosis (an abnormal bacterial environment in the intestines or colon). A long-standing infection weakens the immune system and can cause signs and symptoms quite a distance from the actual infection.

Yeast

Yeast can cause chronic candidiasis, which can lead to myriad symptoms that affect every area of the body. Candidiasis can mimic or be involved in many other conditions, including low blood sugar, autoimmune disorders, allergies, and chronic digestive disorders. Yeast is a normal inhabitant of the gastrointestinal tract, but it can overgrow and proliferate if you are taking antibiotics, steroids, or oral contraceptives; if you eat a high-sugar diet; or if your immune system is compromised.

Parasites

Parasites—including worms and protozoa—are a larger health issue than most people (including doctors) realize. Parasitic infections are common not only in tropical and developing countries, but also here at home. At this moment, 20 to 30 million Americans have pinworms. In one large study, 14 percent of American army recruits were found to be infected with *Toxoplasma,* a protozoa. According to public health experts, up to 25 percent of sexually active Americans may have the sexually transmitted parasite *Trichomonas.* Surveys show up to 5 percent of the American population (over 10 million people) is infected with *Entamoeba histolytica,* a strain of ameba that can cause serious illness. Another 8 to 10 million Americans are infected with *Giardia lamblia,* another intestinal parasite.[17] Parasites are a concern for everyone, but can be deadly for people who are immunocompromised.

Precautions to Take

Some precautions to reduce your exposure to harmful microorganisms include:

- Wash your hands in hot water. With soap. Often. (Same for your kitchen cutting board, knives, utensils, and countertops.)
- Avoid contact with insects that carry disease (ticks, fleas, mites).
- Avoid contact with rodents and their droppings.
- Don't eat raw or undercooked meat, poultry, eggs, fish, or shellfish. Don't buy cooked shrimp that are displayed on the same ice as raw fish. If you drink milk or eat milk products, make sure the milk has been pasteurized. Precook meat and poultry before you barbecue it to make sure it is cooked through. Watch out for hidden sources of raw egg (Caesar salad dressing, homemade mayonnaise, chocolate mousse, eggnog, etc.).
- Avoid medications that kill off the beneficial bacteria in your gastrointestinal tract (such as antibiotics, oral contraceptives, and steroids).
- Keep your intestinal defenses healthy by eating lots of fruits, vegetables, grains, and legumes—but wash (or rinse) them first. (Yes, even the grains.)
- Avoid water that may be contaminated. This includes both ice cubes and mountain streams, which may contain *Giardia*.
- Avoid food that may have become contaminated during its growth or preparation. Avoid reheated foods unless you are certain they were quickly refrigerated in small containers right after they were prepared.
- Make sure your refrigerator is working properly. Bacteria can grow at temperatures above 40 degrees F.
- Use international foods cautiously. Foods that are processed overseas cannot all be tested for the presence of parasite eggs.

At the first sign of illness, there are natural preparations you can take with antiviral, antibacterial, antifungal, or antiparasitic properties. Later chapters will discuss treatment options for different disorders.

HORMONAL DEFICIENCIES AND IMBALANCES

Hormone "balancing" is an extremely important part of returning to and maintaining optimal health and has become a very important part of my practice. Hormonal insufficiency, which plays a role in immune dysfunction, is much more common than people realize and can be difficult to detect. See Chapter 10, Immune System Super Boosters, for a discussion of hormonal health.

DRUGS

My basic rule about drugs is to use them in a comprehensive healing program that addresses the underlying reason(s) why you are sick. I prefer to use more natural, less toxic alternatives if they are available and efficacious. However, sometimes drugs are lifesaving, especially in acute situations. Some of my patients suffer needlessly because they refuse to take a drug that would help them. I encourage these patients to keep an open mind, especially during that period of time when alternative modalities are taking effect. Sometimes a short course of drugs can bridge the gap.

If you must take an over-the-counter or prescription medication, find out how it works, what side effects it can cause, how it should be taken, and what substance should not be taken at the same time. Knowing the correct dosage is most important, as all drugs can be toxic at higher levels. In general, drugs tend to have a much more narrow therapeutic window (and consequently a much larger chance for toxicity) than nutrients.

Do not assume that a medication is safe or appropriate just because a doctor prescribed it for you. Some doctors are misled by pharmaceutical salespeople who give them biased information. Unfortunately, many doctors obtain much of their information about drugs from these salespeople or from advertising. Others base their recommendations on information that is out of date.

In his riveting keynote lecture entitled "Losing the War Against Cancer: Who's Responsible and What to Do About It," given at the American College for Advancement in Medicine conference in the fall of 1994, Samuel Epstein, M.D., drew attention to several carcinogenic drugs, including Flagyl (prescribed for trichomoniasis), Kwell (a lice shampoo containing a highly potent pesticide), clomiphene (a fertility drug associated with ovarian cancer), and tamoxifen (ironically, a treatment for breast cancer). Epstein called tamoxifen "a scientific and ethical travesty," noting that the evidence of its carcinogenicity is overwhelming.

Medications can be very problematic. Many routinely administered drugs can cause health problems. Every class of medication has its potential side effects. Antibiotics alone can cause diarrhea, colitis, liver function abnormalities, and decreased blood cell counts. As a culture, we have to stop using antibiotics to the extent we do because bacteria are becoming more and more resistant. In our search for a stronger and stronger "magic bullet," we are forgetting that real healing comes from the patient's own immune system.

Anti-inflammatory medications can cause gastritis, ulcers, bleeding, and kidney problems. Blood pressure medications can cause impotence and fatigue. Blood thinners can cause abnormal bleeding problems. The Pill is associated with vascular complications (stroke, heart attack, blood clots) and nutrient deficiencies. Steroids suppress the immune system and can allow infections to become more virulent or widespread. Synthetic estrogens are associated with endometrial cancer and breast cancer.

There are far too many medications and too many side effects to mention here. All medications carry a risk/benefit ratio. If I find it necessary to prescribe a drug for one of my patients, I give the smallest effective dose and simultaneously recommend natural immune system boosters. (It should be noted that in certain conditions, such as Lyme disease, the effective dose may be higher than it is for less onerous infections.) In my practice, I always give nutrients and herbs with antibiotics to enhance the immune system and to protect the gastrointestinal tract and the liver.

Medications can:

- Interfere with digestion and with the absorption and utilization of nutrients
- Cause organ strain (different drugs tax different organs, including the liver and the kidneys)
- Elevate your body's need for certain nutrients used in the detoxification process
- Raise your need for antioxidants to combat free radical damage

If you're taking any medication, particularly for an extended period of time, make sure you're eating an optimal diet and getting healthy doses of antioxidants and the specific nutrients and herbs you need to protect the organ(s) that may be affected by your medication. If you must take an antibiotic, see the recommendations in Chapter 9.

Alcohol

Alcohol is a drug, so I need to mention it here. While your body is able to detoxify it in limited amounts, alcohol is in fact poison for every system in your body. In the short term, alcohol depresses your nervous system (causing impaired judgment and lack of coordination), irritates the digestive system, dilates blood vessels in the circulatory system, and suppresses the immune system. Alcohol depletes nutrient reserves, inhibits the functioning of bone marrow, and is dehydrating. Too much alcohol will cause unconsciousness and can result in death. Pregnant women should avoid alcohol because it crosses the placenta and can disrupt normal fetal development.

Long-term use of alcohol can impair brain function; contribute to heart disease, hypertension, and stroke; and result in irreversible liver damage. High alcohol consumption increases the risk of cancer and is often associated with gastritis, pancreatitis, and peptic ulcers. Because heavy drinkers get plenty of calories from alcohol, they often do not eat well and are undernourished.

Despite all the above, I have to admit that an occasional bottle of wine shared with friends or a glass of champagne at a wedding probably does more good than harm. There is some data to suggest that a glass of red wine with dinner can be protective of the heart. Just remember that alcohol contributes to your immune burden, so it is counterproductive to consume alcohol when you are under any kind of stress.

Recreational Drugs

Everybody knows illegal drugs are incompatible with immune system health. People who do drugs have lower nutrient levels than people who don't, and it has been shown that malnutrition and infection go hand in hand.

I hope you are already aware that recreational drugs are not part of an optimal immune health program, but if you need persuasion, consider these facts:

• A cocaine habit invariably leads to poor nutrition, which suppresses the immune system. Malnutrition is associated with a reduced ratio of helper T cells to suppressor T cells.

• Crack can cause high blood pressure and heart attack by placing a demand on the heart it cannot meet.

• Intravenous drug users are particularly at risk for opportunistic infections, including hepatitis and AIDS. In fact, I have recently seen an increasing number of patients in their forties, including many successful professionals, who had used drugs in their younger days and are now discovering they have chronic hepatitis (especially hepatitis C). Some of them find this out when they have blood tests for a routine physical exam or blood work to qualify for life insurance.

Marijuana is not a benign drug and has documented immunity-inhibiting effects. It may inhibit both cytotoxic T cell activity and macrophage activity. Marijuana smoke has toxic, inflammatory, and carcinogenic effects on lung tissue. One study found that regular, heavy use of marijuana is associated with chronic, acute bronchitis and impaired function of the macrophages in the lungs. The study concluded that marijuana smoking may cause airway injury, lung inflammation, and impaired pulmonary defense against infection. In addition, marijuana smoke is even worse for you than cigarette smoke (see page 111). The smoke of one marijuana cigarette led to the deposition of four times as many particles in the lungs as one filtered cigarette.[18]

RADIATION AND ELECTROMAGNETIC FIELDS

Back in Chapter 2, I mentioned that high-energy radiation is clearly dangerous to our health, and that low-energy radiation may well be. At the high-energy end of the electromagnetic spectrum are short-wavelength forms of radiation called *ionizing* radiation. Ionizing radiation can knock electrons out of their orbits around the nucleus of an atom, creating a reactive free radical—an ion that has an electrical charge and can combine with other ions.

A free radical is looking to combine with other atoms to pilfer an electron and regain its neutral charge.

X rays are a form of ionizing radiation. The voltage of the X ray depends upon how far it has to penetrate. A dental X ray, for example, uses less radiation than an X ray of the lungs. Radiation therapy uses X rays that are generated at several million volts.

In high doses, ionizing radiation can kill. Radiation can damage the bone marrow and directly suppress the immune system. By causing mutations in cellular DNA, it promotes cancer.

The effects of ionizing radiation accumulate over your entire lifetime. To limit your exposure:

- Refuse any X rays that aren't absolutely necessary.
- Refuse unnecessary medical procedures that use any form of radiation, including radioactive dyes or radioactive iodine.
- Don't work in an occupation that exposes you to nuclear energy.
- Don't live near a natural or artificial source of nuclear energy (power plant, waste disposal site).

To combat the effects of any ionizing radiation to which you are exposed, take antioxidants.

A little further down the electromagnetic spectrum is ultraviolet light, a component of sunlight. The wavelength of cosmic rays is a little longer than that of ionizing radiation—cosmic radiation is a little less energetic. Even so, ultraviolet radiation is powerful enough to penetrate several feet of the earth's surface and to damage the DNA in our skin cells. Ultraviolet rays are the major cause of skin cancer. Again, to counteract the effects of cosmic rays, take antioxidants.

To limit your exposure to ultraviolet radiation:

- Don't live on the equator, where ultraviolet exposure is highest.
- Live at sea level. (Someone living in Denver, Colorado, at an altitude of 6,000 feet receives more than twice the annual radiation dose of cosmic rays than someone living at sea level.)
- Don't go outside when the sun is at its highest.
- Cover up. Dark colors absorb ultraviolet rays more completely than light colors.
- Wear a hat. Eighty percent of skin cancers occur on the head and neck.[19] Every inch of brim reduces your lifetime cancer risk by 10 percent.
- Wear a sunscreen. It's more effective at blocking ultraviolet rays than clothes are.
- Avoid tanning salons.

COMMONLY ASKED QUESTION NO. 8:

Tanning booths are safer than sunbathing, right?

Wrong. It's hard to determine exactly how much skin cancer is due to tanning salons because most people who use tanning booths also sunbathe. We do know, however, that the ultraviolet light emitted by sunlamps can damage the skin, and this damage eventually can cause cancer.

One woman from northern England who had never sunbathed in her life mystified doctors when she developed cancerous lesions all over her body. It turns out she had been using a tanning booth once or twice a week for three years. She stopped frequenting the tanning salon—but ten years later she was still developing skin cancers.[20]

At the far end of the electromagnetic spectrum are still longer wavelengths, including microwaves, radio and television transmissions, and extremely low frequency (ELF) radiation. It is possible that these forms of energy disrupt electrical currents within the body. Common electrical appliances also subject us to radiation because weak magnetic fields are generated around all wires that carry electricity. Most people aren't troubled by this, but certain sensitive people are able to detect when a microwave or computer is turned on.

To limit your exposure to electromagnetic radiation:

• Don't live near a radio tower, microwave or television transmitter, power transformer, or high-power tension wires.
• Don't sleep with an electric blanket or heating pad. (You can turn it on to warm up the bed, then turn it off.)
• Don't keep an electric clock radio next to your bed.
• Buy a screen for your computer monitor that eliminates any electromagnetic transmissions.
• Reduce your need for electric heat and air-conditioning.
• Use appliances that run on rechargeable batteries.
• Avoid dimmer switches.
• Keep at least 3 feet from the television and computer (when possible).
• Unplug appliances when not in use.

Not all electromagnetic exposure is "bad." For example, electromagnetic fields are generated by the weather, and our own neurons communicate by means of electrical currents.

Some therapeutic uses for electromagnetic fields are currently being researched, using energy levels at far lower frequencies than any of the appliances just listed. (Energetic medicine is discussed in Chapter 10.)

SMOKING

There is a classic story about a medical student—actually, a resident—who was making hospital rounds with the allergist/immunologist who was training him. Believe it or not, the physician was smoking. When the resident asked him to please stop because he was allergic to cigarette smoke, the doctor replied that there has never been a double-blind study that proved cigarette smoke can cause an allergic reaction.

This attitude is almost unbelievable. Cigarette smoke is an irritant that blackens the lungs and causes lung cancer. It is packed with as many as 6,000 chemicals, many of them poisonous. Components of cigarette smoke include cadmium, carbon monoxide, and benzene—all known health hazards. Smoking generates massive amounts of free radicals (a single puff of cigarette smoke can contain up to 100,000 trillion free radicals![21]) and depletes antioxidants and other nutrients from lung tissue.

Cigarette smoke reduces the ability of the blood to deliver oxygen to the heart and brain and is the major preventable risk factor for cardiovascular disease (meaning it sets the stage for heart attack and stroke). Bone fractures take an average of 21 weeks to heal in nonsmokers. In smokers, this figure jumps to 39 weeks—almost twice as long.[22] Obviously, the body's healing systems are adversely affected by smoking.

Smoking also affects problem-solving skills and cognitive performance. In a computer driving simulator, smokers who had just smoked were involved in almost 3.5 times as many rear-end collisions as nonsmokers.[23]

Smoking is also associated with reproductive problems, including reduced fertility in women and sperm damage in men. Smoking may decrease sperm density and increase the risk of impotence. Smoking during pregnancy has a direct biological effect on the fetus and is associated with a significantly increased risk of sudden infant death syndrome.

"Passive" or "secondhand" smoke—smoke from other people's cigarettes—is also dangerous. Nonsmokers who are exposed to secondhand smoke on a daily basis have an increased risk of both fatal and nonfatal cardiac events. Children who are exposed to smoke in their environment have more respiratory illnesses and ear infections than normal. The evidence linking passive smoke to health problems in nonsmokers continues to mount.

For general health as well as immune system health, stopping smoking is probably the most important lifestyle modification I ask my patients to make. The good news is that the human body begins to heal itself as soon as a person quits smoking. Within twenty minutes of the last cigarette, blood pressure and pulse rate drop to normal, and the temperature of the hands and feet increases to normal. Within eight hours, carbon monoxide concentrations in the blood fall to normal levels and oxygen content increases to normal. Within twenty-four hours, the chance of a heart attack decreases. Within seventy-two hours, the bronchial tubes relax and lung capacity increases. Over time, lung function improves, the cilia in the lungs grow back, the risk of infection goes down, and the ex-smoker's energy level goes up.

ENVIRONMENTAL POLLUTION

In this chapter I have repeatedly touched on the subject of pollution. Much of our immune system burden can be traced to toxins in our air, food, water, and home and work environments.

The problem of environmental pollution extends far beyond the scope of this book. Toxic chemicals are used in the manufacturing and maintenance of just about everything we associate with modern life, from running shoes to the space shuttle. As a result, hazardous wastes contaminate our streams and ground water and pollutants fill our air.

Chemical toxins, as we've already seen, accumulate in the body's fat and can cause a wide range of health problems from headaches to cancer to birth defects. I had hoped to include here a rundown of common chemicals and their uses, but the list became so long and complex that I decided to offer instead the same tips I give my patients.

Indoor Air Pollution

A truly modern phenomenon is the "sick building syndrome." Many substances used in a new or refurbished home, school, or office building "outgas" odors that can make us sick. A brand new home can be filled with toxic vapors from the glue, pressed wood, carpets, paints, varnishes, and vinyl floor coverings used to build it. Hermetically sealed buildings with limited access to fresh air also create health problems.

The number one precaution against indoor air pollution is ventilation. In addition:

- Don't let anyone smoke in your home.
- A dehumidifier is a two-edged sword. Lower humidity combats dust mites and water damage that leads to mold, but standing water in the dehumidifier grows mold. Empty your dehumidifier often, or rig it up high with a permanent hose that drains outside.
- If you use a humidifier, use distilled water and clean it daily or it will grow mold and spray microorganisms into your air.
- Central heating/cooling systems can become a breeding ground for contaminants that are then distributed throughout the house. Change filters often.
- Fuel-burning appliances (space heaters, oil furnaces, gas appliances, wood stoves) all give off a range of combustion by-products, including carbon monoxide, which is colorless, odorless, and tasteless. At least 250 people die each year from residential carbon monoxide

poisonings[24] (including the well-publicized death of tennis pro Vitas Gerulaitis due to an improperly installed heater). Therefore, ventilate your appliances correctly, never leave your car idling in the garage, and buy a carbon monoxide detector.

• Radon is a colorless, odorless gas that is released naturally by uranium as it breaks down in rock or soil. Radon exposure causes no obvious symptoms, but long-term exposure is linked to lung cancer. You can check the radon level in your home and correct it.

• Don't store chemicals—especially half-used containers—inside.

• Don't spray or "bomb" your home with pesticides.

• Don't use mothballs, aerosol air fresheners, or room deodorizers.

• Avoid pressed-wood products (particle board, fiberboard, plywood), which outgas formaldehyde.

• Avoid carpets, which contain a potpourri of poisons.

• If asbestos is present in your home, don't disturb it. If you want it removed, hire a professional with much experience in the proper removal methods.

Global Pollution

Herbicides and pesticides have a profound impact on water quality, food safety, and wildlife habitats. Yet one study found that less than 0.1 percent of the 2.5 million tons of pesticides used each year (that doesn't count herbicides) actually reached the targeted pests.[25] The United States alone uses 886 million pounds of pesticides each year to produce foods and crops. (Together, California and Florida account for 25 percent of the nation's total usage.[26]) According to the National Academy of Sciences, pesticide residues on food crops cause 14,000 new cases of cancer each year.[27] The average farmer uses 1.5 to 2 pounds of pesticides per acre. Consumers use as much as 10 pounds per acre on their lawns. Golf courses use 15 pounds per acre.[28]

"In grade school, you learned that water is made of hydrogen and oxygen," reads the advertisement for Pūr water filters. "No one ever mentioned lead, chlorine, or Cryptosporidium." Millions of Americans drink water that does not meet federal health standards. According to the National Resources Defense Council, one in five Americans (over 50 million people) between 1993 and 1994 drank water that violated EPA standards,[29] and each year 7 million people get sick and 1,200 people die from illnesses related to drinking water.[30]

Our water supplies are contaminated with heavy metals, industrial chemicals, sewage, pesticides, herbicides, and parasites. One of life's little ironies is that the chlorine added to drinking water as a disinfectant is itself a health hazard. Long-term consumption of chlorinated water is thought to be associated with an increased risk of rectal and bladder cancer.

The motto of the National Association of Physicians for the Environment (NAPE) is "Pollution prevention is disease prevention." Toxins can directly (and indirectly) affect every system of the body. To limit your exposure to toxins and pollutants:

- Try not to work in manufacturing or in a chemical plant.
- Don't use herbicides, pesticides, or insecticides at home. There are natural alternatives available.
- Don't live near a hazardous waste dump.
- Have your water tested.
- Buy a water purifier. Not just a carafe, or a sink model, but a system that filters toxins out of your shower water as well.
- Eat lower on the food chain, and avoid animal fats. If you eat animal meat, choose free-range, organic chicken or turkey.

Heavy Metals

Heavy metals that we ingest, inhale, or absorb include lead, mercury, cadmium, arsenic, nickel, and aluminum. As I mentioned in Chapter 2, heavy metals can inhibit immune function by preventing enzymes (including antioxidants) from doing their job. They also may activate viruses by blocking the immune mechanisms that keep viruses in check.

Signs and symptoms of heavy metal poisoning include fatigue, headaches, depression, cognitive problems, abdominal complaints, anemia, high blood pressure, liver and kidney disease, and cancer. In modern society, heavy metal poisoning is a hidden cause of illness. Even when the signs and symptoms of heavy metal exposure are apparent, they mimic other disorders and the underlying problem is often overlooked.

To avoid damage to your immune system, limit your exposure to heavy metals and maintain an Immune Empowering Diet that supplies plenty of minerals and antioxidants. Specific nutrients that can be helpful with heavy metal overload include selenium, zinc, glutathione, N-acetylcysteine, vitamin C, vitamin E, and others.

Evidence suggests that there is a bioaccumulation of heavy metals with age. If you know you have been exposed, or if you have reason to believe that heavy metals have accumulated in your body, you can have tests done to evaluate the levels of heavy metals in your tissues. If necessary, chelation therapy can be used to eliminate heavy metals from the body (see Chapter 10, Immune System Super Boosters).

Lead

Lead can cause a wide variety of symptoms, including learning disabilities in children. A study of eight hundred boys attending public school in Pittsburgh found a direct relationship between the amount of lead in their leg bones and aggressive and delinquent behavior. Even after allowing for other predictors of delinquency, boys with higher lead levels were more likely to engage in antisocial behavior.[31] Lead poisoning may have contributed to the fall of the Roman Empire (the Romans drank from lead cups and their water was carried in lead pipes). According to highly esteemed geologist Claire Patterson, Ph.D., *all* modern people are subclinically lead poisoned because the average civilized individual has a body burden of lead a thousand times greater than five hundred years ago.[32] Children are especially susceptible to lead poisoning because they absorb more lead per pound of body weight than adults do. Each year in the United States, about two hundred children die from lead poisoning while another eight hundred suffer permanent brain damage.[33]

We are exposed to lead in lead-soldered pipes, leaded gasoline, food from cans with lead seams, and ceramic pottery with lead-containing glazes. Crops may contain heavy metals because of contaminated soil, as may milk and organ meats from animals grazing in contaminated pastures. In some areas, moonshine is contaminated with lead because it is distilled in lead-soldered equipment. Chips of leaded paint and lead-containing dust are well-known health hazards, but even undisturbed lead paint can react with sunlight and moisture to release tiny, breathable particles into the air. The amount of lead used in household paint and automobile gasoline in this century totals hundreds of thousands of tons and is the equivalent of two mountains.[34]

Lead paint is often regarded as an inner-city problem because so many housing units in urban areas received coat upon coat of lead-based paint in the early years of the twentieth century. However, a newly recognized problem is lead poisoning in middle-class families due to the restoration of older houses, including urban homes, suburban dwellings, and farmhouses. Removing old lead paint by means of sanding, torching, or the use of heat guns produces fine particles of lead that can be ingested or inhaled. Lead fumes that are generated by heat removal are especially dangerous and can cause acute lead poisoning within days or even hours.[35] Even if your home is safe, you may be at risk from a neighbor's renovation of an old house. The more you can do to eliminate your exposure to these sources (and efforts to eliminate several of them have been made in the last twenty years), the less lead you will accumulate.

Mercury

Mercury accumulates in the tissues and is a powerful neurotoxin. (The "mad hatter" in *Alice in Wonderland* was modeled on workers in the nineteenth century who suffered mercury poisoning from dipping felt hats into mercuric nitrate before shaping them.) Mercury also blocks the action of folic acid in the body and is a risk factor for heart attack. Mercury is found in certain fish (especially tuna, swordfish, and nonfatty freshwater fish), in some fungicides (and the grains on which they are used), in wood preservatives, in floor waxes and polishes, in film and photo engraving supplies, in certain pharmaceutical items (remember Mercurochrome?), and in "silver" dental fillings (which are in fact over 50 percent mercury). It is clear that mercury-containing fillings give off vapors, particularly in people who grind their teeth or chew gum, and there is some evidence that they suppress T cell counts.[36] In 1988, scrap dental amalgam—that is, a filling that has been removed from your mouth—was declared a hazardous waste product. Still, the American Dental Association maintains that this kind of dental amalgam has been used safely for 150 years, and the majority of doctors and dentists do not believe it can have negative effects.

While this controversy rages, I have observed certain patients who were undoubtedly sensitive to mercury-containing fillings and who felt much better after their "silver" fillings were replaced. I am also routinely seeing many more patients with unusually high levels of mercury—often not high enough to qualify as mercury toxicity, but definitely high enough to be considered mercury overload. I believe that the extent of the problem of mercury overload in the general population has yet to be fully recognized.

Cadmium

Cadmium, whether it is ingested or inhaled, is toxic to every body system and tends to accumulate in body tissue. Cadmium is an extremely potent immune suppressant, is especially toxic to the kidneys, and can be involved in causing hypertension. We are exposed to cadmium in paint, rubber tires, rubber carpet backing, fungicides, fertilizers, and colored plastics, among many other things. A major source of cadmium is cigarette smoke (including secondhand smoke). As little as one cigarette a day can increase blood cadmium levels.

Arsenic

Arsenic is poisonous whether it is inhaled or ingested. It is a neurotoxin and interferes with detoxification and control of free radicals. Common sources of arsenic include insecticides, weed killers, wood preservatives, ceramics, paint, and tobacco smoke. A major source of arsenic in the environment is copper-smelting factories.

Nickel

Nickel is deceptive because a small amount is necessary for proper cellular functioning. However, inhaled nickel (usually from industrial accidents) can cause nerve degeneration in the brain, cancer of the respiratory tract, and heart attack. Nickel is found in steel and metal alloys and in tobacco smoke. Nickel-containing jewelry can cause contact dermatitis.

Aluminum

Aluminum was not previously considered to pose a significant health risk, but recent evidence suggests the contrary. Aluminum is a neurotoxin. It increases the permeability of the blood/brain barrier, allowing potentially harmful molecules to pass into the brain. Aluminum is associated with memory loss and dementia and also causes softening of the bones. It is present in antacids, antiperspirants, and deodorants; aluminum cans; aluminum foil;

tobacco smoke; and aluminum pots, pans, and coffeepots. Baking powder can contain so-dium aluminum sulfate.

PSYCHOSOCIAL FACTORS

Emotional states are translated by the body into chemicals that have a large and measurable effect on immune response. This means that stress, loneliness, isolation, and anxiety all compromise the immune system. However, it also means that love, joy, and contentment bolster the immune system. This mind/body connection will be discussed in depth in Chapter 8, Stress Management Techniques.

WHAT YOU CAN DO

People are funny. I find that some patients take better care of their cars than they do of themselves. Mothers almost invariably take better care of their children's health than of their own.

A home may be our castle, but the body is our real dwelling place. With a little common sense, a little effort, and a little vigilance, you can make this dwelling a palace.

Please take a few minutes to complete the Immune System Profile starting on page 121. A high score is bad; a low score is good. The highest score you could possibly get is 280; the lowest score you could possibly get is −250. Use the Immune System Profile to discover your high-risk areas and to determine the overall condition of your immune system before you start the Immune System Empowerment Program. Then revisit the profile after three months, and after six months, to measure your progress. If you follow my recommendations in the chapters that follow, I am certain you will be pleasantly surprised with the results.

CRO   *ROSEMARY'S STORY*

Although her story is not typical, my patient Rosemary presents a good example of a completely overloaded immune system. Hers is really the story of the restoration of an immune system—and of a life as well.

When Rosemary first came to see me, she was a sixteen-year-old nonfunctional adolescent. She had been sickly all her life, and at this point she could scarcely go to school. In fact, she missed so much of tenth grade that she had to repeat the year. Rosemary was very dependent upon her parents, as chronically sick children often are, and she basically had no independent life.

"I want to live a normal life," Rosemary told me. The desire was there, but she simply didn't have the health. In our twenty-page self-survey for patients, Rosemary had checked off nearly every symptom. She felt dizzy and dazed, she suffered from chronic headaches and persistent fatigue, she had chronic stomach and gastrointestinal trouble, and she couldn't stand up straight because she felt as if she had "spikes" in her legs. Rosemary's sinuses hurt, her nose was always stuffy, and she had breathing difficulty that she called "icy lungs." She was prone to recurrent respiratory infections, earaches and pharyngitis, and had been on repeated courses of antibiotics.

Questioning revealed that Rosemary had a lifelong history of ear infections, allergies, eczema, rashes, and headaches. As a child she'd had her adenoids taken out and ear tubes put in. She had so many food allergies that eating was difficult, and her nutritional status was questionable. Rosemary was allergic to milk, but stated that all calcium supplements made her legs hurt. She had been getting allergy shots for dust, mold, and pollen, but her food allergies remained a definite problem.

Rosemary's previous doctor had placed her on nystatin for yeast overgrowth and gave her sublingual drops for her allergies. These measures were helpful, but Rosemary still had so many symptoms that she said she couldn't function as a human being. Her Immune System Kettle was overflowing to the point where she no longer knew what it felt like to be even close to healthy.

On examination, I found that Rosemary's thyroid was tender and slightly enlarged (thyroiditis). Subsequent blood work revealed that she had the highest level of autoimmune antithyroid antibodies I have ever seen. The normal range is 1:100; Rosemary's test results were 1:1,638,400.

To help get Rosemary on track, I prescribed a stronger antifungal medicine (Nizoral) for her candida and thyroid medication to give her thyroid a rest and alleviate her thyroiditis. Rosemary's blood work suggested poor nutritional status, but she had sensitivities to so many oral supplements that I decided to start her on intravenous vitamin C with added nutrients. To round out her immune-supporting regimen and to help treat her chronic pains, I referred Rosemary to an acupuncturist near her home.

These therapies were all helpful, and Rosemary's health improved. However, two years later she started running an occasional low-grade fever and began to experience headaches, joint pain, muscle aches, sinus tenderness, aching bones, and chronic abdominal pains. CT scans of her abdomen and pelvis revealed nothing unusual, and Rosemary's Lyme titer test results were negative. Still, she continued to have persistent fatigue, chronic asthma, and various aches and pains. Rosemary was able to complete one fall semester at college, which was a major accomplishment for her, and her allergies were improved—but still she was far from well.

We kept up with Rosemary's regimen—allergy management, thyroid medication, and intravenous vitamin C—until the following June, when Rosemary tested positive for Lyme disease. To combat the Lyme, I placed Rosemary on the oral antibiotic doxycycline for six weeks, making sure she simultaneously took nystatin to help prevent any yeast overgrowth. The antibiotic alleviated many of Rosemary's symptoms, including her headaches and bone aches, but it also caused her candidiasis and gastrointestinal symptoms to worsen.

Encouraged by Rosemary's response to the oral antibiotic—overall her condition did improve noticeably—but mindful of the persistence of some of her symptoms, we decided to try a two-week trial of intravenous Rocephin (another antibiotic). Happily, Rosemary's symptoms almost completely resolved. Her head cleared and her aches and pains, including that persistent bone pain, faded to the point where she stopped taking analgesics altogether.

Four days after she stopped taking Rocephin, Rosemary's symptoms returned. I was reluctant to put her right back on intravenous antibiotics, and we agreed to wait and see how things went. Unfortunately, Rosemary experienced a considerable relapse. By December, she had chronic fatigue and aching bones again. (This deep bone pain—not muscle aches, and not joint pain—was consistently one of Rosemary's most prominent symptoms. I found it somewhat puzzling, but for this patient, "bone pain" was a signal that all was not well.) Rosemary stopped going to school, stopped baby-sitting, cut back on her activities, and even stopped driving. She was housebound.

In February, Rosemary consulted a neurologist at a neurology department of a prominent medical center. He found no neurologic dysfunction and had no explanation for her symptoms. However, he rejected the idea that Rosemary might have chronic Lyme disease, and discounted her treatment for candidiasis. His recommendations were psychotherapy and aerobic exercise (despite the fact that Rosemary was too tired to do her own laundry). Basically this amounted to telling Rosemary that she should somehow just "buck up," since nothing in his medical textbooks could explain her many debilitating symptoms. The neurologist expressed concern about Rosemary's future and intimated that she was overly dependent on her parents in an emotionally unhealthy way.

For my part, I believed that Rosemary had seronegative Lyme disease (that is, Lyme disease that fails to produce a positive blood test result). However, before putting Rosemary back on antibiotics again—which might cause her other symptoms to worsen—I wanted to try some other approaches. To boost her level of health, I adjusted Rosemary's dose of thyroid medication, added additional hormone treatments to her regimen, and prescribed a succession of antidepressants (Rosemary ended up trying several, but none were helpful).

These therapies were not enough. By September, Rosemary was suffering from many chronic problems, including exhaustion, nausea, headaches, and joint pains. She still was troubled by candidiasis, allergies, rhinitis, and thyroiditis. Her immune system was upregulated (which accounted for the allergies and autoimmune problems) and downregulated (underactive) at the same time.

At this point I placed Rosemary on a high dose of intravenous Rocephin. After three weeks, her neurological symptoms abated. After six weeks, she noted a definite overall improvement. By December, she was able to read an entire book and to leave the house. By February, she told me she had "turned a corner." She was cross-country skiing, attending church, seeing friends, and resuming a normal life.

Imagine how shocked the staff was in May when Rosemary arrived for her intravenous treatment and *ran* up the stairs. Jaws dropped! After eight months of treatment, Rosemary was able to bicycle several miles at a time. Eight months is a heck of a long time to be on an intravenous antibiotic, but it took that long to overcome the onerous Lyme spirochete that had been residing in Rosemary's tissues for some time. In addition, all the adjunctive nutrients—both oral and intravenous—helped Rosemary's immune system to restore itself and take charge of her health.

I made further adjustments to Rosemary's medications and started her on enzyme-potentiated desensitization (EPD) for her food, chemical, and inhalant allergies. Little by little her immune system came back into balance and Rosemary was able to leave her symptoms further and further behind. She was able to go out with friends, do yardwork, and work part-time. She could think more clearly and was better able to tolerate substances that used to provoke her sensitivities.

By the following November, Rosemary said, "I finally feel like my blueprint is correct." She had driven herself to the office for her appointment, and she looked like an entirely different person.

In January of the following year, Rosemary took a trip to Utah by herself. Now that she had the energy to pursue her goals, she was pulling down a 3.8 grade point average in college.

A year later, Rosemary had a recurrence of Lyme disease, and her long list of symptoms returned. I placed her on penicillin shots and intravenous hydrogen peroxide therapy, and after four months she had recovered.

Today Rosemary is dating, attending college (driving one hour each way), teaching piano, and working out at a health club. Her allergies are so much improved that she can even eat dairy products, and she says that when she is exposed to viruses and colds, she just doesn't catch them anymore. Rosemary is maintaining her good health with nutritional supplements, homeopathic remedies, and ongoing EPD and intravenous hydrogen peroxide treatments on a periodic basis.

I'm nearly as proud of Rosemary as her parents are, for before my eyes she has grown up to be an energetic young woman. I often think of the neurologist who disapproved of Rosemary's treatments and questioned her aptitude for leading a full and independent life. Using progressive medicine, we were able to rehabilitate Rosemary's immune system, thereby freeing her to live the life she wanted all along.

The Immune System Profile

Following is the Immune System Profile, a questionnaire to help you evaluate the state of your immune system and target ways to lower your immune load. This is not a scientific instrument and it is not intended as a tool to diagnose specific illnesses or disorders.

The scoring is self-evident: a higher total is bad, a lower total is good. Try to avoid the temptation to portray yourself in the best possible light. If you give a frank evaluation of your situation today, you'll be better able to appreciate the improvements you've made when you revisit the Immune System Profile in the future.

Key:
0 Never
1 Occasionally — Not Severe
2 Occasionally — Severe
3 Frequently — Not Severe
4 Frequently — Severe

SYMPTOMS	Score	Score in 3 months	Score in 6 months
1. Headaches			
2. Light-headedness			
3. Dizziness			
4. Insomnia			
5. Red, watery, or itchy eyes			
6. Dark circles under the eyes			
7. Eyes sensitive to light			
8. Earaches, ear infections			
9. Ringing in ears			
10. Stuffy or runny nose			
11. Sinus problems			
12. Coughing			
13. Need to clear throat			
14. Swollen glands			

SYMPTOMS	Score	Score in 3 months	Score in 6 months
15. Sore throat, hoarseness			
16. Canker sores, mouth sores			
17. Hives			
18. Dry skin			
19. Eczema			
20. Hair loss			
21. Hot flashes			
22. Irregular or skipped heartbeat			
23. Rapid or pounding heartbeat			
24. Chest congestion			
25. Bronchitis			
26. Asthma, wheezing			
27. Shortness of breath			
28. Nausea, vomiting			

	Score	Score in 3 months	Score in 6 months
29. Diarrhea			
30. Constipation			
31. Bloated feeling			
32. Belching			
33. Passing gas			
34. Heartburn			
35. Intestinal/stomach pain			
36. Frequent, urgent, or burning urination			
37. Genital itch or discharge			
38. Pain or aches in joints			
39. Arthritis (swelling of joints)			
40. Stiffness or limitation of movement			
41. Pain or aches in muscles			
42. Muscle weakness			
43. Feeling of generalized weakness			
44. Chronic fatigue			
45. Craving certain foods			

	Score	Score in 3 months	Score in 6 months
46. Compulsive eating			
47. Water retention			
48. Overweight			
49. Difficulty losing weight			
50. Underweight			
51. Difficulty gaining weight			
52. Restlessness			
53. Numbness or tingling of extremities			
54. Memory loss			
55. Confusion, poor comprehension, difficulty concentrating			
56. Learning disabilities			
57. Mood swings			
58. Anxiety, fear, nervousness			
59. Anger, irritability, aggressiveness			
60. Depression			
Symptoms: Grand Total			

Personal History and Lifestyle

GENETIC BLUEPRINT

	−10	−5	0	5	10	Score	Score in 3 months	Score in 6 months
Family history of cancer or autoimmune disorders?			Don't know or none	A few family members	Multiple family members			
Family history of longevity?	Most family members die of natural causes over the age of 85	Some family members live to over 85	Don't know or average lifespans (until 70s)	Some early deaths due to illness (not accidents)	Multiple early deaths due to illness (not accidents)			

DIET

	−10	−5	0	5	10	Score	Score in 3 months	Score in 6 months
Do you eat an optimal diet (organic fruits and vegetables, whole grains, low-fat, high-quality proteins)?	Daily	Frequently	Occasionally	Infrequently	Rarely			
Do you eat sugar (candy, sweets, ice cream) and refined carbohydrates (foods made with refined white flour)?	Rarely	Infrequently	Occasionally	Frequently	Daily			
Do you take nutritional supplements (i.e., antioxidants, including vitamin C, vitamin E, and beta-carotene)?	Daily	Frequently	Occasionally	Infrequently	Never			

ALLERGIES/SENSITIVITIES

	−10	−5	0	5	10	Score	Score in 3 months	Score in 6 months
Do certain foods bother you?	Never	Infrequently	Occasionally or not aware of problem	Frequently	Daily			

Question						Score	Score in 3 months	Score in 6 months
Do certain chemical odors bother you (such as perfumes, paint, or cleaning agents)?	Never **-10**	Infrequently **-5**	Occasionally or not aware of problem **0**	Frequently **5**	Daily **10**			
Do certain inhalants (dust, mold, pollen, animal dander) bother you?	Never **-10**	Infrequently **-5**	Occasionally or not aware of problem **0**	Frequently **5**	Daily **10**			
Have you taken steps to avoid the items that trouble you (i.e., food and chemical avoidance, environmental controls)?	I am very careful **-10**	I am usually careful **-5**	I am occasionally careful or not aware of problem **0**	I am seldom careful **5**	I am not careful **10**			

INFECTIOUS AGENTS

Question						Score	Score in 3 months	Score in 6 months
Have you been bothered by recurrent infections (bronchitis, sinusitis, urinary tract infections, sore throats, vaginitis, flu-like symptoms, etc.)?	Never **-5**	Once a year **0**	2–3 times a year **5**	4 or more times a year, or for a prolonged period (6 weeks or longer) **10**				
How would you describe your recovery from acute viral illness (such as the flu)?	Very rapid **-10**	Fairly rapid **-5**	Average **0**	Somewhat slow **5**	Very slow **10**			

DRUGS

Question						Score	Score in 3 months	Score in 6 months
Do you take antibiotics?	Never, or very rarely **-10**	Seldom (less than once a year) **-5**	Once a year **0**	2–3 times a year **5**	4 or more times a year, or for prolonged periods **10**			
Do you take prescription painkillers, muscle relaxants, decongestants/antihistamines, steroids, or antidepressants?	Never **-10**	Seldom **-5**	Occasionally **0**	Several times a week **5**	Daily **10**			

Question	-10	-5	0	5	10	Score	Score in 3 months	Score in 6 months
Do you self-medicate with over-the-counter medications such as Tylenol, Advil, aspirin, cold medications, or antacids? (Exception: aspirin each day for cardiovascular health)	Never	Seldom	Occasionally	Several times a week	Daily			
Do you use recreational drugs (including marijuana or alcohol)?	Never	Seldom	Occasionally	Several times a week	Daily			

RADIATION

Question	-10	-5	0	5	10	Score	Score in 3 months	Score in 6 months
Are you exposed to radiation at work or where you live?	Never	Infrequently	Intermittently	For short periods	For prolonged periods			
Have you had radiation therapy, nuclear scans, or diagnostic X rays (including dental X rays or mammograms)?	Never, or very rarely	Infrequently	An occasional diagnostic X ray	Have had numerous diagnostic X rays and/or numerous nuclear scans	Have had radiation therapy			

SMOKING

Question	-10	-5	0	5	10	Score	Score in 3 months	Score in 6 months
Do you smoke?	Never	Quit at least 5 years ago	Very rarely or quit recently	Occasionally	Daily			

ENVIRONMENTAL POLLUTION

Question	-10	-5	0	5	10	Score	Score in 3 months	Score in 6 months
Are you exposed to hazardous chemicals where you live or work?	Never, or very rarely	Infrequently	Intermittently	For short periods	For prolonged periods			
Do you drink filtered or bottled water?	Daily	Several times a week	Occasionally	Seldom	Never			
Do you have adequate ventilation where you live or work?	Daily	For short periods	Intermittently	Infrequently	Never			

Question	-10	-5	0	5	10	Score	Score in 3 months	Score in 6 months
Do you get daily exposure to natural light or full-spectrum light?	For prolonged periods	For short periods	Intermittently	Infrequently	Never			

PSYCHOSOCIAL FACTORS

Question	-10	-5	0	5	10	Score	Score in 3 months	Score in 6 months
Do you tend to be worried or obsessive (about work, exercise, mistakes, the past, etc.)?	I am flexible and accepting of what life brings	I have a positive attitude and don't worry about what I can't control	I worry occasionally	I worry frequently	I worry constantly, even about little things			
Are you a goal-oriented perfectionist?	I do the best I can and see mistakes as opportunities	I like things done correctly but I can tolerate big mistakes	I like things done correctly but I can tolerate small mistakes	I am a perfectionist about my own actions	I am internally driven and can't tolerate any mistakes			
Have you experienced a significant psychosocial stress in the last six months?			Things are status quo	Moderate (such as loss of job, retirement, purchase of new home, birth)	Severe (such as death of spouse, separation or divorce)			
Do you practice stress management techniques, such as yoga, meditation, biofeedback, or self-hypnosis?	Daily	Frequently	Occasionally	Rarely	Never			
Do you exercise regularly for half an hour (walking, biking, swimming, treadmill, etc.)?	3–5 times a week	1–2 times a week	Active lifestyle, but no regular exercise	Overexercise	Inactive lifestyle			
Is love present in your life?	For prolonged periods	For short periods	Intermittently	Infrequently	Never, or very rarely			

Personal History and Lifestyle Grand Total:

Chapter 5

~

THE IMMUNE EMPOWERING DIET

Let thy food be thy medicine, and thy medicine be thy food.

—HIPPOCRATES

When Charlie Abrahams was born in March 1992, his parents had no way of knowing the difficulties that lay ahead. Charlie had his first seizure before he was a year old, and soon was diagnosed with Lennox-Gastaut syndrome, a severe form of epilepsy. Despite $100,000 worth of drugs, tests, and surgery, Charlie's seizures worsened. Before long his convulsions, which lasted from a few seconds up to forty-five minutes, were occurring up to a hundred times a day, despite a regimen of anticonvulsants that included four different drugs taken simultaneously. If Charlie's epilepsy could not be controlled, he risked mental retardation.

"I was raised to believe . . . that the answers to an illness came in prescriptions," Charlie's father, movie director Jim Abrahams, told *People* magazine in a story about Charlie's illness. "And that just isn't true."[1]

What eventually restored Charlie's health was an unusual high-fat, no-sugar diet that forces the body to burn fat for energy instead of sugar. On day 3 of his new diet, Charlie's seizures stopped.

Obviously, this unorthodox diet is not for everyone, but I mention this story because it dramatically illustrates the power of food. One of my younger patients, like Charlie, also responded only to this nutritional intervention (called the ketogenic diet) for her persistent, recalcitrant seizure disorder. Many, many other patients in my practice have responded to other special dietary modifications, often after conventional drug therapies failed. Food provides energy, but it's a lot more than just calories. What we eat can modify our hormone production, immune responses, and the processes that lead to inflammation. Nutrition is a biological response modifier.

127

FOOD AS FRIEND . . . OR FOE

It has been observed before, but it bears repeating: We are what we eat. Our diet helps determine the makeup of our cells, our internal metabolic processes, the components circulating in our blood, and our immune responses. Nutrition influences cell growth and function, cell-to-cell communication, and the production of extremely influential hormones within the body. Our health is affected on every level by what we do—and do not—put into our mouths.

• **Preventive Nutrition.** When it comes to nutrition, an ounce of prevention is worth at least a pound of cure and possibly a good deal more. A healthy diet contributes directly to our host resistance and can help us ward off a huge spectrum of illnesses, from the common cold to cancer. Because reversing illness, especially chronic diseases, can be difficult, it makes sense for us to do everything in our power to stay well. This chapter will outline the Immune Empowering Diet, which will provide your body with the nutrients it needs to maintain an optimally functioning immune system with a maximum ability to ward off illness.

• **Nutritional Therapy.** As Charlie's story shows, food is also medicine. Manipulating Charlie's diet caused changes in his metabolic processes, which in turn brought about beneficial changes in his brain chemistry. It's also possible to target specific foods that have particular pharmacologic effects. Nutritional intervention can be a powerful tool in overcoming illness. Although the intention of this book is not to provide in-depth treatment recommendations for specific illnesses, the Immune Empowering Diet will act as a cornerstone in any restorative and rejuvenating program.

• **Food as Poison.** Food can be hazardous to your health, and not just because of the chemicals, additives, and contaminants mentioned in the last chapter. The typical Western diet, characterized by lots of processed foods, sugar, and saturated fat, is directly linked to diseases like osteoporosis, rheumatoid arthritis, diabetes, hypertension, atherosclerosis ("hardening of the arteries"), and coronary heart disease. Just as eating the right foods helps keep us well, eating the wrong foods increases our chances of developing chronic illness. This chapter will include guidelines on foods to limit or to avoid.

All food is made up of *macronutrients* (carbohydrates, protein, and fat) and *micronutrients* (vitamins, minerals, and trace elements). Macronutrients provide energy for cells to burn and material with which the body can manufacture and repair cells. Micronutrients do not supply energy, but are needed for normal metabolism (including energy production) and healthy cell functioning. A deficiency of any one of a number of nutrients can impair immune function. This chapter will primarily address macronutrients, while micronutrients are discussed in Chapter 6, Immune System Boosters.

THE IMMUNE EMPOWERING DIET

I define good nutrition as (a) providing the body with all the nutrients it needs, and (b) not burdening the body with substances it doesn't need or might not tolerate well. The Immune Empowering Diet is high in antioxidants; includes abundant amounts of vegetables, fruits, and grains; is low in fat; and provides a reasonable amount of calories. The breakdown looks like this:

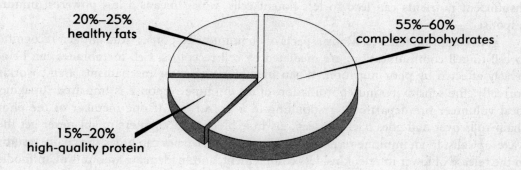

Some people require a diet that is lower in carbohydrates. An appropriate low-carbohydrate diet to meet their needs is discussed separately at the end of this chapter.

Unlike some well-known physicians, notably Nathan Pritikin (who, by the way, died of cancer), I don't recommend consuming less than 20 percent of total calories from healthy fats. Please note the word *healthy*. As you'll see in this chapter, the body needs a constant supply of certain kinds of fats. Insufficient fat intake suppresses the immune system (as does excessive fat intake).

NUTRITION AND IMMUNOCOMPETENCE

The immune system is extremely sensitive to nutrient deficiencies and is more easily damaged by undernutrition than any other system. Researchers have conducted extensive experiments to show why this is so, but the bottom line is that poorly nourished people get sicker—more frequently and for longer periods—than people who are well nourished.

If you think back to Chapter 3, you'll recall all the complex processes that make up an immune response. Nutrient deficiencies can cause decreased or abnormal functioning in an immune response at any step along the way. Expecting your body to make a forceful, well-orchestrated immune response without vital nutrients is like trying to start your car without spark plugs.

Poor nutrition can cause:

• **Decreased cell proliferation and impaired cell differentiation.** Cell reproduction involves the reshuffling of genetic information, and that can occur only if certain nutrients are present.

• **Poorer cell function.** An immune response depends not only on adequate numbers of cells, but also upon the optimal functioning of each type of cell. The effectiveness and resilience of cells depends upon the nutrient building blocks they have at their disposal. Insufficient nutrients can lead to less potent cells, which means a less powerful immune response.

• **Recognition failures.** Many aspects of an immune response, from antigen recognition to cell-to-cell communication, are mediated by cell receptors. Cell membranes can be adversely affected by poor nutrition. When membrane receptor mechanisms aren't working correctly, the sensitivity and coordination of an immune response is impaired. Imagine a local volunteer fire department responding to a 2 A.M. fire. If one member of the phone chain rolls over and goes back to sleep, a whole block of firefighters might never get their wake-up calls. In an immune response, nutritional deficiencies can break the chain, resulting in the release of fewer interleukins, less complement, and inadequate amounts of antibodies.

In addition to cellular mechanisms, immunocompetence also depends upon the correct functioning of different kinds of tissue. As we saw in Chapter 3, the skin, lymphoid tissues, thymus, mucosal linings, and reticuloendothelial system all have an important role in the day-to-day functioning of the immune system. Poor nutrition can undermine the effectiveness of these tissues. (One of the signs of severely compromised immune competence is thymic atrophy.)

Remember the Illness Spiral? Many chronic health problems start small. Often someone who has poor eating habits will develop subtle nutrient deficiencies that eventually lead to immune deficiency. Immune deficiency leads to illness. Illness places extra nutritional demands on the body because of the nutrients that are used up during an immune response. If these extra demands are not met, the immune system is set back even further. If this Illness Spiral isn't reversed, more serious health problems develop—either immune overreaction (for example, an autoimmune disease) or underreaction (for example, tumor growth). In this way, the path that started out with poor nutrition can end up with immune dysfunction.

MALNUTRITION AND UNDERNUTRITION

American multibillionaire Howard Hughes died of malnutrition, so clearly malnutrition can permeate every socioeconomic level of society. Our Western diet is generally inadequate in those nutrients that are needed for a strong immune system. Numerous surveys show that our society is malnourished because of a phenomenon known as "overconsumption undernutrition." That is, we eat foods that are calorie-rich but nutrient-poor—and plenty of them. While I only infrequently see patients who are truly starving, resembling the bone-thin malnourished children of underdeveloped countries, I do frequently see patients who are malnourished—including some who are overweight but definitely undernourished.

Malnutrition is a potential problem for people who either can't or don't eat healthy foods, including alcoholics, anorectics, bulimics, the poor, the elderly, and the chronically ill. Many hospital patients—from 25 to 50 percent[2]—are malnourished. Some enter the hospital that way, while many others become malnourished during their hospital stay. Have you ever eaten hospital food? It's about the furthest thing I can think of from healthy "recuperative" food. (Recall my father's sugar-laden diet when he was in the hospital recovering from pneumonia.) The phenomenon known as "hospital malnutrition" is caused by the cumulative effect of marginal nutrition, illness, and treatments that increase the body's nutrient needs, such as surgery, radiation, and immunosuppressive drugs. There is a direct relationship between nutritional status and resistance to infection. In one study, 23.5 percent of chronically malnourished adults experienced postoperative wound infections, bacteremia (bacteria in the bloodstream), and/or pneumonia, compared to 5.6 percent of well-nourished postoperative patients.[3]

More common in this country than malnutrition is undernutrition. Undernutrition is not only more widespread, but also more subtle. Unlike frank nutrient deficiencies, undernutrition often goes unrecognized. Those at risk for undernutrition include everyone in the categories mentioned above, plus dieters, teenagers (who have notoriously bad eating habits), people with gastrointestinal absorption problems, people with increased nutrient needs (due to illness, advanced age, or drug interactions), people who are losing nutrients due to increased excretion (due to diarrhea, alcohol, vomiting, or drug interactions), and those who have lost their appetite. Wasting diseases such as cancer and AIDS also can cause undernutrition, which can progress to frank malnutrition.

Nutrition expert Patrick Quillin estimates that at least 20 percent of Americans are clinically malnourished, with 70 percent undernourished and only 10 percent optimally nourished.[4] I'm hoping that this book will improve these figures!

DIET AND IMMUNE SENESCENCE

Old age is not a disease, yet many of our elderly are too sick to enjoy their longevity. Even in middle age, many people find themselves slowed down by chronic ailments. I have patients in their thirties and forties who feel years older. Why?

I believe that a lifetime of inadequate nutrition leads to ever-increasing nutrient deficiencies that ultimately undermine immune competence. While there are genetic and environmental components to immune senescence, there is undoubtedly also a nutritional component.

As the immune system ages, it becomes more prone to both overreaction and underreaction. Aging is generally associated with an increase in autoimmune problems and decreased immunity to neoplasia (malignancy).[5] Because food can contribute greatly to immune competence, a healthy diet can have a beneficial effect on these problems.

DIET AND GUT IMMUNITY

Our gastrointestinal tract engages in innumerable immune skirmishes every day. Large clusters of immune cells—in fact, more than 50 percent of all our immune cells—are clustered around the gastrointestinal tract to help fight off the antigens we constantly take in with our food. In addition, secretory IgA in the mucosal lining of the gastrointestinal tract provides an important immunological barrier against food antigens.

Research has shown that undernutrition is associated with low levels of secretory IgA.[6] This could help explain why selective IgA deficiency is the most common immunodeficiency in adults.[7] Many people with IgA deficiency have significant complications.

Low levels of secretory IgA in the gut mean impaired gut immunity, and that can spell trouble. We now know that many systemic illnesses originate with gut disorders. Aberrant function of the gut's lymphoid system is associated with food sensitivities, autoimmune problems, tumors, coronary heart disease, and chronic intestinal infection.[8]

In case you're still not persuaded that gastrointestinal immunity is worth worrying about, consider this: the gut has its own brain, called the *enteric nervous system*, located in tissue that lines the esophagus, stomach, small intestine, and colon. The gut's brain includes 100 million neurons (more than the spinal cord) that send and receive nerve impulses and record emotions and experiences. Researchers in the new field of neurogastroenterology have determined that the head's brain and the gut's brain affect each other. When one gets upset, the other does, too. Most people accept the idea that mental stress can cause gut discomfort, but the relationship between the brain and the gut works the other way, too. For example, patients with bowel problems have been shown to have abnormal REM sleep—so gut health even influences our sleep patterns.[9] (Gut health is discussed in more depth in Chapter 9.)

The Paleolithic Diet

A 1985 article in *The New England Journal of Medicine* raised some interesting questions about the relationship between the major chronic diseases of industrialized society (including heart disease, hypertension, diabetes, and cancer) and the typical modern diet in light of what must have been the typical Paleolithic diet of *Homo sapiens*.[10] Genetically we haven't changed much since the appearance of modern man about 40,000 years ago, but our civilized diet bears little resemblance to that of our nonagricultural forebears.

Early hunter-gatherers primarily ate wild game, fish, roots, beans, nuts, tubers, and fruits. They apparently seldom consumed cereal grains and never ate dairy products. Even without dairy products, however, their calcium intake is believed to have been far in excess of ours because of all the meat they ate. Similarly, even without grains, their fiber intake was probably much higher than ours because of all the fruits and vegetables they ingested.

The Paleolithic diet is believed to have been low in sodium (no added salt!) and high in vitamin C, iron, and folate. Although this diet contained a high level of cholesterol, it would have had less total fat and a higher percentage of the healthier essential fatty acids (see page 151) than today's typical civilized diet.

The Paleolithic diet correlates with the oldest blood type known to man, type O. Naturopathic doctor Peter D'Adamo, building upon the groundbreaking work of his father, proposes that our optimal diet is determined in part by our blood type. Blood type A, according to D'Adamo's research, is a more recent blood type that correlates with an agrarian diet high in complex carbohydrates and low in fat and protein.[11]

I'm not about to endorse a diet high in mastodon meat (or any other meat, for that matter), but I do think it is worth noting that genetically we are more adapted to the Paleolithic diet than to our modern diet—particularly what has now become the typical American diet.

THE TYPICAL AMERICAN DIET

The most commonly eaten foods in America are white bread, coffee, and hot dogs.[12] (Toxicologist Samuel Epstein, M.D., links hot dogs with soaring rates of childhood leukemia and brain cancers.[13]) Each year the average American eats 756 doughnuts, 60 pounds of cakes and cookies, 23 gallons of ice cream, 7 pounds of potato chips, 22 pounds of candy, and 365 servings of soda.[14] Some people undoubtedly eat less—but that means others eat more. If you or I don't eat a single doughnut in a year, then statistically it's possible that someone else eats 1,500!

A survey of 11,000 Americans indicated that on a given day 17 percent ate *no* vegetable, 41 percent ate *no* fruit,[15] and 84 percent did not eat any high-fiber food.[16] As a population, we clearly are not consuming adequate amounts of macronutrients *or* micronutrients.

How to Change Eating Habits

When I ask patients to keep track of what they're eating, they are usually very cooperative. The problem is that often they have trouble taking responsibility for the results when they see them on paper. "It was a bad week," they'll say. "Of course, that business trip [or wedding, or funeral, or deadline, or exam . . .] really threw me off!" You and I both know that there is always *something* going on that has the potential of undermining our good eating habits.

I know that eating habits can be difficult to change. Many patients get a certain look when I outline the Immune Empowering Diet for them. Generally I urge people to make gradual changes (for example, see the Immune Empowering Food Exchanges on page 159) and to watch for the pleasant benefits of eating a better diet, such as increased energy and alertness or decreased bloating and discomfort. Patients who are very ill have the most to gain from adopting the healthiest possible diet and are often very motivated. At the other end of the spectrum are teenagers, who often eat in a hasty, catch-as-catch-can manner (that's why it's called "fast food"!), who are susceptible to advertising and peer pressure, and who basically think they're immortal.

I had a hard time persuading my patient Rebecca that her eating habits were wreaking havoc with her immune system. At sixteen, she already was experiencing fatigue, recurrent yeast infections, and flare-ups of acne. She developed a persistent, deep cough in the winter that seemed more or less permanent.

Even though she didn't see anything wrong with them, Rebecca's eating habits were horrifying. She pretended not to be interested in food and rarely ate in front of other people. She'd skip lunch at school, and whenever she went out to dinner, she would order a salad and then move it around on the plate until everyone else was finished eating. On the other hand, sometimes Rebecca would binge on ice cream and peanut butter cookies in her room at night. Feeling guilty, she then wouldn't let herself eat anything except sugar cubes (!) for the next two or three days.

I knew I wouldn't be able to interest Rebecca in steamed vegetables and brown rice right away, but I did make several "doable" recommendations to get her back on track, including eating regular meals, taking supplements, and choosing better foods. When Rebecca's health and skin improved, she found the motivation to make further changes and started listening to my advice with more interest. Eventually Rebecca fell in with some vegetarians at her high school, and together the group lobbied for a healthier selection of foods in the cafeteria as well as more environmentally friendly procedures (including washable trays instead of disposable Styrofoam, and plastic recyclable juice containers instead of juice boxes). From a rather inauspicious beginning, Rebecca ended up being a wonderful success story.

THE IMMUNE EMPOWERING DIET: 15 TO 20 PERCENT HIGH-QUALITY PROTEIN

Protein is the main structural component of our tissues and organs. We need a constant supply of protein for cell growth and repair. The immune system itself is a protein matrix—antibodies, for example, are proteins, and all cells have proteins. Someone who is protein compromised is also immunologically compromised.

All proteins are made up of amino acids arranged in different orders. Twenty amino acids make up all the proteins in humans. Of these, twelve can be made by the body, but eight "essential" amino acids must be obtained through the diet. Digestion is the process of breaking foods down into usable products—or, as one of my colleagues, nutritional physician Sid Baker, has said, "taking the egginess out of egg."

Protein is available from both animal and vegetable sources, including meat, fish, poultry, dairy products, eggs, nuts and seeds, legumes, and grains. It is not true that you must eat animal products to get all the amino acids your body needs. However, it is true that different people feel better eating different kinds of foods because of the unique ways in which our bodies digest, absorb, and utilize proteins.

High-quality protein provides most, if not all, of the essential amino acids with a minimum of fat and toxins. Beef is protein packed, but personally I can't recommend it as a healthy food (see page 138). Nuts and seeds contain high levels of protein, but they also have a high fat content and should be eaten sparingly. Grains contain protein, but not enough to be optimal protein sources. Legumes (especially soy), eggs (preferably pesticide-free), free-range and organically raised chicken or turkey (no skin), and fish (especially toxin-free varieties) are good protein sources. Shellfish is often contaminated with toxins and its use in the diet should be limited.

The immune system is affected by the amount of protein we eat, the kind of amino acids we take in, and the balance between the different types of amino acids. Some amino acids have specific effects on the body. For example, glutamine is the preferential fuel for gastrointestinal mucosa, and arginine enhances lymphocyte response. In fact, arginine is the only amino acid that is essential for the process macrophages use against tumor targets.[17] (Arginine is sometimes given as a supplement, so I've included it in the next chapter.)

How Much Protein Each Day?

It is possible to eat too much protein. Nobody needs a thick steak that droops over both sides of a dinner plate. An "adequate" intake of protein is the amount you need to maintain your muscle mass. Just how much protein you need depends upon your build and activity level, but the average adult needs 0.4 grams of protein per pound. (For example, someone who weighs 170 pounds would need 68 grams of protein per day.)

Protein is more difficult to digest than either fats or carbohydrates, so it isn't an optimal fuel. Metabolizing protein produces toxic by-products that must be detoxified by the liver and excreted by the kidneys, so too much protein can cause organ strain. Also, excess protein is converted into fat—another reason not to overdo.

Acid/Alkaline Balance

Diets high in protein create acid, which the body counteracts by pulling calcium from the bones. If too much calcium is pulled from the bones, they can be weakened. This is why a high-protein diet (greater than 30 percent of calories from protein) can contribute to osteoporosis.

Some health care practitioners believe that we should make every effort to eat a diet that is more alkaline than acid. Acidity is measured by pH: the higher the pH, the more alkaline (less acid) a substance is. The optimal pH level of blood falls in the narrow range between 7.35 and 7.45. Foods that contain acid-forming elements contribute to a more acid environment within the body. This is important because metabolic processes occur less efficiently in an acid environment. When metabolism is inefficient, less energy is made available and more acid by-products are produced—so a vicious cycle is set in motion.

I don't worry too much about the chemical effects of specific foods on the acid/alkaline balance of the body because the Immune Empowering Diet automatically cuts out many of the worst offenders. Highly acid foods include sugar, beef, fried foods, and processed cheese—none of which, as you'll see, is part of the Immune Empowering Diet. On the other hand, the Immune Empowering Diet is heavy on fruits and vegetables, most of which tend toward alkalinity. (Incidentally, you can't use taste alone to determine whether a food has acid or alkaline effects on the body. For example, limes are alkaline and carrots are acid because of the way they are metabolized by the body.)

Lately I've gotten interested in the health benefits of drinking water that has been made less acid. This water is thought to be beneficial for general health and especially for gastrointestinal health because it affects the acid/alkaline balance of the GI tract. I just bought a Microwater ionizer unit for my office—it turns tap water into less acid (more alkaline) water (to drink) and more acid water (it's okay to wash with and even has mild disinfectant properties).

PROTEIN SOURCES

All foods are cooked, where appropriate

	Quantity	Protein (grams)
Meat/poultry/fish		
Liver	4 oz	30
Hamburger, steak	4 oz	25
Fish, canned tuna	4 oz	25
Lamb	4 oz	20
Chicken	4 oz	20
Dairy products/eggs		
Cottage cheese, uncreamed	1 cup	44
Cottage cheese, creamed	1 cup	31
Cheese—cheddar, Swiss	4 oz	28
Milk, yogurt	1 cup	8
Egg	1	7
Vegetarian		
Chickpeas	1 cup	41
Lentils	1 cup	16
Soybeans	1 cup	14
Black beans	1 cup	12
Tofu	4 oz	10
Green peas	1 cup	7.5
Alfalfa sprouts	1 cup	5
Potato	1 medium	4
Green beans	1 cup	2
Spinach	1 cup	2
Broccoli	1 cup	3
Nuts/seeds		
Peanuts	1 cup	60
Sesame seeds	1 cup	42
Almonds	1 cup	25
Sunflower seeds	1 cup	24
Cashews	1 cup	15
Grains		
Brown or white rice	1 cup	5
Oatmeal	1 cup	5

Animal or Vegetable Protein?

Animal protein is concentrated, whereas vegetable protein comes with carbohydrates and beneficial indigestible fiber. A whole cup of cooked lentils, for example, has 16 grams of protein, whereas just four ounces of chicken has 20 grams of protein. You're more likely to have a protein overload with the chicken—and you'll need to add carbohydrates and fiber to your meal separately.

Personally, I don't eat meat. Although my mother reminds me that I used to love her roast beef, I haven't eaten red meat in twenty-five years. However, as you will see later in this chapter when I discuss the low-carbohydrate diet, there is a certain percentage of people who do better eating a higher protein diet, which may include organic chicken or turkey or even some less fatty red meats, such as venison or buffalo (which are also higher in the beneficial omega-3 fatty acids).

In 1995, beef consumption in the United States was 67.1 pounds per person and rising.[18] That's about five quarter-pound hamburgers per week. When you think of all the saturated fat beef contains, this statistic has large implications for the cardiovascular health of Americans.

In addition to saturated fat, meat of all kinds (beef, pork, lamb, turkey, chicken) from commercially raised animals is likely to contain pesticide, herbicide, and fungicide residues (from chemicals sprayed on their feed), industrial toxins (including PCBs and dioxin), antibiotics (which can retain their potency in meat products), and hormones (which can have estrogenic effects on the consumer). Samuel Epstein, the fellow who alerted us to the dangers of hot dogs, describes the levels of estrogenic hormones in meat as "terrifyingly high."[19] Meat can also contain preservatives, flavorings, and coloring agents. If you must eat meat, buy organic.

There are other reasons to avoid meat as well. "Mad cow disease" had a catastrophic effect on the beef industry in England in 1996. Smoked meat products are carcinogenic because of the process used in preparing them. Often meat products are contaminated with bacteria (for example, *E. coli* in beef and *Salmonella* in chicken) and/or parasites. Ground beef is more hazardous than steak because the grinding process mixes bacteria throughout the chopped meat. Thorough cooking will lessen your immune burden by killing these organisms. Eating raw meat, fish, or eggs is a risk that is not, in my view, worth taking. If you're an avid sushi lover, however, there are a number of natural antiparasitic herbs and preparations you can take with your raw fish, such as paramicocidin (grapefruit seed extract). I have never seen double-blind scientific studies to support this approach, but it makes practical sense to me.

In 1995, Americans consumed 70.5 pounds of chicken per person,[20] nearly a pound and a half per week. Most of the fat in chicken can be stripped away with the skin, which is why I am willing to recommend a moderate portion of free-range, organically raised, skinless chicken (or turkey), prepared in a healthful way (not fried!) as a healthy source of protein.

Dairy Products

Some people are surprised to learn that I recommend limiting dairy products (milk, butter, cheese, ice cream, etc.). Milk products tend to be high in fat, so select low-fat or nonfat varieties. Whole milk derives 48 percent of its calories from fat. So-called 2 percent milk derives 31 percent of its calories from fat, and 1 percent milk gets 15 percent of its calories from fat. Skim milk is the best choice, with less than 10 percent of its calories from fat.[21] (For you superobservant readers, no, I didn't make a mistake. Skim milk is not truly fat-free, for it contains a little less than half a gram of fat per cup.)

The amount of fat you take in from dairy products can add up quickly. According to *Health* magazine, pouring skim milk on your cereal for a year instead of whole milk would cut *10 pounds* of fat out of your diet!

In addition to their fat content, dairy products from commercially raised cows contain—just as beef does—pesticide, herbicide, and fungicide residues, industrial toxins, antibiotics, and hormones. When you buy dairy products, choose organic varieties. Try using soy cheese or goat's milk products once in a while.

Many people are lactose intolerant, meaning they lack enough of the enzyme needed to digest milk protein. (If you experience gastrointestinal upset whenever you eat milk products, consider this possibility.) Dairy products have immunological effects as well. As I mentioned in Chapter 3, milk protein can set the stage for autoimmune problems, and milk is the most common food allergen. Many of my patients who have chronic bouts of bronchitis, sinusitis, asthma, and eczema find that their symptoms abate (or even disappear) when they stop consuming dairy products. The folk wisdom that "milk makes mucus" probably has more to do with undiagnosed milk allergy than any particular property of milk.

Dairy products provide simple sugars that the candida (yeast) organisms living in the gut just love. If yeast overgrowth is a problem for you, stay away from milk products.

The dairy product I'm most comfortable recommending is yogurt. Yogurt is milk that has been cultured with beneficial organisms. The active cultures in yogurt (lactobacillus and others) are good for intestinal flora, and evidence suggests that yogurt is an immune stimulant and that it helps to prevent cancer. While people with true milk allergy should not eat yogurt, those with lactose intolerance are often able to tolerate yogurt better than other milk products. Choose the most healthful brand of yogurt you can find: preferably unsweetened, made with organic (but pasteurized) low-fat milk, and containing plenty of active cultures.

A Word About Soy

As long as you aren't allergic to them, soybeans are a healthy protein source. Protein comprises 36 percent of the soybean. Soybeans are cholesterol-free and low in saturated fat, and they do not stress the kidneys. In addition to protein, carbohydrates, and fiber, soybeans also contain natural plant estrogens called *phytoestrogens*. You may have heard them discussed as *isoflavones*.

Phytoestrogens appear to be protective against prostate cancer in men and against estrogen-related diseases in women, including breast cancer, endometriosis, fibrocystic breast disease, and uterine fibroids.[22] Asian women, who consume thirty to fifty times as much soy as American women, have lower rates of breast cancer. Soy estrogens may also be protective against atherosclerosis and osteoporosis, two other diseases that are influenced by estrogen levels.[23] Research also indicates that soy protein has a beneficial effect on serum cholesterol.[24]

Soy is also a unique dietary source of the isoflavone *genistein*. Genistein was originally considered a phytoestrogen until some of its nonestrogenic properties were discovered. Genistein shows promise as an anticancer agent.

No one has detected any down side to eating soy, and the evidence in its favor is very strong, so my recommendation is to find ways to incorporate soy into your meals. It shouldn't be too hard to find a form of soy you like, since an astonishing array of products are made from soy, including hot dogs and other imitation meat products; soy milk, cheese, and ice cream; and tofu. Contrary to public opinion, there are lots of delicious ways to cook tofu.

SUMMARY: IMMUNE-EMPOWERING PROTEIN SOURCES

Choose:

Legumes (soybeans, lentils, etc.)
Fish
Chicken or turkey (free-range, organically raised, skin removed)
Eggs

Limit:

Dairy products
Shellfish

Avoid:

Beef, lamb, pork
Smoked meats
Raw meat, fish, and eggs

THE IMMUNE EMPOWERING DIET: 55 TO 60 PERCENT COMPLEX CARBOHYDRATES

The body's two main sources of fuel are fats (discussed later) and carbohydrates. *Complex carbohydrates* (whole grains, fresh fruits, and fresh vegetables) are unrefined and contain fiber. *Refined carbohydrates* (such as white flour and white table sugar) are highly processed, contain less fiber (if any), and have fewer nutrients. Carbohydrates that have had their fiber removed are sometimes referred to as *defibrinated carbohydrates.*

Complex carbohydrates are good for you; refined carbohydrates are not good for you. Whole grains are good for you, but bear in mind that the flour products made from them are not equivalent. Once the whole grain is broken down into flour—even whole wheat flour—fiber is lost. Similarly, although vitamin, mineral, and fiber supplements can be helpful, *there is no substitute for eating the real thing.* Large amounts of research indicate that a diet high in whole grains, fresh fruits, and fresh vegetables is extremely healthy. In particular, cruciferous vegetables—cabbage, broccoli, brussels sprouts, and cauliflower—contain special substances, called indoles, that help protect against cancer.

A lifetime of eating refined foods with diminished amounts of natural oils, vitamins, minerals, and trace elements can lead to subtle nutrient deficiencies. These, in turn, can cause enzyme slowdown and cellular and metabolic defects. As I've already noted, eventually these irregularities lead to chronic ailments and disease.

Choosing the right carbohydrates is important not only because we need the nutrients and fiber, but also because carbohydrates can have a profound effect on our blood sugar levels.

Controlling Blood Sugar Levels

Carbohydrates are made up of simple sugars linked together. Simple sugars include glucose (found in grains, cereals, pasta, breads, starches, and vegetables), galactose (found in dairy products), fructose (found in fruit), and sucrose (table sugar), among others. Digestive enzymes break down carbohydrates into simple sugars, which the body converts into glucose, which is burned as metabolic fuel.

Our red blood cells and brain cells need glucose to survive. The body has a system of checks and balances to ensure that a constant supply of glucose reaches our cells. Some circulating glucose is immediately burned for energy. Extra glucose that isn't needed right away can be converted by the body into glycogen, which is stored in the liver and muscles for emergency use. (Later, if needed, fat and glycogen can be converted back into glucose to meet the body's needs.) If glycogen reserves are already filled, extra glucose is stored in the body as fat.

The kind of food we eat has a direct effect on our blood sugar levels. Some foods are almost pure energy and flood the bloodstream with a wave of sugar. Other foods—that is, foods with more complex carbohydrates and more fiber—take longer to digest, so sugar is released into the bloodstream more slowly.

After eating—particularly after eating refined carbohydrates—our blood sugar rises. To counteract this surge of extra glucose, the pancreas secretes *insulin*. Insulin facilitates the movement of glucose into the cells and stimulates the storage of extra glucose as glycogen or as fat. As long as insulin levels are high, the body is in a fat-accumulation mode.

After fasting or exercise, our blood sugar level is low. When the pancreas detects low blood sugar, it secretes *glucagon*. Glucagon stimulates the conversion of glycogen or fat back into glucose for release into the bloodstream. Also, when blood sugar levels get too low, the adrenal glands manufacture adrenaline and cortisol to counteract the effect of the insulin. This explains why fluctuating blood sugar levels can stress the adrenal glands.

When the body's system of checks and balances is working correctly, both high and low blood sugar levels can be corrected so the brain has a constant supply of the glucose it needs. You won't be surprised to hear, however, that this system can both overreact and underreact. Sometimes the body produces too much, or too little, of the correct hormone (insulin or glucagon). Sometimes the correct hormone is produced in the right amount, but the receptor cells are deaf and don't get the message. And, to complicate things further, sometimes the body's timing seems to be off.

- People with *diabetes mellitus* are unable to secrete sufficient amounts of insulin, which throws a curve ball into their carbohydrate metabolism. Diabetics need to constantly monitor their blood sugar levels. People with insulin-dependent diabetes—for example, people who produce no insulin at all—need insulin shots to normalize the amount of sugar in their blood. Some people produce low levels of insulin, but are able to control their blood sugar levels by watching their diet and by taking supplements (such as chromium and certain fatty acids) that improve the responsiveness of their cell receptors to insulin.

- *Hyperglycemia,* or abnormally high blood sugar, can be a consequence of poorly controlled diabetes or excessive sugar intake. Hyperglycemia is characterized by thirst, frequent urination, and the presence of glucose in the urine. Severe hyperglycemia can lead to confusion, disorientation, stupor, and ultimately coma.

- Hyperglycemia that occurs after eating is called *glucose intolerance.* People who are glucose intolerant have abnormally high blood sugar levels after meals, but their disorder is not as extreme as diabetes. However, untreated glucose intolerance can progress to diabetes over time.

- In *dysinsulinism,* the body's release of insulin is out of sync. Blood sugar levels rise too high (the insulin doesn't kick in quickly enough), then fall too low (the insulin response lingers too long). The symptoms of dysinsulinism are more severe than those of glucose intolerance because of this up-and-down effect.

• *Hypoglycemia,* or abnormally low blood sugar, is characterized by mental fatigue, sweating, weakness, hunger, dizziness, trembling, anxiety, headache, and palpitations. Extremely low blood sugar can lead to confusion, "brain fog," "drunken" behavior, and coma. Hypoglycemia can be caused by poorly controlled diabetes. (For example, if a diabetic takes too much insulin relative to what he has eaten and the amount of exercise he's had, this can cause a rapid and/or extreme drop in blood sugar.) Hypoglycemia can also be caused by an organic problem, such as an insulin-secreting tumor.

• People who have *reactive hypoglycemia* have an exaggerated insulin response after eating that sends their blood sugar level plummeting. This condition is not appreciated by many conventional physicians, who often attribute patients' symptoms of low blood sugar to other causes, including psychological problems. (Remember my patient Jeffrey, who was able to throw away his Valium after his reactive hypoglycemia was correctly diagnosed?)

• People who experience *insulin resistance* have high insulin production *and* high blood sugar levels. In this case, the insulin is being produced, but the target cells don't respond correctly. Insulin resistance causes hyperglycemia because the blood sugar levels don't go down as they should, even though the body keeps producing more insulin in an attempt to get the proper effect. Insulin that doesn't bind to glucose can hasten the conversion of carbohydrates into fat, which helps explain why some people gain weight even on a low-fat diet. Their bodies are busy converting simple starches into fat because of elevated insulin levels. Insulin resistance is one cause of *hyperinsulinism* (the overproduction of insulin).

There are several ways to diagnose blood sugar problems. It's useful to measure the blood sugar level first thing in the morning before eating (known as the *fasting blood sugar level* because you haven't eaten all night). An unusually low fasting blood sugar level can be a sign of an insulin-secreting tumor. Another common test is the glucose tolerance test, in which the patient is given a large, measured dose of glucose, and insulin and blood sugar levels are checked for the following six hours (see graph).

There's a lot we can do to control our insulin and blood sugar levels. This is important because insulin and blood sugar levels influence many internal processes.

Let's suppose you go out for a celebratory lunch at noon. You have a glass of wine, a big plate of pasta with bread, and a special dessert. This meal creates a surge of sugar, which your pancreas counteracts by pumping out insulin. By three o'clock you're probably feeling tired because the insulin has done an effective job of packing away any extra glucose as glycogen. So you eat a snack for energy, which again raises your blood sugar and again prompts an increase in insulin secretion. This time, however, your glycogen reserves are filled up already, so any extra glucose is converted into fat. Even if all you ate for a snack was fat-free rice cakes, you'd end up storing fat.

I can see you wincing as you read this, and you probably don't want to hear it, but it's true. The fat-free snacks currently being marketed are mostly refined carbohydrates, and high-sugar foods can contribute greatly to increased fats in the blood and obesity. This in turn creates adverse immunological effects.

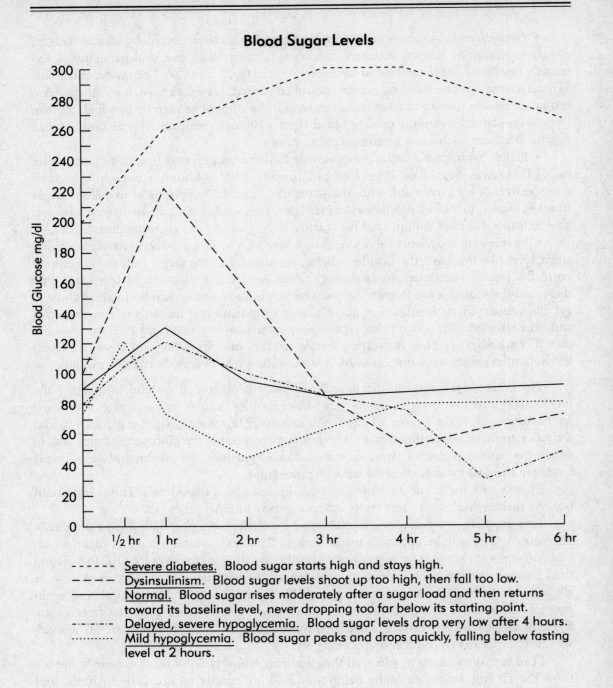

Blood Sugar Levels

- - - - - <u>Severe diabetes.</u> Blood sugar starts high and stays high.
- - - - <u>Dysinsulinism.</u> Blood sugar levels shoot up too high, then fall too low.
———— <u>Normal.</u> Blood sugar rises moderately after a sugar load and then returns toward its baseline level, never dropping too far below its starting point.
-·-·-·- <u>Delayed, severe hypoglycemia.</u> Blood sugar levels drop very low after 4 hours.
·········· <u>Mild hypoglycemia.</u> Blood sugar peaks and drops quickly, falling below fasting level at 2 hours.

The way to avoid this yo-yo blood sugar scenario and to circumvent fat accumulation is to eat complex carbohydrates and to avoid high-sugar foods. Starchy carbohydrates like rice (especially white rice), potatoes, bread, and corn elevate your blood sugar faster (that is, they have a higher glycemic index) than an assortment of fiber-rich fruits and vegetables such as lentils, asparagus, and apples (foods with a lower glycemic index). Next time, consider having yogurt and a salad!

Fiber

We Americans eat a lot of high-calorie, low-fiber foods, when what we really need is the opposite: low-calorie, high-fiber foods.

Fiber is the part of plant foods that passes through our digestive system pretty much unchanged. Although we don't have much effect on fiber, it has a big effect on *us*.

• Fiber keeps the gastrointestinal tract from becoming sluggish and has a healthful effect on what is known as *transit time*. By keeping things moving, fiber helps prevent the accumulation and absorption of harmful substances (toxins, heavy metals, bacterial and fungal metabolites, and carcinogens) into the mucosal lining of the GI tract and from there into the bloodstream. (This is why fiber detoxifies the colon.)

• Fiber slows the rate at which sugar enters the bloodstream, which helps to maintain steady blood sugar levels.

• Fiber helps with weight control. Eating fiber-rich foods is more filling (and more work for your digestive system) than eating a cream puff, which goes down in a flash and has far more calories.

᠀᠊᠀

COMMONLY ASKED QUESTION NO. 9:

What's the difference between soluble and insoluble fiber?

Fiber comes in two varieties: soluble and insoluble. The classic example of soluble fiber is the gooey part of cooked oatmeal. Cooked lentils, on the other hand, are high in insoluble fiber, and can be boiled and boiled without turning to mush. Both kinds of fiber are healthful because they dilute the contents of the bowel.

Soluble fiber has implications for cardiovascular health because it binds with cholesterol in the gut. Insoluble fiber is associated with colon health and correcting bowel problems. Both kinds are good for you.

᠀᠊᠀

To add more fiber to your diet, start with whole grains. Eat several pieces of fresh fruit each day, plus some raw or lightly steamed vegetables. Find a legume dish you like (for example, chili, beans and rice, chickpea salad, or lentil soup). If you haven't been a big fiber consumer in the past, start adding fiber to your diet slowly to avoid discomfort (such as abdominal bloating and gas). Also, increase your water consumption—fiber in the gut absorbs water.

Avoiding Sugar

The total amount of sugar normally present in our bloodstream is approximately *1 teaspoon.*[25] When we eat table sugar—pure energy, no fiber, the supreme example of what is known as "empty calories" (calories without nutrients)—our blood sugar soars, and our body has to work hard to get it down to a normal level again.

In addition to stressing the body, sugar suppresses the immune system. In one study, test subjects were divided into five groups. The first group was the control group. The second group was given a sweetened drink that contained 6 teaspoons of sugar. The other groups consumed drinks with 12, 18, and 24 teaspoons of sugar. Blood samples were taken from each group over a period of five hours and incubated with staphylococcus bacteria.

When viewed under the microscope, each white blood cell of the control group engulfed an average of 14 bacteria. In the group that consumed 6 teaspoons of sugar, the average number of engulfed bacteria per white blood cell was 10. In the 12-teaspoon group, this number went down to 5.5 bacteria; in the 18-teaspoon group, the average was 2; and in the 24-teaspoon group, the average number of bacteria destroyed by each white blood cell had dropped to *1.* The greatest immune-suppressing effect occurred from one to two hours after sugar consumption, but depressed immunity was evident for up to five hours afterward.[26] Think of this the next time you have a cold and reach for that sweet!

Okay, so sugar stresses our glands and compromises the effectiveness of our white blood cells. What else does it do?

• Excess sugar can be converted by the body into saturated fat, which has implications for our weight and cardiovascular health (see page 147).

• In his book *Optimal Wellness,* Ralph Golan, M.D., refers to sugar as a "metabolic freeloader." Sugar contributes no nutrients to the diet, yet nutrients are used up to metabolize it.

• Sugar aggravates hypoglycemia and complicates the control of diabetes and other blood sugar problems.

• Sugar feeds *Candida albicans* in the gut, contributing to yeast overgrowth.

• Cancerous tumors are sugar feeders. A high blood sugar level means that there is a constant supply of tumor fuel circulating throughout the body. Sugar also promotes cancer because insulin is associated with the production of the immune-suppressing hormone prostaglandin E_2.[27]

• High blood glucose levels have a detrimental effect on the conversion of fatty acids (see the discussion of fats following) and can be associated with low levels of healthful fatty acids in the blood.

• A high-sugar diet may accelerate aging through oxidative damage.[28]

• A spoonful of sugar doesn't just help the medicine go down. Along with sugar, we usually take in other harmful substances, such as refined flour and saturated fat. Because sugary, processed foods have so little fiber, we can eat a lot of them before we feel full. By the time we stop, we've consumed a large number of empty calories that many of us will convert into fat (using up valuable nutrients in the process).

To cut down on sugar intake, avoid obviously sweetened foods (soda, cookies, desserts, breakfast cereals). Be alert for hidden sugar lurking in processed foods (canned soups, ketchup, salad dressing, peanut butter, bread, yogurt). Substitute fruit or frozen apple juice concentrate for table sugar. For some people, honey, maple syrup, and other natural alternatives to sugar do not trigger the same cravings as table sugar. (They'll still raise your blood sugar level, but you may not be inclined to eat as much.) Sugar is addictive, so giving it up can be hard. You may feel worse before you feel better, but believe me, you *will* feel better—

SUMMARY: IMMUNE-EMPOWERING CARBOHYDRATES

Choose:

Fiber-rich fresh fruits and fresh vegetables
Legumes
Whole grains

Limit:

Starchy carbohydrates

Avoid:

Sugar and sweets (soda, cookies, candy, pastries, etc.)
Alcohol
Anything made with white flour
Processed, commercially prepared foods

and you'll experience long-term benefits as well. Give your sugar-detox program at least a week. By then you'll be ready to turn your back on sugar permanently.

THE IMMUNE EMPOWERING DIET: 20 TO 25 PERCENT HEALTHY FATS

Dietary fats affect immunocompetence. The right fats are immune enhancing, while the wrong fats are immune suppressing, so it's important to know which are which.

We need an adequate supply of fats and oils for several extremely important reasons:

- We burn fats for energy.
- Certain important vitamins (including A, D, E, and K) are fat-soluble (not water-soluble).
- Fats are necessary for our internal production of extremely influential hormones called *eicosanoids*.
- Fats are used as a structural component of cells, which are the basic component of all living things. Cell walls need to be waterproof, so they contain oil.

The quality of the fats we eat affects the quality of our cell membranes. This sounds relatively simple, but cell membranes are important in myriad complex ways.

- Cell membranes are the basis of all-important cellular receptor mechanisms. Information presented and detected by cell membranes is a critical aspect of many intracellular processes. Two cells can be compared to two prisoners who communicate by knocking on the walls of their cells.
- As I mentioned earlier, cells need to be malleable. Just as we need to be flexible in our everyday life to meet our constantly changing environment, so do our cells need healthy, flexible cell membranes to meet their constantly changing environment and to be able to squeeze through tiny spaces.
- Flexible cell membranes allow the optimal transport of nutrients into (and waste products out of) each cell.
- Little pumps within the cellular membrane maintain the proper mineral balances within cells.
- Cellular membrane pumps are also responsible for maintaining the proper electrical charge of cells.

The fats we eat are incorporated into our cell membranes, so it's important to give our cells an adequate supply of "healthy" fats to work with—and to limit the amount of unfavorable fats at their disposal.

I should add that eating too much fat is never a good idea. Even if you choose healthy fats, too much fat circulating in your blood can lead to the formation of plaques (fat deposits) inside your arteries. Excess fat in the diet can also contribute to high blood pressure, diabetes, and cancer. Women who eat a lot of fat have high estrogen levels in their blood, which may contribute to estrogen-related diseases like breast cancer.

The Structure of Fats

Fats are made up of fatty acids and glycerol. Fatty acids, in turn, are made up of carbon, hydrogen, and oxygen. The number of hydrogen molecules on the carbon sites (see illustration below) determines whether a fatty acid is *saturated, monounsaturated,* or *polyunsaturated.* Fats that have no double bonds are called saturated because they are saturated with the maximum amount of hydrogen. Fats that have a single double bond are called monounsaturated (*mono* means "one"). Fats that have several double bonds are called polyunsaturated (*poly* means "many"). The three types of fats appear together in food, but usually one type is predominant.

The Structure of Fats

Each carbon atom has four binding arms that can attach to other elements:

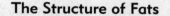

Hydrogen has one binding arm. In fats, hydrogen attaches to carbon atoms like this:

$$-\underset{\underset{H}{|}}{\overset{\overset{H}{|}}{C}} - \underset{\underset{H}{|}}{\overset{\overset{H}{|}}{C}} - \underset{\underset{H}{|}}{\overset{\overset{H}{|}}{C}} - \underset{\underset{H}{|}}{\overset{\overset{H}{|}}{C}} -$$

All four of a carbon atom's binding arms must be attached to something. Some of the carbon binding arms do not have hydrogen attached to them. In this case, the carbon binds twice to the next carbon. This is called a double bond (=).

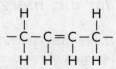

The number of double bonds determines whether a fat is saturated, monosaturated, or polyunsaturated.

Saturated Fats and Trans-Fatty Acids

Saturated fats are solid at room temperature. Butter, cheese, and cream are all high in saturated fat, as are meat and meat products and the so-called tropical oils (coconut, palm, and palm kernel oil).

Saturated fats increase the amount of "bad" cholesterol (low density lipoprotein, or LDL) in the blood, causing atherosclerosis, heart disease, and the restriction of blood flow. When saturated fats are incorporated into cell membranes, the membranes tend to become rigid and less flexible, which in turn can affect their receptor mechanisms. This may explain why saturated fats are associated with insulin resistance. In addition, diets high in animal fat are associated with colon cancer.[29] Saturated fats also depress the phagocytic activity of the reticuloendothelial system, which affects the efficiency with which immune complexes are removed from the blood.[30] Saturated fats are also associated with decreased cytotoxic function.[31] Clearly, this kind of fat is bad for the immune system.

Hydrogenated (or *partially hydrogenated*) *fats* are liquid oils that have been artificially saturated with hydrogen to create a solid fat with a longer shelf life that stays stable at higher temperatures. Margarine and vegetable shortening are examples of this highly unnatural type of fat. It's possible to start with an oil that's good for you and create a hydrogenated product that's bad for you.

Although hydrogenated fat is harmful, we eat plenty of it. One study indicated that Americans consumed 28 pounds of hydrogenated oil per person per year.[32] Hydrogenated and partially hydrogenated oils are used *extensively* in commercially prepared foods, including peanut butter, mayonnaise, baked goods, margarine, and chocolate. If you are serious about cutting back on your fat intake, especially harmful fats, you'll need to make a point of staying away from these hidden fat sources.

Hydrogenated and partially hydrogenated fats are not only saturated, but also contain *trans-fatty acids*, a type of fatty acid that is not created in the body and is rarely found in

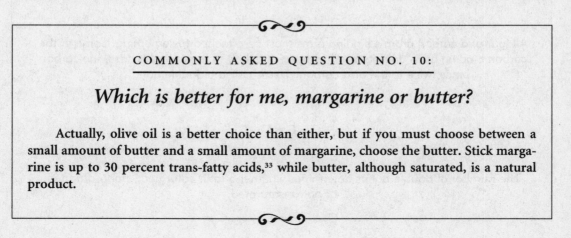

COMMONLY ASKED QUESTION NO. 10:

Which is better for me, margarine or butter?

Actually, olive oil is a better choice than either, but if you must choose between a small amount of butter and a small amount of margarine, choose the butter. Stick margarine is up to 30 percent trans-fatty acids,[33] while butter, although saturated, is a natural product.

nature, but is created when oils are hydrogenated (heated and chemically treated). Trans-fatty acids are found in all fried foods, as well as in commercial brands of liquid oils, which are extracted using heat.

Trans-fatty acids increase serum levels of "bad" cholesterol (low-density lipoprotein, or LDL) and decrease the "good" cholesterol (HDL), and are associated with coronary heart disease. They have been shown to adversely affect metabolic processes in cardiac tissue. Trans-fatty acids can be incorporated into cell membranes even though they are not normal components of tissue. When this occurs, they can interfere with the function of the cell membranes, making them less flexible and blocking natural biochemical pathways.

Monounsaturated Fatty Acids

Monounsaturated fats are usually liquid at room temperature, but may solidify in the refrigerator. The lower the temperature at which solidification occurs, the greater the degree of unsaturation. Monounsaturated fats contain a high proportion of *oleic acid*, a fatty acid that can be synthesized by all mammals, including humans.

Monounsaturated oils include olive oil, peanut oil, avocado oil, and canola oil. These oils are not used by the body to manufacture eicosanoids and they have no effect on insulin levels. Because they aren't harmful, they can be considered healthful. Long-term consumption of these oils (especially olive oil) in several southern European countries is associated with low overall mortality rates and low incidence of coronary heart disease. Olive oil is an important part of the centuries-old "Mediterranean diet," a diet that is making a comeback, as you'll see when we discuss the low-carbohydrate diet later in this chapter.

Olive oil is 72 percent monounsaturated, canola oil (actually extracted from rapeseed) is 65 percent monounsaturated, and peanut oil is 48 percent monounsaturated. Canola and peanut oils are likely to contain chemical residues from the way the plants were raised. Avocado oil is extremely expensive. Your best choice is olive oil—preferably cold-pressed and unrefined ("extra virgin").

These days it's common to go to a restaurant and find a basket of bread with a dish of olive oil for dipping. By choosing olive oil instead of butter, you avoid the hazards of saturated fat. By choosing olive oil instead of vegetable oil, you avoid the immune-suppressing effects of the more harmful oils (see below).

Polyunsaturated Fatty Acids and Essential Fatty Acids

Safflower, sunflower, corn, sesame, and soy oils are all polyunsaturated fatty acids (PUFAs). Even though they are cholesterol-free and low in saturated fat, these oils are still problematic. They are very unstable and susceptible to oxidation, both outside the body and inside it. Outside, they go rancid. Inside, lipid peroxidation creates free radicals that can damage DNA, alter cell membranes, and promote cancer.

The breakdown of polyunsaturated fatty acids produces more oxidants than the breakdown of other types of fats. This is because of the multiple double bonds in polyunsaturated fats. Each double bond provides an opportunity for oxidation. The more polyunsaturated an oil is, the more double bonds there are, and the more potential there is for lipid peroxidation and free radical formation.

Safflower oil is the most unsaturated vegetable oil, and as such can cause significant immune suppression. This is surprising news to many consumers who were told that polyunsaturated oils were part of a healthy diet.

Polyunsaturated fatty acids can be divided into two classes: omega-3 fatty acids and omega-6 fatty acids. Because of the different ways in which the body converts them, omega-3 fatty acids are *generally* immune enhancing, while omega-6 fatty acids are *generally* immune suppressing. Because an omega-3 fatty acid cannot be converted into an omega-6 fatty acid, and vice versa, we need to pay attention to our consumption of each variety. Depending upon how your body utilizes polyunsaturated fatty acids, you may derive healthful benefits from supplementing your diet with either omega-3 or omega-6 fatty acids.

What further complicates this discussion is the fact that the body can manufacture some fatty acids but not others. *Essential fatty acids* must be included in the diet. Many people are deficient in essential fatty acids (an extreme example would be an infant fed only skim milk), and essential fatty acid deficiency is often part of a larger clinical picture that involves immune overreaction or underreaction.

One of my patients, Kevin, is a fifty-five-year-old photographer with coronary artery disease. Kevin read about the low-fat, high-complex-carbohydrate diet recommended by Dean Ornish, M.D., and took it to an extreme. He avoided *all* fats. When Kevin came to see me, he had developed dry skin, constipation, increased thirst, brittle nails, and dry hair—all signs of essential fatty acid deficiency. We liberalized Kevin's diet to include more healthful fats and added essential fatty acid supplements as well. We were able to resolve Kevin's symptoms without compromising his heart condition—and he felt a whole lot better.

The essential fatty acids are building blocks for prostaglandin hormones (so far researchers have identified over thirty), which affect myriad body functions. Prostaglandins are intercellular messengers used on the local level. They can be very short-lived but nonetheless have extremely powerful biologic effects. Prostaglandins are made by every cell (in order to communicate with other cells) and are present in the entire body. Prostaglandin E_1 (PGE_1) and prostaglandin E_3 (PGE_3) are important for good health. Prostaglandin E_2 (PGE_2), however, suppresses killer cell activity and is associated with immune suppression as well as high blood pressure, allergies, heart attacks, and stroke.

You can affect your prostaglandin levels by modifying your diet. Saturated fat, transfatty acids, alcohol, and sugar all block the production of favorable prostaglandins. (So do stress, aspirin, diabetes, and aging, but we're talking about diet here.) Consuming the wrong fatty acids can overactivate the biochemical pathways that synthesize immune-suppressing prostaglandins (type PGE_2). Including the right fatty acids and metabolic cofactors (such as zinc and vitamin B$_6$) in your diet can have the opposite effect and enhance your production of favorable prostaglandins (types PGE$_1$ and PGE$_3$), with their subsequent beneficial effect on immune function.

Cellular proteins are genetically determined, but the polyunsaturated fatty acid composition of cell membranes is largely determined by diet. So, while we can't do much about our genes, we certainly can pay attention to what we eat, and give our immune system a boost in the process.

The Omega-6 Fatty Acids

The omega-6 fatty acids include:

- Linoleic acid (LA), an essential fatty acid
- Gamma-linolenic acid (GLA)
- Dihomogammalinolenic acid (DHGLA)
- Arachidonic acid (AA)

Linoleic acid can be converted by the body into gamma-linolenic acid, which can convert *either* to the favorable PGE$_1$ *or* to arachidonic acid and from there to the unfavorable PGE$_2$. Because arachidonic acid converts to PGE$_2$, it is a particularly unfavorable moderator of the immune system.

The eicosanoids derived from omega-6 fatty acids are generally inflammatory and weak vasodilators, and some promote clotting. High levels of the omega-6 fatty acids are associated with chronic overproduction of PGE$_2$, increased incidence of tumors, suppression of interleukin-2 synthesis, inhibition of T cell proliferation, and suppression of macrophage activity.

Linoleic acid is present in vegetable oils, including corn, safflower, sunflower, and soy. Linoleic acid—which can be a precursor of arachidonic acid—is the predominant polyunsaturated fatty acid in the Western diet.[34] Arachidonic acid is present in meat in high levels, which is another reason to avoid meat. Gamma-linolenic acid is present in evening primrose oil, borage oil, and black currant seed oil.

The Omega-3 Fatty Acids

The omega-3 fatty acids include:

- Alpha-linolenic acid (ALA), an essential fatty acid
- Eicosapentaenoic acid (EPA)
- Docosahexaenoic acid (DHA)

The body can convert alpha-linolenic acid into both eicosapentaenoic acid and docosahexaenoic acid. All of the omega-3 fatty acids have healthful effects.

The eicosanoids derived from omega-3 fatty acids are generally anti-inflammatory and strong vasodilators, and interfere with clotting. (Blood that clots too readily can interfere with blood flow and can cause circulatory problems.) Omega-3 fatty acids promote lymphocyte and phagocyte function. These fatty acids do not convert into the unfavorable PGE_2, and actually favor the production of PGE_3. They also encourage the conversion of gamma-linolenic acid into PGE_1. Omega-3 fatty acids are believed to protect against cardiovascular diseases, arthritis, and other autoimmune disorders, hypertension, stroke, cancer, and diabetes.

Omega-3 fatty acids are necessary for normal growth and development throughout the life cycle, even before birth. They protect against degenerative changes in cells and tissues. When omega-3 fatty acids are added to the diet, they replace omega-6 fatty acids in cell membranes of practically all cells.[35] My colleague and friend Neil Orenstein, Ph.D., a nutritional consultant, refers to this process—which takes four to twelve weeks—as an "oil change." This cuts back on the presence of arachidonic acid, which in turn inhibits the production of PGE_2.

Docosahexaenoic acid is abundant in the retina and may affect visual acuity. It is also one of the most abundant structural lipids in the brain,[36] so it may affect brain development, IQ, and cognitive function. This also may help explain why a deficiency of omega-3 fatty acids is associated with depression.[37] One of the nutritional treatments for depression includes the administration of omega-3 fatty acids.

Omega-3 fatty acids can be found in flaxseed (flax meal, flax oil), hemp oil, purslane (a wild green), pumpkin seeds, walnut oil, and fish oil. Plant sources of omega-3 fatty acids are high in alpha-linolenic acid, which needs to go through several metabolic steps before it converts to the favorable PGE_3. However, the omega-3 fatty acids in fish oil are closer to the end product of fatty acid metabolism and require fewer metabolic steps.

Leukotrienes

Leukotrienes are powerful intercellular messengers, similar to prostaglandins. Like prostaglandins, different leukotrienes are derived from different fatty acids, and some leukotrienes are more favorable for immune health than others.

Arachidonic acid converts to leukotriene B_4 (LTB_4), which is extremely pro-inflammatory. Eicosapentaenoic acid and docosahexaenoic acid convert to leukotriene B_5 (LTB_5), which is neutral. However, if the LTB_5 displaces LTB_4, then the relative change is actually a decrease in inflammation. So again, the fatty acids you eat have a profound effect on the processes taking place within your body.

The Importance of Metabolic Pathways

As we've seen, essential fatty acids can be converted into other kinds of fatty acids, and fatty acids can be used to manufacture different types of prostaglandins and leukotrienes. The body is constantly busy transforming and converting the substances it has at its disposal to meet its needs, and some end products are more favorable to immune health than others.

The omega-6 fatty acids convert like this:

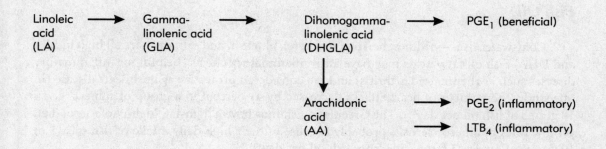

The metabolic step from LA to GLA is weak in humans. Saturated fat, trans-fatty acids, alcohol, sugar, stress, high blood pressure, diabetes, and aging all can block the conversion of LA into GLA. We can bypass this block by ingesting foods or supplements rich in GLA, such as primrose oil or borage oil. Once you ingest GLA, it usually converts to PGE_1 in the body.

Insulin enhances the conversion of DHGLA into AA (instead of into PGE_1). This is an important point, in that it connects hyperinsulinism (increased insulin levels) with immune system effects. Knowing this, we can take steps to control our blood sugar levels and thereby modify our production of prostaglandins.

Eating a diet rich in AA stacks the deck in favor of PGE_2 synthesis. On the other hand, omega-3 fatty acids selectively inhibit the conversion of AA to PGE_2. The essential fatty acids EPA and DHA inhibit the conversion of AA into PGE_2 by displacing the AA on the enzyme that makes this conversion occur.

The omega-3 fatty acids convert like this:

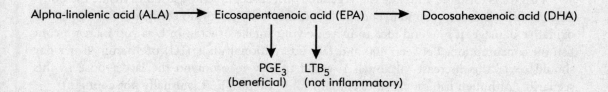

If a metabolic block exists at the first step, we can bypass it by ingesting EPA-rich foods. The metabolic step from ALA to EPA is weak in humans and is susceptible to the same influences mentioned above. This helps explain why people with high blood pressure or diabetes have a limited ability to make EPA and DHA from ALA.[38] When the metabolic step from ALA to EPA is blocked, using flaxseed oil (a source of ALA) would not help to boost EPA or DHA levels. However, we can get around this metabolic block by ingesting foods or supplements rich in EPA and DHA, such as fish oil.

Fish Oil

Cold-water fish—sardines, herring, mackerel, bluefish, and salmon—are all high in EPA and DHA. Fish oil fatty acids may have anti-inflammatory effects (helpful for inflammatory diseases such as rheumatoid arthritis) and are considered protective against heart disease (in one study, the number of heart attacks decreased by 41 percent in a group of subjects given 10 grams of fish oil per day[39]). The Greenland Eskimos have a high-fat, high-cholesterol diet, yet low rates of atherosclerosis, probably because of their high daily intake of fish oils (5 to 10 grams of omega-3 fatty acids from fish oil per day[40]).

Studies regarding the effectiveness of fish oil sometimes yield conflicting results because they use products of unequal quality (rancid fish oil, for example, would do you more harm than good), in different doses (some doses are too small to be effective), for varying amounts of time (generally it takes from twelve to twenty-four weeks before improvement is noted). One of the studies that showed fish oil to be effective against arthritis used high doses—the equivalent of twenty-one 1,000-milligram capsules per day of fish oil, each containing 180 milligrams of EPA and 120 milligrams of DHA (as well as small amounts of oleic acid, linoleic acid, and other fatty acids).[41]

To get the most healthful benefits, purchase high-quality fish oil supplements (not the cheapest) and refrigerate them. If you take cod liver oil (some people prefer this to fish oil capsules), be aware that it also contains vitamins A and D. Depending on how much cod liver oil you use and what other supplements you're taking, you could be getting too much of these vitamins. An alternative is devitaminized cod liver oil.

Vitamin E

Fish oil is unstable and, like the vegetable oils, susceptible to oxidation inside the body. Because fish oil does not contain enough fat-soluble antioxidants to compensate for potential oxidative damage, it's a good idea to increase your intake of vitamin E as you increase your fish oil consumption. Between 400 and 800 international units (IU) of vitamin E per day should cover this increase, although I would usually recommend the larger dose in this scenario. (Although fish oil capsules contain some vitamin E, it is usually not enough.)

One study compared subjects who were given fish oil supplemented with a low dose of vitamin E (0.3 IU/gram) with subjects who were given the same fish oil supplemented with a higher dose of vitamin E (1.5 IU/gram). The low-dose group actually experienced a drop in serum vitamin E, plus a 122 percent increase in malondialdehyde (a reactive free radical produced during lipid peroxidation). Both remained normal in the high-dose group.[42]

Remember how prevalent DHA is in the brain? Taking antioxidant vitamin E may protect these lipids from oxidation, which not only lets them stay where they are in the cell membranes, but also cuts down on the damage caused by free radicals. Oxidative stress in the brain may have untoward effects, and in fact may be associated with neurodegenerative disease, such as Parkinson's disease and Alzheimer's.

SUMMARY: IMMUNE-EMPOWERING FATS

Choose:

Nonfat or low-fat products (2 percent milk is not low-fat)
Cold-water fish (salmon, herring, mackerel, sardines)
Olive oil (expeller-pressed, extra-virgin)

Recommended essential fatty acid supplements:

Flaxseed or flax meal (1 to 3 tablespoons per day)
Flax oil (unrefined, cold-pressed, refrigerated; 1 to 2 tablespoons per day)
Fish oil (1 tablespoon of cod liver oil per day, or three to six 1,000-milligram capsules of EPA/DHA per day)
240 milligrams of GLA (either borage oil, evening primrose oil, or black currant seed oil)

Limit:

Vegetable oils and products made or cooked with them
High-fat foods (avocados, nuts)

Avoid:

Foods that contain saturated fat (meat, butter, cheese)
All products made with vegetable shortening, margarine, tropical oils, and hydrogenated or partially hydrogenated oils
Fried foods (including chips, even from the health food store—try the baked variety)

CHOOSING NUTRIENT–DENSE FOODS

Instead of counting calories, we need to learn to make each calorie count. Nutrient-dense foods—fresh fruits and vegetables, whole grains, legumes, low-fat protein sources—have large quantities of nutrients per each 100 calories. If you make it a general rule to eat only nutrient-rich foods, this will automatically add immune-enhancing foods to your diet and eliminate sugary, processed ones.

Juicing, believe it or not, is somewhat controversial. Juices made from fresh fruits and vegetables contain many of the vitamins, minerals, and enzymes of the original food, but eliminate most of the fiber. (This can be a problem for patients with carbohydrate intolerance because of the effect on blood sugar levels.) If you enjoy doing your own juicing, go right ahead—but don't forget to eat whole foods as well. There are numerous alternative cancer treatment programs, such as the Gerson Program, that include large amounts of daily juicing as one of the mainstays of their therapeutic approach.

Although vitamin and mineral supplements are helpful and will be discussed in the next chapter, I encourage all my patients to start with the Immune Empowering Diet before expecting miracles from supplements. *There is no substitute for eating whole foods,* for they contain accessory nutrients such as bioflavonoids that work hand in hand with the better-known vitamins and minerals. The micronutrients in whole foods have a synergistic effect that is impossible to completely duplicate by taking man-made supplements. I emphasize to all my patients that we can't afford to forget about diet.

It's important to eat a wide variety of foods and not get stuck on a few favorites. Different kinds of foods provide all manner of nutrients and micronutrients, some of which may have health benefits we don't even know about yet. Also, rotating foods is the best way to prevent food allergies. People who are stuck in a food rut often have undiagnosed food allergies.

Finally, one more recommendation: to get the most nutrients possible from your foods, buy seasonal, locally grown organic produce. Because it is grown in better soil, organic produce is on average 87 percent higher in minerals than nonorganic produce.[43] (It also reduces your exposure to immune-suppressing chemical residues.)

PREPARING FOOD IN A HEALTHFUL WAY

This isn't a cookbook, but I would like to mention that some ways of preparing food are better for your immune health than others. Here the rule of thumb is to eat foods in as close to their natural state as possible.

We've already seen that heating oils to a high temperature creates free radicals. In general, choose foods that are baked, steamed, poached, stewed, or boiled rather than fried, stir-fried, barbecued, grilled, or broiled. Some nutritionists even caution against eating melted cheese.

IMMUNE-EMPOWERING FOOD EXCHANGES

Instead of:	Substitute:
Whole milk	Skim milk
Sour cream	Nonfat yogurt
Ice cream	Nonfat frozen yogurt
Ricotta cheese	Tofu
Sugar	Frozen apple juice concentrate
White rice	Brown rice
White flour	Whole wheat flour
White bread	Whole grain bread
Doughnut	Nonfat muffin
Butter	Olive oil, or oil/butter blend
Margarine	Butter
Fried egg	Poached egg
Hamburger	Tuna sandwich
Bacon	Turkey bacon
Hot dogs	Tofu hot dogs
Shrimp	Salmon
Peanuts	Popcorn
Dry-roasted sunflower seeds	Dry-roasted almonds or cashews
Fried chips	Baked chips
Soda	Iced herb tea
Coffee	Herb tea

The worst way to cook a vegetable is to cut it into small pieces and boil it in a large amount of water for a long time. The best way, according to researchers at Cornell University, is to microwave vegetables with very little water. This method preserves 50 to 100 percent of the original nutrients.[44] For those of you who have resisted getting a microwave, steam vegetables in a small amount of water.

Even a properly cooked food will lose its nutritive value if it's not eaten promptly. One study showed that a boiled potato retained 53 percent of its vitamin C. However, after it was kept in the refrigerator for three days, its vitamin C dropped to a mere 5 percent.[45] (The study also showed that a baked potato retained 80 percent of its vitamin C.)

Canned vegetables have little to recommend them. Canned peas, for example, lose 30 percent of their vitamins when they are cooked at the plant and 25 percent during the sterilization process. Another 27 percent are discarded with the liquid, and 12 percent are lost when you heat the peas after you open the can. That leaves 6 percent of the original vitamins![46]

The optimal meal is a vegetable soup, or whole grains with vegetables and/or beans, with perhaps some herb tea. Small meals are better than large, and don't skip breakfast. Purists would say that it isn't a good idea to eat fruits and vegetables at the same time because different enzymes are required to digest them. As this idea may be helpful to some of you, I'll pass it along.

While it's not a good idea for anyone to overeat, I've found that it isn't necessary to count calories while on the Immune Empowering Diet. If you stick closely to this diet, you'll be eating only healthy foods, and your appetite for unhealthy foods will diminish. The calorie issue takes care of itself.

CAFFEINE

I'm not an anticaffeine crusader—for example, sometimes I drink coffee when I'm driving long distances to help me stay alert—but caffeine is *not* part of the Immune Empowering Diet. Caffeine is a stimulant, so it taxes the adrenal glands, elevates blood sugar levels, and revs up the central nervous system. This can lead to increased blood pressure, an increased heart rate irregularity (or heart arrhythmia), irritability, anxiety, and insomnia—as well as rebound fatigue when your system calms down. Caffeine is also associated with fibrocystic breast disease.

We drink a lot of caffeine in the form of coffee. Coffee beans often contain pesticides and herbicides that are used only outside the United States, so if you must drink coffee, buy organic. Because chemical solvents are used to decaffeinate commercial coffees, buy organic water-processed decaffeinated coffee beans. These can be found in gourmet coffee stores, health food stores, and even grocery stores these days.

Caffeine is present in tea, certain kinds of soda, and in cocoa and chocolate, as most people are aware. It's also an ingredient of many common medications, including Anacin, Excedrin, Midol, Vanquish, Cafergot, and Fiorinal, among others.

Caffeine can be addictive, as anyone who has experienced caffeine withdrawal knows. Get a headache every time you sleep late? Caffeine could be the culprit.

Decaffeinated coffee has about 5 milligrams of caffeine per cup. A cup of hot cocoa has about 10 milligrams. A 12-ounce Coca-Cola has 50 milligrams of caffeine, which is less than instant iced tea, which has about 70 milligrams per cup. The amount of caffeine in brewed tea and in coffee varies, depending upon how the beverages are prepared, and averages about 150 milligrams per cup. Don't go by taste alone—some of the gourmet coffees taste strong, but have *less* caffeine than truck-stop coffee.[47]

DIET AND BIOCHEMICAL INDIVIDUALITY

Each of us has unique nutritional needs because of the way we are genetically programmed. In addition, many people have food allergies and intolerances they need to take into consideration when planning their meals and snacks. In most cases, it is not necessary to alter the proportions of the basic Immune Empowering Diet.

• People who are **lactose intolerant** have trouble digesting the milk sugar lactose and should limit their consumption of dairy products. Commercially produced foods often contain milk derivatives (for example, whey and casein) in unexpected places (for instance, in lunch meats). Because yogurt is fermented, it contains less lactose and therefore some lactose-intolerant people are able to eat it without symptoms. Supplemental lactase pills can be helpful for people with lactose intolerance who can't avoid dairy products completely.

• People who have a **gluten intolerance** (in extreme form, this is known as celiac disease) react to the gluten in wheat, barley, rye, oats, and millet. (Gluten is the gluey substance in certain grains that helps bind bread products together.) In serious cases, the lining of the gastrointestinal tract becomes irritated and even scarred, which impairs nutrient absorption. People with celiac disease need to read labels carefully (wheat derivatives are especially common) and can usually substitute corn, rice, potatoes, and legumes for gluten-containing foods. I suspect that mild gluten intolerance is much more prevalent than commonly thought.

• If you have a **yeast sensitivity,** you need to eat foods that nourish you, but not the yeast in your gastrointestinal tract. Yeast is a sugar-feeder, so avoid sweets, fruit juice, alcohol, and refined carbohydrates. Choose unrefined, fiber-rich carbohydrates and low-starch vegetables. (The classic example of a high-glycemic vegetable—that is, one that gets metabolized to sugars quickly—is the potato.) You may need to increase your consumption of high-quality protein as well. People with a **yeast or mold allergy** should eliminate foods that contain yeast or mold, including yeasted breads, brewer's yeast, and fermented foods, including vinegar and aged cheeses.

The Low-Carbohydrate Diet

Many Americans have a **carbohydrate intolerance.** Estimates of the incidence of carbohydrate intolerance range from 25 to 60 percent. Based on my clinical experience, probably one in three Americans has some degree of carbohydrate intolerance. Signs of carbohydrate intolerance include trouble losing weight, bloating after eating, fatigue after meals, trouble concentrating after meals, and cravings for carbohydrates and sweets. Carbohydrate intolerance mimics many other conditions and thus may be mistaken for other disorders.

With carbohydrate intolerance, it is important to alter the breakdown of the Immune Empowering Diet. In his best-selling book entitled *The Zone,* Barry Sears, Ph.D., recommends that carbohydrate-intolerant people eat a diet that is 30 percent healthy fats, 30 percent protein, and 40 percent complex carbohydrates with plenty of fiber. Because carbohydrate-intolerant people shouldn't eat as many carbohydrates as others, they need to burn more calories from fats (preferably monounsaturated fatty acids). Fats also slow the rate at which sugar is absorbed from the intestines. In addition, carbohydrate-intolerant people have higher protein requirements, and may even need to eat meat to feel their best. This is one of those situations in which meat, because of individual metabolic uniqueness, may be a necessary and helpful component of the diet. (Generally I would recommend the other high-quality proteins mentioned earlier.)

As we've already seen, some carbohydrates flood the body with sugar more quickly than others. If you are carbohydrate-intolerant, you'll probably feel better if you avoid bread products (bagels, cookies, cakes), pasta (even whole wheat pasta), corn, and potatoes—all carbohydrates that have a high glycemic index (meaning they are quickly absorbed into the bloodstream as glucose). In this diet, all the carbohydrates you eat should be replete with fiber, as this usually results in a lower and healthier glycemic index. Avoid as much as possible foods that have had their fiber removed.

One of my patients, Dennis, responded remarkably to a low-carbohydrate diet. When Dennis first came to see me, he had mild hypertension that had been escalating for the past couple of years, plus elevated cholesterol, low HDL (good cholesterol), and increased triglycerides. Dennis had a family history of hypertension, heart disease, and stroke on both sides of his family, so now that he was pushing fifty, he felt he needed to "do something— maybe start taking a medication."

Dennis was actually careful about his health. He didn't drink or smoke, he avoided fats and cholesterol, and he consumed coffee only occasionally. He did admit to a weakness for salty foods as well as sweets, and he ate a doughnut or sweet roll at least once a day.

Dennis's job as a backhoe operator had its stressful moments, but he meditated regularly. At 6 feet tall and 235 pounds, he was a big man. He'd put on weight over the last five years without any change in his eating habits, and he found it difficult to take off the extra weight. Dennis also complained of fatigue or "lack of spunk."

In addition to giving Dennis supplements to boost his general state of health and herbs to help his blood pressure, I also placed him on a moderate-protein, low-carbohydrate diet. His response was wonderful to see. In the first three months his blood pressure dropped significantly, he lost 13 pounds, and his energy level was greater. He described his libido as "excellent."

After eight months on the low-carbohydrate diet, Dennis looked (and felt) like a new man. He had dropped a total of 32 pounds, his cholesterol and triglyceride levels had fallen, and he told me that his little grandson had recently asked him, "Grandpa, how come you never used to play with me like this before?"

ERIN'S STORY

All of my patients combine the Immune Empowering Diet with other therapies, but dietary changes were certainly at the heart of Erin's recovery. Before she got sick, Erin was a healthy teenager and an avid tennis player. She had won the girls' Section VII singles title in 1994, and was so good that she then competed the next year on the boys' team and was ranked boys' no. 1 all-star. By the next year, however, Erin was too ill to compete.

Her problems started in May, when she came down with a flu-like illness that included headaches, fever, cough, and unsteadiness. Other students in her school were sick, but Erin was sicker. When she tried to go back to school, the fever, headaches, and dizziness recurred. Erin's local doctor found nothing remarkable about her blood work (with which he ruled out mononucleosis, anemia, and hepatitis), but he placed her on an antibiotic for possible sinusitis.

By the middle of May, Erin was still unwell. A different doctor ruled out sinusitis and advised bed rest. By late May, Erin was no better. Although she kept trying, she couldn't handle going to school. She felt dizzy and was sleeping far more than usual. At the end of May, she was placed on meclizine, a prescription medication used to treat vertigo, but it didn't help.

After a CT scan and chest X ray failed to turn up anything noteworthy, Erin and her parents consulted a neurologist. By this time—early June—she was suffering from headaches, persistent fatigue, and dizziness. She constantly felt like fainting and sometimes would actually pass out. Suspecting ongoing basilar migraine (a migraine related to circulation at the base of the brain), the neurologist placed Erin on Periactin, a prescription antihistamine-type medication that blocks histamine and serotonin.

After two doses of Periactin, Erin was in a wheelchair. She later said that she believed the medication put her "out on the couch for two months." It is unclear whether the medication contributed to her lack of mobility. That summer, Erin couldn't walk and couldn't even sit without support. Tennis seemed a lifetime away. This certainly is an unusual response to this drug, and although there was no medical corroboration, Erin attributed her deterioration to the medication.

Eventually the neurologist ruled out basilar migraine, and Erin consulted an infectious diseases doctor who raised the possibility of chronic fatigue immune dysfunction syndrome (CFIDS). Erin was referred to a nearby medical center, where she consulted an ear, nose, and throat doctor. A battery of tests—including an MRI, tilt test, stress test, and echocardiography—all turned out normal. Everyone was at a loss.

By February, after ten months of illness, Erin and her mother came to my office. Erin suffered from light-headedness and dysequilibrium, head and neck pain, blurred vision, sensitivity to certain kinds of lights, chest pains, and burning fingertips.

Erin's medical history up until the time she fell ill was unremarkable. She'd had frequent ear infections and bouts of tonsillitis when she was younger and had often been placed on antibiotics. She had a history of migraine headaches, and at one time had been diagnosed with irritable bowel syndrome. Erin craved junk food, and her favorite foods were pizza, cheesecake, and chocolate.

We ran some new tests. Erin did not have elevated titers for either Epstein-Barr virus, cytomegalovirus, or Lyme disease. Her human herpesvirus 6 (HHV6) results were low-positive. Her thyroid tests were normal. Intradermal skin testing revealed sensitivities to yeast, mold, and milk.

As it turned out, her bed was on the other side of the wall from a shower and near a damp cellar, so one of the first environmental changes we advised her to make was to move her bed to get away from any mold that might be contributing to her problem.

Erin's glucose tolerance test results were unusual. Even after drinking the intensely sweetened liquid used for this test, her blood sugar level never rose above her fasting blood sugar level, indicating a phenomenon sometimes called *flat-curve hypoglycemia*. Most doctors would not be concerned with this result and would even consider it "unremarkable," but it definitely is not normal and frequently is associated with fatigue and apathy.

My diagnosis was CFIDS and immune dysregulation due to viral illness. I suspected Erin might also need treatment for yeast overgrowth, and made a note to come back to that later.

Erin received nutritional counseling at our office and was placed on an Immune Empowering Diet that excluded sugar (because of her hypoglycemia and also the yeast overgrowth) as well as dairy products and yeast (because of her allergies). This diet was a big change for someone who craved pizza and cheesecake, but I felt strongly that it was essential for Erin's recovery.

I also placed Erin on a number of immune system boosters, including a special multivitamin/mineral for chronic fatigue plus supplemental vitamin C, vitamin B_6, CoQ10, calcium, magnesium, probiotics (including acidophilus and bifidus) and prebiotics (to support the probiotics), essential fatty acids, and nutrients for adrenal support.

After a month on her modified Immune Empowering Diet, Erin told me she felt better, at least as well as she had felt before the Periactin treatment. I started Erin on intravenous vitamin C for immune modulation and on the antifungal medication nystatin to treat the yeast overgrowth. By May—the anniversary of her illness—she was back in school full-time. By July, Erin was running and playing tennis again.

Erin's return to the tennis courts was written up in the local newspaper in an article that noted her "completely new diet." Her father noted, "It [Erin's illness] puts sports in perspective. You appreciate being able to walk across the room and being able to get through the day without a big headache."

Erin still takes several nutritional supplements and receives intravenous vitamin C each month, and she is a candidate for more allergy testing and possibly enzyme-potentiated desensitization (EPD) immunotherapy. Even so, her recovery has been an inspiration to her family, friends, and teammates, who have all seen firsthand what a tremendous difference diet can make.

Chapter 6

❦

IMMUNE SYSTEM BOOSTERS

If you are ill or just not feeling up to par, you should know
that in most circumstances you have the power to create your
own health. You can do it with simple lifestyle changes and
dietary supplements.

—MICHAEL JANSON, M.D.
The Vitamin Revolution in Health Care[1]

Recently my wife and I had a houseguest for a few days who couldn't get over how
many capsules and tablets I take. In addition to my high-dose vitamin and mineral
supplement (the daily dose is divided into six pills and includes beneficial green plant
extracts), I also down a handful of additional antioxidants with breakfast and dinner. I have
a family history of heart disease and a stressful schedule, I'm exposed to many illnesses, and
I eat many of my meals away from home, especially when I'm traveling and lecturing, so I
also take essential fatty acids and some other immune-stimulating and cardiovascular-
protective nutrients.

I take lots of supplements because I know so much about their beneficial effects. Also,
I have easy access to them because we have special formulas made up for distribution
through our health centers. Most people don't take as many supplements as I do, and although I think a certain amount of supplementation is helpful for everyone, I don't expect
all of my patients to follow such an intensive supplement program because of the inconve-
nience and the cost.

Sometimes I compare selecting a supplement program to buying a car. Which one you
choose depends upon your needs, priorities, tastes, and bank account. A complex and expensive regimen isn't possible for everyone, and I often spend a considerable amount of time
creating an individualized program for a patient, taking into account all the variables I just
mentioned.

In my experience, most people are happy to take a moderate number of safe, affordable,
high-quality supplements to help their health. Patients who are ill usually require more
intensive supplement programs and are more willing to follow them.

In this chapter, I'll focus on those supplements that have the greatest effect on immune system function, and I'll recommend a beneficial general regimen of supplements for all readers. At the end of the chapter, I'll make some recommendations for modifying this basic regimen in special circumstances (for example, if you're sick, stressed, or have a family history of cancer).

Often my patients say to me, "But Dr. Bock, you never mentioned ginseng [or Cat's Claw, or L-carnitine, or whatever]. Isn't *that* good for you?" Many times my answer is, sure, it's good for you. But it would be extremely difficult—and prohibitively expensive—to take every possible supplement that could conceivably help your health. In this chapter I've narrowed the field to certain immune system boosters that I know are safe and effective and that apply to a wide variety of circumstances.

Although the focus of this chapter is getting started on an everyday regimen of supplements, I also include other immune system boosters here and elsewhere. Chapter 7, Alternative Therapies, includes a discussion of Chinese herbs, and Chapter 9, Gut and Liver Function: What's the Story? contains information on probiotics (such as acidophilus and bifidus). Additional supplements and techniques that require the advice or assistance of a health care practitioner are included in Chapter 10, Immune System Super Boosters. Super Boosters are not for everyday use. I reserve them for people who are sick and need immune system rehabilitation.

MICRONUTRIENTS AND IMMUNOCOMPETENCE

How well your immune system functions is, as we've already seen, closely linked to nutrition. To complete each step of an immune response, the body needs an adequate supply of the correct nutrients. A deficiency of even a single nutrient can impair our immune defenses.

Numerous studies have linked illness and weakened immune function to vitamin and mineral deficiencies, as well as to deficiencies of amino acids and essential fatty acids. On the other hand, other studies have shown that dietary supplements can stimulate and enhance immune function.

Let's say, for example, your diet is low in vitamin B_6 (pyridoxine). This vitamin is needed for cell reproduction, so low levels of vitamin B_6 translate into lowered cell reproduction and, in turn, lowered antibody production. Without an adequate supply of B_6, your body will not be able to turn out as many antibodies during an infection, and you'll have an acquired immunodeficiency. Fortunately, you can reverse this problem by getting a sufficient amount of vitamin B_6, either through dietary changes or, more likely, by taking supplements.

Single-nutrient deficiencies are common. One survey found that 88 percent of a U.S. hospital population had at least one deficiency.[2] No doubt the principal reason for this staggering statistic is the typical American diet, compounded by the horrors of hospital food and the increased nutrient demands associated with illness and recuperation. Knowing what we do about nutrition and immunocompetence, I can't help wondering how many of the patients included in this survey could have avoided ending up in the hospital if they'd gotten optimal levels of nutrients in the first place.

Surviving Versus Thriving

You'll remember from Chapter 2 that the recommended daily allowances (RDAs) for different nutrients were established to prevent deficiency diseases such as rickets (too little vitamin D), beriberi (insufficient vitamin B_1), scurvy (vitamin C deficiency), and pernicious anemia (vitamin B_{12} deficiency) in mass populations. These minimum requirements were never really intended to guide all nutritional enterprises in this country, and they have little to do with optimal immune status.

Most people can survive for many years on just 10 international units (IU) of vitamin E per day, but 100 IU of this vitamin per day lowers the risk of heart disease, and 800 IU per day has been shown to elevate immune function.[3] This being the case, who could argue that the RDA of 15 IU is truly sufficient? To achieve and maintain peak immune performance, I recommend ingesting certain nutrients at levels that can significantly exceed RDA guidelines.

Note the wide margin we are able to work within when we take supplements. With prescription medications, there is a narrow band of efficacy between a dose that is too low to do any good and a dose that is too high and causes side effects or toxicity. While it's true that very high levels of some nutrients can be toxic, in general we have far more leeway (sometimes called the "therapeutic window") with dosages of natural preparations, especially those that are water-soluble.

Symptoms of a frank vitamin or mineral deficiency take months or years to develop. By the time they're apparent, optimal immune function has been lost and body processes have started to break down. The sequence goes like this: First, tissue stores of the nutrient are used up. Next, biochemical processes are adversely affected because enzymes can't do their jobs without the proper cofactors. As deficiency deepens, symptoms develop and immune function deteriorates. After a prolonged period, classic deficiency diseases can be observed and diagnosed.

Taking in optimal amounts of nutrients over the long term is more beneficial than suddenly reaching for the multivitamins when you don't feel well. As you can see from the sequence above, optimum immune function is lost well *before* symptoms develop. This fact is not meant to terrorize you, however. If you start taking beneficial supplements today, some aspects of your immune function will improve in as little as two weeks, and you'll experience even greater effects after three months. I tell all my patients when they start their supplements not to expect too much too soon. It takes up to three months for supplements to become part of our cells and to effect significant changes.

There's a broad spectrum between optimal nutrient status and frank deficiency. If you're not getting an optimal amount of micronutrients, then you may have an insufficiency, but not a classic deficiency. Frank deficiencies are more easily recognizable but significantly less common than relative insufficiencies. Although they are more common, insufficiencies are more subtle and less readily appreciated.

Let's say you're relatively healthy, but you have a suboptimal level of several antioxidants. If nutrients were money, you wouldn't have enough to send your child to a good college, but you'd have too much to qualify for financial aid.

There is an important distinction between basal (resting) nutrient needs and functional (working) needs. You may have enough of a particular nutrient to meet your basal need, but if you don't have enough reserves of that nutrient to meet an increased demand as it occurs, then you have a functional insufficiency. For example, you may have enough B vitamins to maintain health until you experience a significant stress, which increases your B vitamin needs to the point where your supply becomes functionally insufficient.

The first step in getting abundant nutrients is to eat a good diet. The Immune Empowering Diet outlined in the previous chapter consists of many different nutrient-rich foods, preferably those that are fresh, organic, locally grown, and prepared in a manner that preserves as many nutrients as possible. Eating fresh foods ensures that we are getting adequate levels of a variety of nutrients, including those that haven't even been isolated and studied yet. Will this wholesome diet provide us with all the nutrients we need? Unfortunately, no.

WHY ISN'T A WHOLESOME DIET SUFFICIENT?

The argument most commonly used against supplements is that we get adequate levels of nutrients from our food. This is a little like the "if God meant for us to fly, he'd have given us wings" argument. Not being able to fly, we invented airplanes. Not being able to get all the necessary nutrients in adequate amounts from diet alone, we invented supplements.

Biochemical Individuality (Again): Differing Nutrient Needs

Each of us has unique nutrient needs. Earlier I mentioned a study that proved we all have different vitamin C requirements. An amount that is sufficient for me may not be sufficient for you. This means all of us may need a boost in certain nutrients.

In an ideal world, everyone would be tested for his or her own biochemical profile. We would all know our metabolic type and our unique needs for different amino acids, fatty acids, vitamins, and minerals. This specialized testing can be quite costly and therefore is not available to most people. However, we know there are certain nutrients with which we should generously supply our bodies in order to make sure we are meeting our individual biochemical needs.

Medications Affect Nutrient Needs

If you're taking a medication regularly—including birth control pills, heart or blood pressure medication, painkillers, and antidepressants—this can affect your nutrient needs (see the chart). Short-term courses of therapy—including antibiotics, radiation, and chemotherapy—can also change your nutrient needs. Drugs can interfere with the digestion, absorption, transport, excretion, and/or utilization of vitamins and minerals. Often it is difficult to know just how long-term use of a medication will affect your nutrient needs. It's safe to assume that while taking drugs, we probably have an increased need for one or more nutrients and that supplementing our diet with safe levels of vitamins and minerals will help ensure that these increased nutrient needs are being met.

HOW MEDICATIONS AFFECT NUTRIENT NEEDS

Condition	Medication	Increased nutrient needs
Birth control	Oral contraceptive	Vitamin B_6 and folic acid
High blood pressure, congestive heart failure	Diuretics	Potassium and magnesium
Bacterial infections	Antibiotics	Probiotics for gastrointestinal health and possibly liver-protective nutrients
Inflammation (arthritis, etc.)	Nonsteroidal anti-inflammatory drugs (NSAIDs)	Glutamine and aloe vera liquid to protect stomach lining (natural anti-inflammatories, such as the omega-3 fatty acids, can lessen the need for NSAIDs)
Fungal infections	Antifungals (such as Diflucan, Nizoral, Sporanox)	Liver-protective nutrients and herbs
Autoimmune disorders, allergic and inflammatory conditions	Potent corticosteroids (such as prednisone)	Calcium, antioxidants, chromium, glutamine, probiotics, magnesium

Scarce Nutrients

Some nutrients are difficult to obtain in sufficient amounts from diet alone. Vitamin E, for example, is an extremely beneficial antioxidant, but it is impossible to get an optimal amount of vitamin E from the food we eat.[4] It is also unlikely that people get enough CoQ10 (see page 197) from their diet. Selenium (see page 189) is theoretically available in our food supply, but much of the world's soil that is used for agriculture has been depleted of selenium, so the food that is produced is low in this mineral. And, as I discussed in the previous chapter, much of our food is of poor quality, having been grown in poor soil, often harvested before it was ripe, treated with chemicals, transported long distances, and processed or cooked beyond recognition.

Other nutrients are in short supply because we can't manufacture enough of them internally. Sometimes we are slow converters, and sometimes we are missing important cofactors that are necessary for the entire process to occur.

Humans can't synthesize vitamin C at all. Guinea pigs and monkeys can't, either—but they eat more vitamin-C-rich foods than most of us do! It's possible to get plenty of vitamin C from diet alone, but most people don't make the effort.

Malabsorption Problems

How much mileage you get out of the food you eat depends in part upon how well your gastrointestinal tract is functioning. Poor absorption of micronutrients from the digestive tract can be caused by many factors, including infections (bacterial, viral, fungal, or parasitic), rapid transit time (not enough time to absorb beneficial nutrients), and antibiotics. Supplements help ensure that you obtain adequate amounts of micronutrients. (It's also possible to bypass digestive problems and administer vitamins by injection or intravenous drip. Because this kind of therapy requires a doctor, I've included it in Chapter 10, Immune System Super Boosters.)

Detoxification Requires Nutrients

The body uses up micronutrients when it breaks down toxins. As we've already seen, toxins can arise internally, or they can enter the body from outside. A buildup of toxins in the body can poison the immune system (which, by the way, has given rise to a new field called *immunotoxicology*). Today we are exposed to so many more toxins, pollutants, and carcinogens than before that we have an increased need for certain nutrients that are helpful in detoxifying poisons and supporting tissues.

Remember Mr. Benedi, who needed a liver transplant after taking Tylenol Extra Strength with wine? We know that alcohol depletes the body's stores of glutathione (an antioxidant discussed on page 200). We also know that without adequate glutathione, the liver has a hard time detoxifying acetaminophen. In addition, some people need extra gluta-thione because they are genetically sluggish detoxifiers. It's interesting to speculate whether Mr. Benedi's story might have had a different outcome if he'd been taking supplementary glutathione and other nutrients to help keep his detoxification pathways functioning better.

Why We Need Antioxidants

As I described in Chapter 4, the dual processes of oxidation and reduction are the key to our cellular existence. During oxidation, the body burns carbohydrates and fats inside our mitochondria (little "factories" inside each cell) by combining them with oxygen to produce energy. This process is catalyzed and controlled by special enzymes, and the energy that is released is stored as ATP. The unfortunate by-product of oxidation is highly unstable oxygen free radicals that have an unpaired electron in their outer shell. In their zeal to stabilize themselves, free radicals will grab an electron from a neighboring molecule—which solves their problem, but creates another. This "hot potato" effect accounts for the different kinds of free radical damage I described earlier, including harm to cell membranes and to the fragile genetic material inside our cells. Degenerative diseases like heart disease, arthritis, cancer, and Parkinson's disease are all associated with free radical damage.

Tissues of the central nervous system may be especially vulnerable to free radical dam-age because of their high rate of oxygen consumption and their high mitochondrial density. The mitochondria produce free radicals during the normal processes of oxidative metabo-lism (see Chapter 11), and these free radicals can do local damage within the cell. If the mitochondrial DNA is damaged, the cell's metabolic processes may become flawed, leading to greater free radical damage and ultimately neurodegenerative disease.

The body has ways of handling oxidative stress, but if these systems are overwhelmed, the balancing act between oxidation and reduction can be disrupted. Living things survive only as long as their antioxidant power is sufficient to counterbalance oxidative stress. If there is too much oxidative stress, or too few antioxidants, damage can proceed unchecked.

Vigorous exercise generates free radicals because oxidative processes go into high gear and free radical production accelerates. Phagocytes use free radicals to kill infectious organ-isms, and run the risk of hurting nearby cells as well as themselves. (These self-inflicted wounds are known as *auto-oxidative damage*.) Dietary factors, drinking, smoking, drugs, alcohol, medications, pollution, radiation, infection, surgery, inflammation, and stress all increase the level of free radicals within the body. Modern life places burdens upon our bodies that didn't even exist when our parents were growing up. What can we do? Take antioxidant supplements. The greater your free radical burden, the more antioxidants you should take. Diet alone is not enough.

Study after study has determined that it is beneficial to our health to have an excess of antioxidants held in reserve, and that antioxidants can have profound benefits for the immune system. During reduction, antioxidants give away their electrons to satiate free radicals and to stop their pillaging. In addition to helping prevent free radical damage, antioxidants stimulate phagocytes and help the body neutralize toxins.

Important antioxidants include vitamin C, vitamin E, beta-carotene, glutathione, CoQ10, selenium, and zinc. There are also *antioxidant enzymes*, most notably two types of superoxide dismutase (SOD), one of which protects mitochondrial membranes; glutathione peroxidase (GP), which helps minimize lipid peroxidation; catalase, which breaks down hydrogen peroxide (a by-product of lipid peroxidation) into water and oxygen; and glutathione reductase, which helps recycle antioxidant molecules after they have been oxidized. Antioxidant enzymes need certain cofactors (vitamins, minerals, and/or amino acids) to function. Provided they have their appropriate cofactors, antioxidant enzymes can neutralize huge quantities of free radicals. (For example, it's theorized that one molecule of catalase can neutralize a million molecules of hydrogen peroxide.) Antioxidant enzymes also can increase in number when the body is challenged by a higher level of free radicals.

Antioxidants work together synergistically to replenish one another and amplify their effectiveness. Taking supplementary vitamin C is good, but taking a variety of antioxidants is even better.

The "ideal" antioxidant affects oxidative stress both directly and indirectly. Beneficial qualities in an antioxidant include:

- The ability to quench a variety of free radicals
- Both water-soluble and fat-soluble properties
- Ready bioavailability
- The ability to regenerate other antioxidants (such as glutathione and vitamins C and E)
- The ability to get where it's needed and to build up a level of concentration in tissues, cells, and/or extracellular fluid
- Metal-chelating activity (certain metals induce the formation of free radicals, including the "transition metals" copper and iron, and the heavy metals cadmium and mercury)

Generations of mothers have urged their children to eat their vegetables. Today we need not only to eat our vegetables, but to take our antioxidants as well. Unfortunately, medical doctors are among the last people to recognize this fact. When my father was in the hospital in Florida with a severe respiratory problem, eating very poorly and being given very high concentrations of continuous inhaled oxygen (which can add to oxidative stress), I asked his attending physician to give him some antioxidants. The doctor became very uncomfortable and loudly replied, "We don't do that stuff here! You can do whatever you want once he gets out." It disturbs me that it is acceptable to give a hospitalized patient with these problems a high-sugar, low-nutrient diet, but it is not acceptable to give him vitamins C and E.

THE IMPORTANCE OF ANTIOXIDANTS

1. Antioxidants protect cells from free radicals that are generated during oxidation, thereby helping to prevent the development of degenerative diseases associated with free radical damage.
2. They also protect us against free radicals from other sources, including diet, stress, radiation, lifestyle choices such as smoking, and occupational hazards such as chemical exposure.
3. Antioxidants boost immune system function.
4. They help the body neutralize toxins and process medications.
5. They protect cell membranes (and the integrity of cell membranes is vital in cell-to-cell communications of all kinds).
6. They aid in cell and tissue renewal.
7. Antioxidants replenish one another.

In addition to all the qualities on this list, we now know that antioxidants can also have regulatory effects on gene expression. Antioxidants affect the transcription of proteins that different genes encode for. These include proteins that affect cell regulatory functions and proteins that are involved in growth and metabolism. It is becoming more and more recognized that various nutrients, including antioxidants, can have an effect on gene expression.

THE MOST EFFECTIVE WAY TO TAKE SUPPLEMENTS

For the foundation of your supplement program, find a high-quality, high-potency, balanced multivitamin and mineral supplement (for dosage levels, see the summary list at the end of this chapter, on p. 206). Choose a formula without iron unless you have a documented iron deficiency or are a menstruating woman. It should contain a minimal amount of inert ingredients (fillers, artificial flavors and colors, etc.), as these can actually compete in the body with the nutrients you need.

Buy supplements that are produced by a reputable company, preferably recommended by a knowledgeable practitioner who can vouch for their quality. Paying a lot of money doesn't guarantee high quality, but very low cost almost always guarantees poor quality.

Hypoallergenic supplements (typically made without corn, wheat, yeast, soy, milk, or egg) are preferred. Even if you don't have any food allergies you're aware of, you could have hidden allergies. Exacerbating them every day with a nonhypoallergenic formula could hinder your recovery.

I generally favor capsules over tablets, but most of the high-quality, high-potency multivitamins are tablets. Tablets are highly condensed, like little rocks, and they can go right through some people who have poor digestion. (If this happens to you, it's an indication that you need to either change your supplement or take a closer look at your digestive processes!) When choosing a specific supplement, find out if you can which type is most readily absorbed.

If you have a touchy stomach, take your supplements after you eat, or even in the middle of your meal. Some supplements are better tolerated than others, so if you can't tolerate one type, you may be able to take a related form or brand. Ask your health care practitioner to recommend a supplement that his or her other patients with this problem have successfully tolerated.

It's true that ideally certain supplements should be taken separately. For example, some experts recommend taking selenium and vitamin C at different times for maximum absorption. I find that for my patients, this just isn't convenient. In most cases, worrying about which supplement combinations are right or wrong ends up creating stress, which is counterproductive. However, it is a good idea to take fat-soluble nutrients (such as CoQ10) with a meal that contains some fat (to enhance absorption), and to take water-soluble nutrients (such as vitamins B and C) with liquids (to get proper dispersal in the body).

Do take your supplements in divided doses over the course of the day. This will help your body maintain steady-state levels of nutrients. If you take huge quantities of nutrients all at once, your body will excrete much of what you don't need, leaving less available for later.

When you first start your new regimen, take the multivitamin/mineral supplement first and see how you tolerate it. Wait one to three days before introducing each additional supplement. Each time you take a new product, watch for any ill effects. If you have any problems, test to see if they're just coincidental by waiting four days, then reintroducing the supplement. Or, to find out which one is the problem, stop them all and reintroduce them one at a time every fourth day.

The Immune System Boosters described in the pages that follow are team players. No one nutrient will make you entirely healthy, but a combined regimen of vitamins, minerals, and other substances will work together to enhance immune function and well-being.

Of course, there are limits. One grandfather boasted to his granddaughter that the first vitamin pill he takes in the morning makes him strong, the second makes him wise, and the third makes him handsome. After a pause, she responded, "That last one doesn't work very well, does it?"[5]

VITAMINS

We've known for a long time that vitamins are important to good health. However, recent studies are revealing new ways in which vitamins affect immune function.

Vitamin A (Retinol)

A fat-soluble vitamin, vitamin A plays an important role in immune system function. Vitamin A:

- Helps maintain the surfaces of the skin and the mucosal immune system, important barriers against infection
- Promotes the production of mucous secretions and lysozyme (a protein that destroys bacteria) in saliva
- Aids in cell differentiation and proliferation
- Has been shown to reverse precancerous lesions

High levels of vitamin A:

- Enhance macrophage function
- Stimulate cytotoxic T cells
- Enhance resistance to infection and carcinogens
- Prevent the immune suppression that commonly follows surgery

Vitamin A is essential for bone growth and reproduction, helps wound healing, and prevents night blindness. This vitamin is used up more rapidly when we are under stress.

The body lacks efficient mechanisms for getting rid of extra vitamin A, so excessively high doses—100,000 IU per day or more—may be immune suppressing and can cause toxicity and liver damage. Some cancer patients are treated with extremely high doses of vitamin A without showing signs of toxicity, but in general, healthy individuals should avoid megadoses of vitamin A.

One of my patients, an actress named Simone, consulted a doctor who recommended a variety of supplements, including potent vitamin A drops. Simone mistakenly took the wrong dose (one dropperful instead of one drop) for a period of weeks and developed signs of toxicity, including headaches, vomiting, blurred vision, and vertigo. Her doctor attributed these symptoms to yeast die-off (a phenomenon that can occur with a new regimen, but usually after days or weeks, not months). Simone's condition continued to worsen to the point where she could no longer function. When she came to my office, we went over her regimen together and discovered that vitamin A toxicity was the source of her problem. It took Simone months to recover from her overdose of vitamin A.

I don't want to scare you away from vitamin A, however. An article in the *Lancet* notes that "vitamin A deficiency clearly has profound effects on the immune system."[6] Vitamin A deficiency causes impaired antibody and lymphocyte responses, increased susceptibility to infection and to some tumors, and slower wound healing. It also causes neurological degeneration; dry skin; gastrointestinal, genitourinary, and respiratory problems; anemia; and night blindness.

Vitamin A is found naturally in animal products including liver, fish liver oil, egg yolks, and dairy products. Unlike the water-soluble vitamins, vitamin A can be stored in the liver and retrieved by the body as needed.

The body can manufacture vitamin A from beta-carotene (see below), but in certain situations this conversion process (which occurs in the intestines) may be sluggish. Patients with diabetes and hypothyroidism have an impaired ability to convert beta-carotene to vitamin A. I see impaired conversion in my cancer patients as well.

I frequently recommend 10,000 IU of vitamin A per day in a multivitamin along with supplemental beta-carotene (see below). Doses of vitamin A up to 25,000 IU are generally well tolerated. Higher doses can be beneficial in certain circumstances (such as with acute or recurrent respiratory infections), but if you're taking over 25,000 IU of vitamin A per day for an extended period of time, you should be monitored for signs of toxicity by a nutritionally oriented physician. (If necessary, vitamin A levels in the blood can be followed.) For an acute respiratory infection I sometimes recommend 100,000 IU daily for five days. This will be helpful and won't be a problem during this short period. Avoid doses over 5,000 IU per day during the first three months of pregnancy. If you are pregnant, or trying to get pregnant, it is prudent to consult your physician for an appropriate supplement regimen.

Carotenoids and Beta-Carotene

There actually are over six hundred carotenoids found in nature,[7] but the most familiar (as well as the most predominant) is beta-carotene, which gives the yellow color to many fruits and vegetables. Beta-carotene, a fat-soluble nutrient and powerful antioxidant, affects immune function by:

- Enhancing lymphocyte production
- Increasing macrophage cytotoxicity and cytotoxic T cell activity
- Helping detoxify pollutants
- Enabling the growth and development of cells
- Maintaining the membrane receptors that are essential for immune function
- Modulating the release of prostaglandins and leukotrienes[8]

In addition to its antioxidant and immune-stimulating properties, beta-carotene is necessary for protein metabolism. It also has anticancer effects. One study found that subjects with the lowest beta-carotene level were 4.3 times more likely to develop lung cancer than those with the highest level of beta-carotene.[9] In another study, beta-carotene prevented the development of precancerous lesions in the mouth.[10]

Beta-carotene is a precursor of vitamin A, but it has effects that vitamin A does not. It is a far more powerful antioxidant than vitamin A, it is more beneficial than vitamin A in the formation of healthy skin cells, and it appears to have immune-stimulating properties that vitamin A does not. Eating plenty of beta-carotene helps ensure that the body manufactures enough vitamin A. Overproduction of vitamin A is not a problem, however, because a feedback mechanism prevents this from occurring.

Although consuming high levels of beta-carotene may tint your skin yellow, you can't take too much beta-carotene because toxic levels do not build up in the body. Many, many studies have shown that a diet rich in carotenoids is associated with a lower risk of cancer and heart disease.

In 1996, beta-carotene supplementation received a lot of bad press when two studies failed to determine that beta-carotene was protective against cancer or heart disease. Dr. Richard Klausner, director of the National Cancer Institute, was quoted in *The New York Times* as saying, "I can see no reason that an individual should take beta-carotene."[11]

Personally, I believe that beta-carotene is most effective when it is used as part of an integrated program that includes a healthy lifestyle and supplementation with other nutrients, including other carotenoids and other antioxidants. The idea that beta-carotene was, by itself, a "magic bullet" was unrealistic. Recent evidence suggests that carotenoids may be most beneficial when taken together, as they appear in nature.

One of the disappointing beta-carotene studies followed the health of a large number of Finnish men who smoked heavily. Some were given beta-carotene supplements and some weren't. Researchers were shocked to find that the beta-carotene-supplemented group actually had a higher incidence of lung cancer and higher death rates. This implies that something about supplementing strictly with beta-carotene could be toxic. As a consequence of high oxidant stress, it's possible that oxidized beta-carotene built up (becoming a pro-oxidant) because there were not enough fellow carotenoids or other antioxidants to reconvert it (or, technically, to reduce it) back to its antioxidant form.

This study raises other questions as well. Perhaps we need to rethink the way in which we conduct nutritional studies. Is it reasonable to isolate a single nutrient that does not appear alone in nature? And does it really make sense to apply the findings from a study of heavy smokers to healthy nonsmokers? In this case, beta-carotene supplementation may simply have been too late. Antioxidants may be more helpful in the prevention of disease than in its reversal.

Beta-carotene is found in most dark green and deep yellow fruits and vegetables. Marine algae is also a good source of carotenoids. I recommend supplementing with 15,000 to 50,000 IU of mixed carotenoids (along with other antioxidants) per day. I am not at all worried about toxic effects from beta-carotene when it is taken in this manner.

The B Vitamins

There are several different nutrients in the B complex, including:

B_1 (thiamine)
B_2 (riboflavin)
B_3 (niacin)
B_5 (pantothenic acid)
B_6 (pyridoxine)
B_{12} (cobalamin)
Folic acid
Biotin
Choline
Inositol
Para-aminobenzoic acid (PABA)

The B vitamins, which are water-soluble, are involved in metabolic processes and cell proliferation. Each nutrient in the B family makes its own unique contribution to good health, but all the B vitamins work together synergistically. They are important for immune system strength because antibody-producing cells can't replicate without them.

Vitamin B_6 is particularly important for immune function. It is not only necessary for protein synthesis, but also stimulates antibody response. A deficiency of vitamin B_6 can cause a decreased lymphocyte response, an impaired antibody response, and atrophy of lymphoid tissue. Because vitamin B_6 is used up when hormones are metabolized by the liver, B_6 deficiency is common in women of childbearing age, women who have had multiple pregnancies, and women who have taken birth control pills without supplementary B_6. (This last is a classic example of a medication creating an enhanced need for a specific nutrient.)

Vitamin B_{12} is essential for nucleic acid synthesis, which means it is needed for cell growth and division. This helps explain why a deficiency of vitamin B_{12} causes an impaired lymphocyte response. Because vitamin B_{12} is needed for normal red blood cell production, extreme B_{12} deficiency causes pernicious anemia.

Like vitamin B_{12}, **folic acid** is also essential for the production of red blood cells. During pregnancy, folic acid plays an important part in the development of the nervous system and blood cells of the fetus. A deficiency of folic acid can cause anemia as well as impaired neutrophil function, impaired cytotoxic T cell function, impaired antibody response, and impaired lymphocyte response. Low folic acid levels may also promote cancer. One possible explanation is that without enough protective folic acid, the DNA of cells is more vulnerable to attack.

It's a little off the subject, but I'd like to mention here that in addition to their role as immune system boosters, vitamin B_6, vitamin B_{12}, and folic acid also are important for heart health because they help "mop up" serum homocysteine (a harmful by-product of protein metabolism). High levels of homocysteine in the blood may be a more significant factor in heart attacks than serum cholesterol, and elevated levels of homocysteine may explain why many people who have none of the traditional risk factors for cardiovascular disease still experience cardiovascular events. It's likely that older people are more vulnerable to heart attacks because they have trouble absorbing B vitamins from their food, which in turn contributes to elevated homocysteine levels.

So much attention has been paid to cholesterol that other risk factors for cardiovascular disease—such as homocysteine, lipoprotein A [Lp(a)], fibrinogen, and ferritin—tend to be overlooked. In our offices, we have assembled a cardiovascular panel (blood test) that we use to evaluate all these risk factors so we can recommend appropriate nutritional interventions when indicated. The main modifiers of these risk factors are nutritional, rather than pharmaceutical—which may help to explain why these risk factors are not more routinely assessed.

Vitamin B_6 is found in many foods, including blackstrap molasses, meat, potatoes, bananas, and wheat germ. Vitamin B_{12} is present only in animal products, including liver, kidney, and dairy products. Strict vegans—who eat no dairy products, red meat, poultry, or seafood—run an increased risk of B_{12} deficiency.

It's a little more difficult to obtain a sufficient amount of folic acid from diet alone. Prenatal vitamins always include folic acid to ensure pregnant women get enough. Sources of folic acid include liver, black-eyed peas and other legumes, spinach, peanuts, artichokes, asparagus, romaine lettuce, and sunflower seeds.

⟨⟩

COMMONLY ASKED QUESTION NO. 11:

Why do vitamin pills turn my urine yellow?

The answer is vitamin B_2 (riboflavin). The body takes what it needs and excretes the rest, causing the urine to turn bright yellow or gold.

Some crusaders use the "expensive urine" argument to denigrate the value of supplements. My feeling is that a supplement may have many beneficial effects before it is fully processed by the body and excreted. Also, because it's impossible to know exactly how much you need of a given nutrient, providing abundant amounts ensures that you're getting enough—particularly of the water-soluble substances that don't build up in the body.

⟨⟩

I generally recommend B vitamins in the following daily doses:

B₁	50 to 100 mg
B₂	25 to 50 mg
B₃	100 to 200 mg
B₅	150 to 500 mg
B₆	25 to 100 mg (50 to 100 mg for birth control pill users)
B₁₂	100 mcg
Folic acid	800 mcg
Biotin	300 mcg
Choline	50 to 150 mg
Inositol	25 to 100 mg
PABA	50 mg

Vitamin C (Ascorbic Acid)

Dr. Linus Pauling, a brilliant scientist and two-time winner of the Nobel prize, was an outspoken advocate of vitamin C supplementation. Whereas the RDA for vitamin C is 60 milligrams, Dr. Pauling recommended megadoses in the range of 10 grams per day or more. He took 18 grams a day—and, incidentally, he lived to be ninety-three years old.

Was Dr. Pauling correct? Here's what we know.

Vitamin C, which is water-soluble, is ubiquitous inside our cells. Vitamin C has myriad important immune functions, including:

- Enhancing the movement of phagocytes (which affects both antigen presentation and microbe killing)
- Stimulating the reproduction and maturation of lymphocytes
- Improving natural killer cell function
- Increasing the release of interferon
- Protecting the liquid parts of cells with its antioxidant effects
- Regenerating the reduced form of vitamin E
- Increasing tissue levels of glutathione[12]
- Helping to convert toxins to water-soluble, inert substances

Lymphocytes naturally use vitamin C to fight viruses. This cellular vitamin C, in a concentration that is ten times that in most other cells, needs to be constantly replenished. During an infection, the amount of vitamin C in these cells rapidly decreases.

Vitamin C is also important in cell repair and in the formation of collagen, which means it helps with the healing of wounds and fractures. In addition, vitamin C is involved in the synthesis of neurotransmitters and in the metabolism of cholesterol and lipoprotein A.

Vitamin C reduces the toxic effects of radiation therapy by protecting the skin and bone marrow. Interestingly, it does not protect the tumor that is being irradiated.

Not all studies support the claim that megadoses of vitamin C will help prevent colds, but we all know individuals who swear vitamin C supplements work for them. One of my nurses started taking 8 grams of vitamin C a day after coming to work for us and was amazed when she went through an entire New York winter without a single sinus infection. At the very least, vitamin C has been shown to reduce the severity and duration of upper respiratory infections. Regular intake of vitamin C seems to be more helpful than suddenly taking vitamin C supplements when cold symptoms appear. However, I suggest to my patients that they increase their intake of vitamin C at the first sign of an infection by several grams and maintain this increased dose for at least a week.

Vitamin C deficiency is associated with immune suppression, including decreased inflammatory response, impaired cytotoxic T cell activity, and impaired phagocyte function. This helps explain why low levels of vitamin C are associated with lowered resistance to infection, increased susceptibility to dental cavities, poor wound healing, and increased occurrence of cancer and heart disease. Extreme vitamin C deficiency results in scurvy, which can be fatal. (Up until 1753, scurvy killed more people than war.[13] Then it was demonstrated that sailors could be prevented from developing scurvy on long voyages by eating lime juice—hence the term *limeys*.)

Scurvy is characterized by generalized tissue disintegration at all levels. Interestingly, it is also accompanied by undifferentiated cellular proliferation. Taken together, these processes resemble the development of cancer—a fact that may not be just a coincidence.

In a lecture entitled "Vitamin C and Cancer" sponsored by the American College for Advancement in Medicine, Gladys Block, Ph.D., an expert on public health, presented a roundup of studies that all indicated vitamin C has a statistically significant protective effect against many types of cancer. Linus Pauling tried to tell us the same thing back in 1979 in his book *Cancer and Vitamin C*, written with Ewan Cameron, M.D. The two men also collaborated on a review paper entitled "Ascorbic Acid and Cancer" that emphasizes the importance of vitamin C not only in boosting the immune system and helping the body detoxify carcinogens, but also in maintaining the integrity of the intercellular matrix and its ability to resist infiltration. Vitamin C is also required for the formation of collagen that the body uses to help encapsulate tumor cells.[14] (For information about using high doses of vitamin C to treat cancer, see Chapter 10.)

While the National Cancer Institute recommends three or more servings of vegetables per day and two or more servings of fruit per day (which together would provide at least 200 milligrams of vitamin C), Dr. Block pointed out that only 9 percent of the U.S. population actually eats this way. Clearly many millions of Americans have vitamin C intakes at levels associated with an increased risk of cancer.

A study focused specifically on the effect of vitamin C on natural killer cells found that there was a sharp increase in NK activity eight hours after the administration of vitamin C (at a dose of 60 milligrams per kilogram of body weight). The activity was further increased at twenty-four hours before dropping back again after forty-eight hours. An enhancement of NK cytotoxic activity may be one way through which vitamin C exerts its anticancer effects.[15]

Another study, which involved 730 elderly subjects, found that low levels of vitamin C are associated with stroke. In this study, the vitamin C level was as strong a predictor of death from stroke as diastolic blood pressure (the lower number in a blood pressure reading).[16] It seems likely that the presence of vitamin C in tissues and cells helps prevent the free radical reactions that initiate degenerative diseases, including cerebrovascular disease. Vitamin C intake at 300 milligrams per day is associated with an extra six years of life in men.[17]

So what is the right dose of vitamin C? Some scientists feel that if we had not lost the ability to synthesize vitamin C millions of years ago, our livers today would be producing 10 to 30 grams of vitamin C per day. If we look at the amount of vitamin C that animals manufacture, and adjust this amount to the size and weight of humans, we come up with a daily requirement of approximately 5 to 15 grams per day (not allowing for illness or stress, which would require an increased dose).

Another point of view derives from the "Paleolithic diet" I mentioned in the previous chapter. It is estimated that our ancestors consumed 400 to 2,000 milligrams of vitamin C per day. Although our modern diet would be unrecognizable to a caveman, our metabolic processes are much the same as they were thousands of years ago when vitamin C intake was higher.

Along with numerous other nutritionally oriented physicians, I often employ the "bowel tolerance" approach to vitamin C dosage, especially for cancer, chronic infections, and allergies. This means you increase your vitamin C intake until you develop gas and/or diarrhea, then back off a little until these effects disappear. (This gastrointestinal upset is not harmful, just uncomfortable.) People who have an increased need for vitamin C—for example, those with cancer or a chronic infection—require and are able to tolerate a higher dose of vitamin C than healthy individuals. Usually a dose over 10 grams per day brings on diarrhea, but people with an infection often can ingest up to 30 grams a day without ill effects,[18] presumably due to their increased need (and I've had severely ill patients who have tolerated even larger doses than this).

In 1996, researchers at the National Institutes of Health recommended an optimal daily intake of 200 milligrams of vitamin C, based on the results of a study that involved seven young, healthy men. At doses over 200 milligrams per day, the young men absorbed less and excreted more vitamin C. At doses over 1,000 milligrams (1 gram), their urine was found to contain oxalate, a breakdown product of vitamin C that can be associated with kidney stones. (This theoretical risk can be minimized by taking magnesium and B complex supplements.) Dr. Mark Levine, who directed the study, was quoted in *The New York Times* as saying, "This means Linus Pauling was all wrong."[19]

I don't think so. I am not convinced that the results of a study involving seven young, healthy men who lived in a hospital ward for four to six months should be applied to, say, a forty-five-year-old mother of three who works in a manufacturing plant and has a family history of cancer. Many, many previous studies found that the benefits of supplemental vitamin C became most evident at doses of 1,000 milligrams or more per day—and no harmful side effects were noted.

Vitamin C is abundant in fresh fruits and vegetables. One navel orange, for example, has 80 milligrams of vitamin C, but red chili peppers top the list, followed by guavas, red and green sweet peppers, kale leaves, collard leaves, turnip greens, broccoli, and brussels sprouts. Vitamin C is destroyed by exposure to air, so eat those fresh fruits and vegetables promptly. In addition to eating fresh fruits and vegetables, I recommend taking at least 3 grams of vitamin C per day (the "buffered" variety is better tolerated), preferably in divided doses throughout the day. Taking vitamin C steadily over the course of the day helps to keep cells saturated.

Most multivitamins do not contain high enough amounts of vitamin C, so you'll need to find a supplement. Ester C is a considerably more expensive form of vitamin C that is theoretically better utilized, but studies have not definitely proved this to be so. My patients have had good results with buffered vitamin C products.

Vitamin D (Cholecalciferol)

A fat-soluble substance, vitamin D is sometimes referred to as the "sunshine vitamin" because we produce it when our skin is exposed to sunlight (or to artificial ultraviolet light). Ironically, the fact that we can manufacture our own vitamin D by means of this photochemical process means that the substance we call vitamin D isn't really a vitamin, or even a nutrient, at all.

Vitamin D is not directly immune enhancing, but it does affect good health. Although vitamin D is itself biologically inert, it is converted by the body into a steroid hormone that affects the use of calcium (for example, for bone growth or lactation). It also helps the body maintain the correct calcium balance inside cells (sometimes called "whole body calcium homeostasis") and helps maintain those nerve and cell functions that depend upon calcium.

The relationship between vitamin D and calcium is intimate. Interestingly, vitamin D deficiency can be triggered by low calcium intake (or malabsorption of calcium). Low calcium levels can lead to the destruction of vitamin D, which helps explain why rickets (vitamin D deficiency disease) is common in areas of the world where people get plenty of sunshine but not much dietary calcium.

Although dietary supplementation of vitamin D can help offset vitamin D deficiency, most people generate enough vitamin D through photochemical synthesis. It's just that they destroy what they make because of an underlying problem with calcium. A 1995 article in the *Lancet* questioned whether the long-term fortification of processed foods (such as milk and breakfast cereal) with vitamin D is a good idea, and pointed out that "evidence from domestic animals suggests that persistent feeding of dietary vitamin D may be associated with the development of chronic vascular disease."[20] The article went on to point out that orally administered vitamin D is so potent that it is currently used as rat poison!

There are few natural foods that supply vitamin D in any substantial amount, but a notable exception is fish liver oil. Because vitamin D is fat-soluble, it can accumulate and thus be toxic if taken in excessive doses. Signs of vitamin D toxicity include anorexia, nausea, thirst, diarrhea, muscle weakness, joint pains, kidney failure, calcification of soft tissues, and loss of bone. I seldom recommend vitamin D supplementation, except perhaps for elderly patients who are not exposed to direct sunlight and for women who are approaching (or who are in) menopause. Because osteoporosis (loss of bone mass) is a concern for women as they age, I advise women over thirty-five to take supplementary calcium and magnesium with a small amount of vitamin D (plus some vitamin C as well). The multivitamins that I have made up for our offices include 50 to 100 IU of vitamin D as not everyone, including adult males, needs the 400 IU present in many multivitamins, an amount that I consider to be too high.

Vitamin E (Tocopherol)

You'll recall from the previous chapter that vitamin E is a major fat-soluble antioxidant. There are actually eight compounds in the vitamin E family, but d-alpha-tocopherol has the highest biological activity and is the most widely available form in food.[21]

Vitamin E is important for immune system function because it:

- Accumulates in cell membranes and protects them from free radical damage
- Makes cell membranes more stable (which has a beneficial effect on cell-to-cell communication)
- Inhibits the production of inflammatory prostaglandins
- Protects against environmental toxins

The cell-protecting effects of vitamin E extend to nuclear and mitochondrial membranes, nervous system cells (i.e., in the brain and spinal cord), and immune system cells (which are highly susceptible to the harmful effects of free radicals). The antioxidant properties of vitamin E are protective against heart disease and cancer—but bear in mind that these "silent" diseases take time to develop, so vitamin E should not be thought of as a "quick fix."

In one study, healthy volunteers were divided into two groups. One group received vitamin E supplements, while the other received a placebo. After several days, blood samples were taken. It was found that the LDL cholesterol in those who had been taking supplements seemed protected from being oxidized, with a rate of oxidation only half that of the placebo group. This is important, because oxidized LDL cholesterol is associated with atherosclerosis.[22]

Vitamin E is also believed to inhibit platelet aggregation—put more simply, it makes cells less sticky. This, too, has significant implications for good circulation and for cardiovascular health.

High levels of vitamin E are immune stimulating. Supplemental vitamin E enhances both humoral and cellular immunity and augments phagocyte efficiency. Vitamin E also works synergistically with selenium (see page 189) to enhance antibody response.

Vitamin E deficiency is associated with depressed T cell and B cell response. Low levels of antioxidants, including vitamin E, are consistently implicated in heart disease. Acute vitamin E deficiency causes neurodegeneration as well as impaired neutrophil and macrophage activity (which in turn allows tumor cells to grow faster).

Vitamin E deficiency is not uncommon. A population survey of older Americans revealed that over 40 percent of elderly men and women had intakes of vitamin E two thirds below the RDA[23] (and, as you know by now, the RDA of vitamin E is hardly the optimal amount for immune strength). This figure could help explain why aging is associated with a decline in immune response and an increase of disease.

Vitamin E is found primarily in vegetable oils, leafy green vegetables, egg yolks, whole grains, seeds, and nuts. However, it is not possible to obtain enough vitamin E from diet alone.

I usually recommend 400 to 800 IU of vitamin E per day. Read labels carefully, and be sure to choose d-alpha-tocopherol, or, even better, mixed natural tocopherols, including d-alpha with d-beta, d-delta, and especially d-gamma. D-alpha-tocopherol acetate is a derivative of natural vitamin E with a longer shelf life. D-alpha-tocopherol succinate, another derivative of natural vitamin E, is used in dry products and appears to penetrate cells more efficiently, where it can have beneficial effects on the cellular organelles, including mitochondria. This is important for people with defective mitochondrial function. (Characterized by chronic fatigue and muscle weakness, reduced mitochondrial activity may be more common than previously thought.)

I do not recommend the synthetic form, dl-alpha-tocopherol, which is 50 percent less active than the natural form. It's also less expensive, so buyer beware—a good deal on vitamin E might not be such a great deal after all.

If you are elderly or if you regularly take essential fatty acids such as borage oil or fish oil supplements, add another 400 IU per day. Too much vitamin E—over 1,200 IU per day—occasionally can cause high blood pressure and headaches, but in my experience this is uncommon. I have a number of patients taking up to 1,600 IU per day, and even occasionally 2,000 IU for specific illnesses (including Parkinson's, thrombophlebitis, and multiple sclerosis), who have shown no toxic effects at these doses.

MINERALS

Many minerals affect our bodily health and well-being, including:

Boron	Magnesium	Silicon
Calcium	Manganese	Sodium
Chromium	Molybdenum	Sulfur
Cobalt	Nickel	Tin
Copper	Phosphorus	Vanadium
Iodine	Potassium	Zinc
Iron	Selenium	

The minerals that are particularly important for immune system strength are copper, iron, magnesium, selenium, and zinc, so those are the ones I'll focus on here.

Copper

Copper is essential for immune function. Copper deficiency is associated with suppressed function of the reticuloendothelial system and enhances susceptibility to microorganisms such as *Salmonella*.[24] Copper deficiency also appears to impair the maturation of lymphocytes, and has been reported to inhibit T cell activity (resulting in more infections).

Copper and zinc together are mineral cofactors for one type of the essential antioxidant enzyme superoxide dismutase. (The other type of superoxide dismutase is dependent upon manganese.)

Copper and zinc (see page 190) are balanced in the body, so an excess of one can cause a relative deficiency in the other. One of my patients had read in various magazines that zinc is good for you, so every time he read this, he added more zinc to his daily regimen. Unfortunately, he never read anywhere that it's important to supplement with copper at the same time. By the time I saw him, he had increased his zinc supplementation to 250 milligrams a day, and he had induced a copper deficiency.

I recommend a 10:1 ratio of zinc to copper (for every 10 milligrams of zinc, take 1 milligram of copper). If you take 30 milligrams of zinc, include 3 milligrams of copper. We used to recommend a zinc/copper ratio of 14 or 15 to 1, but today there is greater appreciation of copper deficiency. This concern is in contrast to the work of Carl Pfeiffer, M.D., Ph.D., in the early 1980s, who led many to believe that copper excess was a very common occurrence. Note: People with copper pipes get additional copper in their drinking water (unless they're drinking bottled water), so they are less likely to be deficient. However, they may get too much copper, a situation that can be ascertained with testing.

Iron

Most of the iron in the body is located within red blood cells as a part of hemoglobin, the molecule that carries oxygen to all our cells. Many of us grew up listening to advertisements warning us about the effects of "iron-poor blood." It's well known that iron deficiency can cause anemia, which in turn causes listlessness and fatigue.

Iron is also necessary for cell proliferation (it is needed during DNA synthesis), and it is a cofactor for the activity of many enzymes. Iron deficiency is immune suppressing: it impairs the activity of phagocytes, causes lymphocyte depletion, causes decreased antibody production, depresses T cell and B cell function, and inhibits cytokine production. This all adds up to increased susceptibility to infection. In fact, response to tetanus toxoid and herpes simplex antigens is low in iron-deficient people, and supplemental iron results in a significant improvement in the response.[25]

Low iron levels have also been linked to impaired learning, perhaps because of a relationship between reduced body iron and reduced levels of certain chemical messengers in the brain. Iron is also a mineral cofactor for the antioxidant enzyme catalase.

Don't reach for the iron pills yet, however. Too much iron is also immune suppressing. It impairs the proliferation of cytotoxic T cells and helper T cells and enhances suppressor T cell activity. Iron also can stimulate the production of free radicals, thereby amplifying free radical damage. In addition, excess iron is used by bacteria and yeast for replication and can contribute to the virulence of an infection. Long-term, excess iron is associated with heart disease and cancer.

Iron is found in meat, kelp, blackstrap molasses, raisins, and dark, leafy greens. Many processed foods are iron-fortified. Because iron is a two-edged sword, I do not recommend iron supplements unless a patient has a documented iron deficiency. Most multivitamins include iron, but ironically the majority of people don't need it. Those least likely to need supplemental iron in general are men and postmenopausal women. Those most likely to need added iron are menstruating or pregnant women, undernourished children, and some elderly (due to malnutrition). Any major loss of blood—for example, due to surgery or injury—also raises the body's need for iron. When a patient needs iron, I usually recommend 18 milligrams a day. In our offices, we carry several multivitamin/mineral combinations that include iron.

Magnesium

The importance of magnesium is often overlooked, but this mineral plays an important role in many biochemical functions. Magnesium helps with muscle function (including the heart), with neurologic function (including the brain), and with the metabolism of fats. Magnesium reduces heart arrhythmias, is an important part of bone, and is a cofactor in over three hundred enzyme systems,[26] including reactions involving energy, protein, and nucleic acid metabolism.

Serum levels of magnesium are not as important as its concentration in tissues. Only 1 percent of total body magnesium circulates in the blood, while the rest is inside cells, mostly bones and muscles. However, the body will do whatever it can to keep the circulating level of magnesium within a strict range, including pull magnesium from the tissues, so it's possible to have normal serum levels of magnesium but still be deficient intracellularly. (The blood test can still be valuable for determining low serum magnesium. Different labs have different cutoff points, so what is "normal" for one could be "low" for another.)

Magnesium helps elevate immune activity. It is crucial for lymphocyte growth and transformation. Magnesium deficiency is associated with lowered levels of immunoglobulins and a reduced number of antibody-forming cells. Magnesium deficiency also favors free radical production and lipid peroxidation.

Magnesium deficiency, which is common, can cause a wide variety of puzzling symptoms, from muscle cramps to light sensitivity to constipation to premenstrual syndrome. Sid Baker, M.D., who lectures frequently on the subject of magnesium deficiency, believes there may be a connection between our current magnesium deficiency epidemic and the increase in the presence of agoraphobia. Patients who suffer from anxiety, insomnia, and emotional distress do not have a "Xanax deficiency," notes Dr. Baker, nor do they need to be treated with "Valium and condescension." They may have a genuine (and reversible) magnesium deficiency.

Low levels of magnesium can be caused by diuretics and by the overconsumption of caffeine, alcohol, or sugar. Diabetics are often magnesium deficient. Also at risk for magnesium deficiency are the acutely or chronically ill.

Good natural sources of magnesium include kelp, wheat bran, wheat germ, almonds, cashews, blackstrap molasses, buckwheat, Brazil nuts, peanuts, millet, and tofu. I recommend taking at least 500 milligrams of magnesium per day. I often recommend higher doses—up to 1,200 or even 1,500 milligrams a day—for specific conditions, such as muscle spasms, fibromyalgia pain, premenstrual syndrome, cardiac arrhythmias, and chronic fatigue immune dysfunction syndrome.

It's generally a good idea to take as much magnesium as you do calcium, or even more magnesium than calcium. Many multivitamins have more calcium than magnesium—twice as much or more. Find a multivitamin that has the correct ratio—500 milligrams of each—or take a supplement to even out the doses.

Selenium

Selenium is an antioxidant that protects our cells from the free radicals that are generated during phagocytosis and other cell-killing processes. Selenium is also a precursor of the extremely important antioxidant enzyme glutathione peroxidase. Working in tandem with vitamin E and beta-carotene, selenium protects cell membranes from lipid peroxidation.

Selenium deficiency is immune suppressing. Low levels of selenium have been shown to impair antibody responses and reduce lymphocyte proliferation.

Even a moderate increase in selenium can be immune enhancing, for selenium increases the killing capacity of phagocytes. High levels of selenium are associated with a reduced risk of cancer and heart disease. However, selenium does have the potential for toxicity. Signs of selenium toxicity include hair loss, dizziness, fatigue, and dermatitis.

Good natural sources of selenium include wheat germ, Brazil nuts, barley, shellfish, and oats. Keep in mind, however, that selenium-poor soil cannot yield selenium-rich foods. I generally recommend 200 micrograms of selenium per day. The formulas we make up for our offices include organic selenium bound from kelp and sodium selenite. We avoid yeast-based selenium because so many of our patients are sensitive to yeast.

I sometimes recommend higher doses of selenium (up to 400 or 500 micrograms a day) for certain patients—for example, those with chemical sensitivities, cancer, heavy metal toxicity, or heart disease—but I monitor their blood levels of selenium to maintain it within a normal range.

Zinc

Zinc stabilizes cell membranes and is necessary for DNA synthesis, cell division, protein metabolism, and carbohydrate digestion. According to a 1995 overview of zinc in *Nutrition*, zinc acts as a mineral cofactor in approximately three hundred enzyme systems.[27] In addition to being a cofactor for other enzymes, zinc is a cofactor (with copper) for the antioxidant enzyme superoxide dismutase. Because of its role in cell growth, zinc is important in everything from normal development to wound healing to lymphocyte production.

The effects of zinc deficiency are well documented and include stunted growth, skin changes, and delayed wound healing. Zinc deficiency can compromise the immune system on many fronts. It can cause thymic atrophy (which can cause a reduction in the number of mature T cells), decrease NK cell activity (which is important for tumor surveillance), and promote the secretion of immune-suppressing corticosteroids. No wonder zinc deficiency is associated with increased susceptibility to infection!

Zinc is a potent immunostimulant, and its role in immune function has been studied widely. High levels of zinc are associated with increased circulating lymphocytes and increased antibody production.

However, with zinc, more is not necessarily better. Excessively high levels of zinc—over 300 milligrams per day—are immune suppressing and have been shown to depress neutrophil and macrophage motility and to depress phagocytosis.

Zinc is not stored in the body, and zinc levels can be depleted by increased excretion (due to diuretics, alcohol, and/or stress), by the presence of heavy metals, and by an excess of copper (which can act as a zinc antagonist). Many Americans have low zinc intake. People who may need extra zinc include the elderly, the chronically ill, strict vegetarians, pregnant or nursing women, and anyone who has sustained tissue damage. Happily, adding zinc to a zinc-deficient diet can restore normal immune function in as little as two weeks.[28]

The highest natural source of zinc is oysters. Other top sources include lamb, pecans, dried split peas, Brazil nuts, beef liver, and egg yolks. For general use, I recommend 20 to 30 milligrams of zinc per day, along with 2 to 3 milligrams of copper. Occasionally I recommend higher doses of zinc, up to 100 milligrams, along with enough copper to maintain a zinc/copper ratio of 14 or 15 to 1.

Zinc sulfate is a common form of zinc, but it is my least favorite because it is less well absorbed than other forms. Zinc picolinate is believed to be the optimal form for absorption, although zinc gluconate and chelated zinc are also okay.

Lozenges containing zinc gluconate appear to be a promising treatment for the common cold, although researchers have not yet determined if their success is due to underlying zinc insufficiency in susceptible people or to some direct effect zinc has on rhinoviruses.

OTHER IMMUNE SYSTEM BOOSTERS

In addition to vitamins and minerals, there are other supplements you can take to maximize your immune function.

Alkylglycerols

The oil from the liver of the ratfish is an ancient remedy among fishermen along the west coasts of Norway and Sweden.[29] In 1992, some substances were discovered in this oil that may account for its healthful effects. Called *alkylglycerols,* these substances—which are also found in the liver oil of the Greenland shark, among other places (including mother's milk and bone marrow)—can now be synthesized artificially and are being studied as possibly playing a role in the treatment of solid cancers. Natural alkylglycerols have been shown to elevate the production of all types of white blood cells, which makes them a general immune stimulant.

I prescribe alkylglycerols to my cancer patients, especially those undergoing chemotherapy and radiation, to counteract the decreased white blood cell and platelet counts that are frequently associated with these treatments. I use doses of alkylglycerols in the form of natural shark liver oil from 300 milligrams per day to as high as 1,200 milligrams per day.

Amino Acids

As we saw in Chapter 5, amino acids—the building blocks of protein—are essential for cell growth and repair throughout the body. I would prefer to have you get your amino acids from eating high-quality protein, but in certain circumstances it may be beneficial to take individual amino acid supplements, some of which have immune-boosting effects. I usually recommend amino acid supplements in combination, generally to treat patients with malnutrition, chronic viral infections, metabolic imbalances (such as hypoglycemia), and heart disease. The appropriate dose depends upon the health of the individual and the condition that is being treated.

Arginine

Arginine is important for cell growth and wound healing and becomes essential during periods of growth, illness, or stress. It strengthens the immune system and helps protect against tumors by enhancing natural killer cell activity, by causing the production of increased numbers of lymphocytes, and by stimulating lymphocyte responses. In postoperative surgical patients, arginine enhanced T cell responses and contributed to resistance against infection. Supplementary arginine is associated with reduced hospital stays after major operations. Arginine also can enhance growth hormone secretion and is sometimes regarded as a "muscle builder," but in the present context I prefer to focus on its immune-stimulating effects.

Arginine is a precursor of nitric oxide, which in turn helps open up arteries because it is an arterial wall muscle relaxant. Supplementary arginine can be helpful for people with hypertension and coronary artery disease. It also may help people with asthma by relaxing the muscles of the bronchial airways.

I recommend arginine for severe burns, major surgery, major trauma (such as injuries due to a car accident), high blood pressure, angina, and coronary artery disease. I also use arginine as part of a protocol (along with enzyme-potentiated desensitization) for chronic-fatigue immune-dysfunction syndrome. The usual range for arginine supplementation is 1 to 3 grams per day, and occasionally 6 grams per day. Studies with severely ill, hospitalized patients have used much higher doses.

Very high levels of arginine can activate the growth of certain viruses. Arginine acts as an antagonist for lysine, another amino acid that tends to keep the herpes simplex virus in check. This is another illustration of the concept of balance in nutrient intake.

Carnitine

Carnitine is sometimes referred to as the body's "fat carburetor" because it is necessary for the metabolism of fat in the cells. Carnitine enables fatty acids to pass through the mitochondrial membranes so they can be burned for energy. By enhancing the body's use of fat, carnitine stimulates the metabolism of fatty acids, lowers the amount of fat circulating in the blood (which may be protective against arteriosclerosis), and reduces the body's dependence on glucose for fuel (which can improve energy and stamina in athletes). Carnitine also may make it easier for some people to lose weight.

Carnitine can be transformed by the body into acetyl L-carnitine (ALC), which has received attention because of its ability to boost mitochondrial activity, defend against lipid peroxidation, and protect against neurodegeneration. In one study, patients with probable Alzheimer's were given 2.5 grams per day for three months, then 3 grams per day for another three months. After six months, the ALC-supplemented group demonstrated significantly less deterioration than the nonsupplemented group.[30]

Carnitine is not an essential amino acid because the body is capable of synthesizing it from other amino acids, but sometimes production is slow (especially when we are sick). I recommend carnitine (either carnitine or ALC) for elevated triglycerides, cardiomyopathy, myocardial ischemia, and for some patients with chronic fatigue, usually in doses up to 1,500 or 2,000 milligrams per day. Recently I have also started to use higher doses, especially of ALC, for some neurological and neurodegenerative disorders, including Alzheimer's disease.

Cysteine

Cysteine enters into various detoxification pathways, so it is helpful in neutralizing and excreting toxins and heavy metals that otherwise might accumulate and poison the immune system. It is able to do this because of its sulfur-containing thiol group. (*Thiol* indicates the presence of a sulfur and a hydrogen atom bound together.) Ever since the Greeks used garlic, elemental sulfur has been used in remedies for many kinds of disorders.[31]

Cysteine helps the liver metabolize alcohol, acetaminophen, and carbon tetrachloride, and it protects us against free radicals, mutagens, and carcinogens. In addition, cysteine boosts the synthesis of glutathione.

Lab experiments have demonstrated that cysteine supply strongly influences the proliferation of lymphocytes and the activation of cytotoxic T cells. Cysteine's antioxidant effects protect cells of the immune system from self-inflicted damage when they release free radicals while fighting infectious organisms.

Cysteine is related to, but should not be confused with, homocysteine, the by-product of protein metabolism mentioned earlier that is a risk factor for heart disease. Also, oxidized cysteine can form cystine, an amino acid with a different chemical structure than cysteine.

I recommend 200 to 500 milligrams of N-acetylcysteine (NAC) per day, as this cysteine derivative is more effective. For certain disorders, such as chronic obstructive pulmonary disease and elevated lipoprotein A [Lp(a)], I employ 1,500 to 4,000 milligrams per day. It's important to take zinc and copper along with cysteine supplements because cysteine leaches these metals from the body. Also, take vitamin C to help prevent the oxidation of cysteine into cystine.

Glutamine

Glutamine has been called the "essential nonessential" amino acid due to its important roles. The body puts glutamine to work in many ways. Glutamine helps build muscle and hastens wound healing, and it also can be used by the brain as an alternative fuel when glucose levels are low. Glutamine also can be converted by the body into glutathione (see page 200).

Glutamine is important for any rapidly dividing cells, including gastrointestinal mucosal cells and immune cells. It is specifically helpful for immune function because it is necessary for lymphocyte proliferation. In addition, lymphocytes and macrophages burn glutamine for energy. Most important, glutamine is the favorite fuel of the cells that line the digestive tract (especially the upper GI tract), so it contributes greatly to the immunologic integrity of the gut by enhancing the levels of secretory IgA. Glutamine can be helpful in correcting gastrointestinal disorders (specifically gastritis and duodenitis), "leaky gut" syndrome, the gastrointestinal effects of alcoholism, and food allergies, just as lack of sufficient glutamine can contribute to these problems.

I generally recommend glutamine for patients with the gastrointestinal disorders mentioned above, those who are losing muscle mass due to weight loss from illness, and those who need immune boosting. Doses can range from 500 milligrams to 12 grams per day. Glutamine has been used in clinical trials at doses as high as 40 grams per day for patients undergoing bone marrow transplants and for patients who are HIV-positive.[32]

Taurine

Taurine can be made in the body from cysteine, but we don't always make an optimal amount. Phagocytic cells carry a high amount of taurine to protect them from one of their own cytotoxic substances (hypochlorous acid, which happens to resemble bleach). This is the antioxidant function of taurine. The liver uses taurine to convert fat-soluble compounds into water-soluble complexes that the body can excrete. Taurine also plays a role in balancing sodium and potassium in the heart muscle (and other cells), so it is sometimes taken to help with heart rhythm problems and heart muscle problems such as congestive heart failure and cardiomyopathy. Taurine has recently been added to infant formula due to its importance in maintaining health.

I generally recommend up to 1,500 milligrams of taurine per day, and occasionally employ up to 2,000 milligrams per day in more serious circumstances (such as cardiomyopathy).

Bioflavonoids

Bioflavonoids are naturally occurring phytochemicals (plant chemicals). They are basically pigments that act as antioxidants. Unlike other antioxidants, some bioflavonoids can be both water- and fat-soluble. The human body cannot produce bioflavonoids, so they must be supplied in our diet.

In addition to their antioxidant role, bioflavonoids also can be potent anti-inflammatory, anti-allergic, anticancer, and antiviral agents. In addition, bioflavonoids strengthen the blood vessels and support the actions of vitamin C. Ten years ago, bioflavonoids were relatively obscure and few people recognized their importance. Today we know that they are extremely important in many biological pathways and processes.

Many bioflavonoids are available in the form of supplements, although nature packages many more in fruits and vegetables. For example, the white stuff inside citrus peel is loaded with bioflavonoids.

For everyday use, I recommend up to 1,500 milligrams of mixed bioflavonoids per day. For patients with certain types of cancer or with allergic, inflammatory, or autoimmune disorders, I sometimes recommend doses that are somewhat higher, and/or I'll recommend a higher dose of a particular bioflavonoid.

Genistein (see page 140) is a bioflavonoid found in soy products that is associated with lowered cancer risk. It also has purported cardiovascular benefits and can be helpful in decreasing the symptoms of menopause, fibroids, and fibrocystic breast disease. Eating soy is healthy, and it's also possible to take isolated soy isoflavones in supplement form. Treatment doses of soy isoflavones can be from 100 to 300 milligrams a day. Usually I recommend them because of their phytoestrogen effects for menopausal patients or for patients with certain types of cancer (including breast and prostate cancer).

Proanthocyanidins, found in grape seeds and in other plants, are potent antioxidant bioflavonoids. Although they are water-soluble, they can stay in the body for a few days (longer than other water-soluble antioxidants). Proanthocyanidins were formerly called *pycnogenols,* but they now have more specific names. Proanthocyanidins that are bound together are collectively known as *proanthocyanidin oligomers,* or *PCO.* PCO can be incorporated into cell membranes and also protects against both fat-soluble and water-soluble free radicals, making it a more potent antioxidant than vitamin C or E. Research also indicates that proanthocyanidins enhance NK cell cytotoxicity.[33] In addition, they can have anti-inflammatory and anti-allergic effects. I generally recommend 50 to 150 milligrams of proanthocyanidins per day. In certain situations I use doses of up to 300 milligrams per day.

Quercetin helps to stabilize the membranes of mast cells, preventing the release of histamine, which can cut down on allergic symptoms. Quercetin also has antiviral, antitumor, and antioxidant effects. Based on clinical results I'm seeing, I recommend quercetin for allergic and autoimmune disorders such as asthma, inflammatory bowel disease, and arthritis. Usually I recommend a dose of 900 milligrams a day, although for some patients I will use up to 2,400 milligrams per day.

Ginkgo biloba, long used in Chinese medicine, has been shown to dramatically improve circulation to the extremities and the brain, thereby improving memory, enhancing concentration, and even relieving depression. Ginkgo relaxes the smooth muscles in arteries and also inhibits platelet aggregation (cell stickiness). These effects help explain why ginkgo supplementation diminishes the risk of stroke and heart attack. Ginkgo extract actually contains a variety of bioflavonoids that act as antioxidants and free radical scavengers. For memory loss, problems with peripheral vascular circulation, or cerebrovascular circulatory problems I generally recommend 120 to 240 milligrams of ginkgo biloba a day (one or two capsules, 40 milligrams each, three times a day).

Bovine and Shark Cartilage

Cartilage is tough, elastic tissue found in most animals and humans. One of its interesting characteristics is that it does not have a blood supply because it contains a substance that inhibits the development of blood vessels (a natural process called *angiogenesis*). It has been theorized that this antiangiogenic substance may interfere with the blood supply of tumors, but this effect is currently the subject of some debate.

John F. Prudden, M.D., discovered in the 1950s that bovine cartilage promotes wound healing as well as tumor shrinkage. Over the forty years since then, bovine cartilage has been shown to be effective with multiple types of cancer as well as with inflammatory autoimmune disorders (including arthritis, ulcerative colitis, and scleroderma) and immunological skin disorders (such as psoriasis).

The use of bovine cartilage for both cancer and autoimmune problems may seem paradoxical, for as we've seen, cancer is due to an underactive immune system, and autoimmune disorders are associated with an overactive immune system. However, bovine cartilage appears to act as an *adaptogen.* Adaptogens are substances that work in accordance with each individual's needs to preserve a healthy steady state and to normalize immune function. Adaptogens are not so much *anti* anything as they are immunorestorative.

Many of the biological response modifiers being researched and tested today (including the interferons, interleukins, and tumor necrosis factor) can actually disrupt the critical balance of the immune system because of the large doses that are required and the way these substances artificially promote one kind of immune response at the expense of another. Bovine cartilage, on the other hand, can stimulate the immune system to resist cancer and viruses as well as downregulate the immune system in the presence of rheumatic diseases.

Interestingly, bovine cartilage resembles a type of undifferentiated fetal tissue called *fetal mesenchyme* from which muscles, bones, tendons, ligaments, and bone marrow develop.

This resemblance suggests that bovine cartilage may contain powerful molecular "bio-directors" that could account for its normalizing effects.

Bovine cartilage contains mucopolysaccharides (complex sugar molecules not unlike the immune-enhancing polysaccharides discussed on page 201), which are believed to block the cell division of tumor cells. They are also thought to activate macrophages, cytotoxic T cells, and B cells. Usually, but not invariably, an increase in NK cells has also been noted. Dr. Prudden is currently preparing a paper on his research regarding 120 cancer patients treated with bovine cartilage.[34] I do not give bovine cartilage to all my patients by any means, but to those for whom I think it would be helpful, I generally recommend a treatment dose of up to 9 grams per day (3 grams three times a day).

Probably more people have heard of shark cartilage than bovine cartilage because of all the media attention it has received. The main mechanism proposed for shark cartilage is its antiangiogenic properties, but there is some question whether the large protein molecules responsible for this effect actually can survive digestion when shark cartilage is taken orally. Disadvantages of shark cartilage include the dosages (you need to take large quantities), the strong fishy odor and taste, and the expense. Because of these drawbacks, people sometimes take shark cartilage at suboptimal amounts that are of questionable effectiveness. Also, in high therapeutic doses, shark cartilage delivers a huge calcium burden to the body, far in excess of the U.S. RDA. However, despite all of the above, I have patients who prefer shark cartilage. I usually use shark cartilage in doses of up to 1 gram per kilogram of body weight (which is basically ½ gram per pound of body weight).

I generally recommend higher doses of cartilage when treating cancer. For arthritic conditions, lower doses of either kind of cartilage can be employed.

CoQ10 (Ubiquinone)

CoQ10 is a coenzyme, meaning it is a substance that is necessary for the proper functioning of certain enzymes. It is present in every cell (its ubiquitous nature contributed to its name) and plays an essential part in the energy production of each cell. CoQ10 is critical to the optimal functioning of all cell types, and all metabolically active tissues are highly sensitive to any deficiency of CoQ10.

The body absorbs CoQ10 from food, yet dietary deficiency of CoQ10 is common. We also can manufacture CoQ10 in the liver, but the seventeen-step process involved is complex and requires many cofactors, so we can't always make enough to meet our needs, especially when we need extra CoQ10 for healing.

CoQ10 is an immune stimulant. High levels of CoQ10 enhance the ability of immune cells to kill bacteria and also elevate antibody response. Several studies have demonstrated the immune-enhancing effects of CoQ10. It has been shown to increase the phagocytic activity of macrophages, increase proliferation of granulocytes, and increase the survival rates of infected lab animals. In a study of chronically ill patients, a dose of 60 milligrams per day of CoQ10 was associated with significant increases in serum IgG levels.[35] However, you don't have to be chronically ill to benefit from CoQ10 supplementation.

CoQ10 has a beneficial effect on T cells and anticancer properties as well. In one study involving high-risk breast cancer patients whose cancer had spread to axillary lymph nodes, CoQ10 was associated with tumor regression. The thirty-two subjects were put on a regimen that included antioxidants (beta-carotene plus vitamins C and E), essential fatty acids, and 90 milligrams of CoQ10 per day. None of the patients died during the 18-month treatment period, and none showed signs of further metastases. Six patients had an apparent partial remission. In one of these six cases, the dosage of CoQ10 was increased to 390 milligrams per day, and the tumor vanished in two months.[36] Additional anecdotal evidence also supports the use of CoQ10 in cancer treatment.

During a viral infection, the CoQ10 levels in white blood cells plummet. Blood levels of CoQ10 diminish with age, which may help explain the decrease in immune response we see with aging. In the United States, as many as 75 percent of people over fifty years old may be deficient in CoQ10.[37]

CoQ10 is essential in converting food into energy. It acts as a catalyst in the production of ATP, the stored energy within each cell. Insufficient CoQ10 means less ATP is produced, and low ATP stores translate into insufficient energy to keep body processes running efficiently. Cells that have a high demand for energy—including the cells of the heart, muscles, and immune system—have a greater need for CoQ10. Therefore, it is not surprising that CoQ10 deficiency is associated with heart problems, muscle weakness, lethargy, and impaired immunity. Research has shown that Parkinson's disease is associated with a deficiency of certain enzymes that depend upon CoQ10, and studies are currently under way to see if CoQ10 can help reverse degenerative brain diseases.

In addition to its other vital roles, CoQ10 is a very effective fat-soluble antioxidant. It protects cell membranes and is effective in preventing the oxidation of LDL cholesterol, which in turn helps prevent heart disease. CoQ10 also contributes to cardiovascular health by reducing blood viscosity, which allows blood to flow more easily through the arteries and veins, eases the burden on the heart, and reduces the likelihood of clot formation.

CoQ10 is naturally present in small amounts in a wide variety of foods. Organ meats (heart, liver, kidney) are high in CoQ10, as are beef, sardines, and mackerel. However, you'd have to eat a pound of sardines to get 30 milligrams of CoQ10! I generally recommend supplementing with 50 to 150 milligrams of CoQ10 per day, preferably divided into three doses throughout the day. In patients with cardiomyopathy or advanced cancer, I will frequently use much higher doses in the range of 300 to 400 milligrams per day, and have even increased this amount to 600 milligrams per day in a few of my most seriously ill patients. Because CoQ10 is fat-soluble, absorption is improved when it is taken with a fat-containing food.

COMMONLY ASKED QUESTION NO. 12:

If CoQ10 is so effective, why isn't it more generally recommended?

CoQ10 has been extensively studied and used, especially in Japan. I've been recommending it for years, and lately have been using higher doses. Recently the benefits of CoQ10 have started to penetrate the cardiology literature, and cardiologists are starting to trumpet their "new" discovery.

Traditional medicine is focused on treatment more than prevention, so the idea of taking CoQ10 preventatively is outside the paradigm of most physicians. Also, CoQ10 is not patentable, so the pharmaceutical companies, lacking a big profit incentive, are not interested in producing it. In addition, the current distributors of CoQ10 are not in the business of physician education, as the drug companies are. This kind of education is very costly and is undertaken only when there is some assurance of a hefty profit from a patent-protected product.

Traditional doctors would argue that not enough studies have been done to prove the efficacy of CoQ10, and that its long-term effects are not known. In fact, CoQ10 was first identified in 1957, and there have been eight international symposia on CoQ10 since 1976. How many studies, over how many years, are "enough"? Many prescription drugs have been put into circulation with less scrutiny than CoQ10 has received.

Garlic

Garlic is a wonder food! Don't underestimate the healthful effects of this common little bulb. There's nothing New Age about garlic, which has been used for medicinal purposes for centuries. Garlic is rich in antioxidants, vitamins, and minerals. Close cousins of garlic include onions, chives, and scallions.

An immune system stimulant, garlic increases the activity of natural killer cells, which in turn helps check the spread of cancer. In fact, high garlic intake is associated with a lowered risk of stomach cancer. Garlic is also a potent natural antimicrobial substance, known to inhibit the growth of infectious microorganisms such as bacteria, viruses, fungi, and parasites. For this reason, garlic can be helpful in cases in which an organism has become resistant to conventional antibiotic therapy.[38] Some folk remedies call for applying garlic directly to the skin, but I can't recommend this technique because there are documented cases of chemical burns caused by crushed fresh garlic (not to mention the smell).

Garlic also helps boost the immune system by detoxifying carcinogens, and its antioxidant effects help protect the liver and brain cells from free radical damage. In addition, garlic protects against cardiovascular disease and the formation of blood clots by decreasing platelet aggregation, lowering LDL cholesterol (and raising HDL cholesterol), and lowering blood pressure.

Cooking garlic will inactivate its antimicrobial effects, so to get the full range of garlic's benefits, either use more fresh garlic in your meals or use tablets or capsules prepared from fresh garlic. The odorless variety won't give you garlic breath. I frequently recommend two garlic capsules per day, 350 to 500 milligrams each, in divided doses. For the conditions mentioned above, I recommend six, and sometimes up to nine, capsules per day in divided doses.

Glutathione

A water-soluble tripeptide antioxidant, glutathione consists of glycine, cysteine, and glutamic acid. It is an essential component of the important antioxidant enzymes glutathione peroxidase and glutathione reductase. Glutathione combats free radicals and the by-products of lipid peroxidation, improves immune function, stabilizes red blood cells, and helps protect the body from external toxins. The liver has high levels of glutathione, which it uses to detoxify estrogen hormones, toxins, and certain medications such as acetaminophen by making them water-soluble and easier to excrete. Low glutathione levels stress the liver and can contribute to liver damage.

Phagocytes and lymphocytes both need glutathione. Phagocytes carry high levels of glutathione, which they use to protect themselves from the free radicals they use to kill infectious microorganisms. Because glutathione protects phagocytes, there is a direct link between this nutrient and our immunocompetence.

Intracellular glutathione is depleted when cells are exposed to oxidative stress. In fact, the glutathione status of a cell is indicative of the cell's general state of health, for glutathione depletion is followed by functional and structural breakdown.[39]

Studies have shown that high glutathione levels correspond with good health, and low glutathione levels are associated with chronic conditions such as heart disease, arthritis, and diabetes. Insufficient amounts of the amino acids that the body uses to make glutathione—including cysteine—can contribute to low glutathione levels.

I usually recommend 50 to 150 milligrams of glutathione per day. I use the higher doses to help alleviate chemical sensitivities and liver detoxification problems. Depending upon the severity of the situation, I may recommend even higher doses, in the range of 225 to 300 milligrams per day.

Immune-Enhancing Polysaccharides

Polysaccharides are just complex groups of sugars. Different polysaccharides can have different effects, and many of the actions of Chinese herbs (see Chapter 7) have been traced to particular types of polysaccharides. I use various types of commercially prepared concentrated polysaccharides for their immune-enhancing effects.

Arabinogalactan, a long, densely branched polysaccharide, is present in different plants, including echinacea and the larch tree. Most commercial arabinogalactan is produced from Western larch. Arabinogalactan enhances NK cell activity by influencing cytokine production. It also has anti-inflammatory effects and antiviral properties, and helps prevent cancer from metastasizing (that is, establishing itself in a new site), especially to the liver.[40] A maintenance dose of arabinogalactan is 1 teaspoon per day. For a mild viral illness, I generally recommend 1 to 3 teaspoons per day. When metastatic cancer is possible or present, the dose can go as high as 10 to 14 teaspoons a day.

Echinacea was the most widely used medicinal plant of the Native Americans in the Great Plains region, so it has been in use for hundreds of years. As mentioned above, echinacea contains arabinogalactan. It increases the number of white blood cells, enhances the activity of phagocytes, and enhances the production of interferons. It is used for a wide variety of disorders, but especially for mild viral infections. Echinacea is available in capsules or tinctures and in varying strengths, so the dosage varies with the preparation. I generally use several hundred milligrams (approximately 20 drops of tincture) three to four times a day for seven to ten days for viral infections.

Lectins are proteins commonly found in highly nutritious foods. They have several effects based on their interaction with membrane substances, including sugar proteins (*glycoproteins*) and sugar lipids (*glycolipids*). One of these effects is to help prevent cancer from metastasizing to the liver. The reticuloendothelial system of the liver contains lectins, which bind to galactose residues on the surface of cancer cells. Unfortunately, this may allow the cancer cell to take up residence in the liver, which of course creates a problem. On the other hand, when circulating lectins bind with cancer cells, they create a complex that is not only less likely to metastasize but also more likely to be recognized by the immune system and subsequently dealt with appropriately.

Modified citrus pectin is a soluble component of plant fiber derived from citrus fruit. Modified citrus pectin does not affect primary tumor growth, but it has been shown to help prevent cancer metastases in animal studies and in studies of human cancer cells. Modified citrus pectin works by interfering with the adhesion of cancer cells to endothelial cells. For cancer to metastasize, it first needs to adhere to a new location. Modified citrus pectin binds with the surface of human prostate cancer cells, breast cancer cells, and melanoma cells so they are less "sticky" and less likely to implant themselves elsewhere.[41] I generally recommend 1 teaspoon of modified citrus pectin three times a day (up to a total of 3 teaspoons per day) for my patients with metastatic cancer. Some patients who have cancer that has not yet metastasized, or who have been "successfully" treated for cancer, choose to take modified citrus pectin as well.

Maitake mushroom—sometimes called "the king of mushrooms"—has been known for its beneficial health effects in Japan for centuries. Recent research indicates that it is the most potent immunostimulant of all mushrooms. The active ingredient of maitake mushroom is a beta 1,6 glucan polysaccharide known as maitake D-fraction, which is currently being studied for its antitumor effects. Maitake mushroom activates macrophages, NK cells, and helper and cytotoxic T cells. It also enhances cytokine production, including IL-1 and IL-2. In addition to its immune-stimulating effects, maitake appears to lower blood pressure and serum glucose levels as well.

Lipoic Acid

When it was first discovered, lipoic acid (also called thioctic acid) was thought to be a vitamin because it is absorbed from the diet. We now know that it can be produced by the body, and it can be made synthetically as well. Researchers have been aware of lipoic acid for years, but new information about its different roles continues to emerge.

Lipoic acid quenches free radicals and is therefore helpful with all of the problems associated with oxidative stress, including LDL oxidation, cataracts, apoptosis (programmed cell death), diabetes, and neurodegenerative diseases. One study showed that lipoic acid helped to reverse the effects of constant low-level radiation exposure in children living in areas affected by the Chernobyl nuclear reactor accident.[42] It also appears to be somewhat protective against cigarette smoke. Because it functions as both a fat-soluble and water-soluble antioxidant, lipoic acid has both intracellular and intercellular effects.

The reduced form of lipoic acid is called dihydrolipoic acid (DHLA). Lipoic acid is rapidly converted to DHLA in many tissues, which accounts for its initial effects. However, DHLA has its own roles, both as an antioxidant and as a reducing agent. Supplementation with lipoic acid actually involves the effects of both lipoic acid and DHLA.

DHLA acts synergistically with other antioxidants and thereby increases their effectiveness. It regenerates vitamin C and (indirectly) vitamin E from their inactive forms in a process known as "antioxidant recycling." In animal studies, lipoic acid supplementation has been shown to be protective against the symptoms of vitamin C deficiency and vitamin E deficiency. In addition, DHLA causes an increase of intracellular glutathione, which—as you just read—is essential to proper cellular functioning. Because there is always some question regarding the absorption and utilization of oral glutathione, lipoic acid could play an important role in maintaining optimal glutathione levels in the body.

Both lipoic acid and DHLA have metal-chelating activity. They bind to the transition metals, iron and copper, which in turn has antioxidant effects, and they are of clinical value in the treatment of mercury and cadmium poisoning.

In addition to all these effects, lipoic acid has an absolutely vital role in metabolism. It is a necessary cofactor in mitochondrial activity, and in fact the Germans consider it a rate-limiting factor for oxidative metabolism. (For more on metabolic processes, see Chapter 11.)

Lipoic acid also appears to be protective of the liver. There is not universal agreement on this, but Burton Berkson, M.D., Ph.D., has had very notable success administering intravenous lipoic acid for mushroom poisoning, alcoholic liver degeneration, and primary biliary cirrhosis.[43] In cases of mushroom poisoning, the lipoic acid does not interfere with the toxin itself, but increases the metabolism of the healthy cells of the liver, which enhances regeneration. I use lipoic acid in numerous situations that tax the liver, including infections, use of certain medications, and exposure to toxins.

Because lipoic acid may affect the genes that are involved in normal growth and metabolism, it may play a role in the nutritional modulation of genetic expression. It also holds promise for the treatment of AIDS. In cultured cells, lipoic acid and DHLA prevented the replication of HIV (the virus that causes AIDS). In studies involving HIV-positive individuals, lipoic acid improved the antioxidant status, increased the number of helper T cells in six out of nine subjects, and improved the helper T cell/suppressor T cell ratio in six out of ten subjects.[44]

When all of these effects are considered together, it becomes clear that lipoic acid may be helpful for a wide variety of conditions, including liver problems, diabetes, heavy metal poisoning, radiation damage, AIDS, memory loss, and numerous degenerative conditions that may be related to mitochondrial dysfunction (see page 344). In Germany, high doses of lipoic acid are used to treat diabetic polyneuropathy. I generally recommend 100 to 300 milligrams of lipoic acid per day for its antioxidant effects, and up to 1,000 milligrams per day (in divided doses) for serious problems.

Melatonin

Melatonin, which has received a lot of attention lately, is a hormone naturally secreted by the pineal gland (located at the base of the brain) only during darkness. Whether or not you're sleeping is irrelevant, but the amount of light perceived by your eyes is critical. Melatonin secretion may also be affected by electromagnetic fields.

Melatonin is used to reset the body's "clock" (our circadian rhythms). It can be helpful in treating jet lag, sleep disorders (including insomnia), and seasonal affective disorder (SAD). Melatonin secretion diminishes with age, and melatonin supplementation is thought to slow aging, perhaps because of its antioxidant effects.

Most important for our purposes here, melatonin is believed to be immune enhancing.

By observing the effects of low melatonin levels, researchers have deduced that melatonin has potent anticancer properties. It appears to have a stimulating effect on natural killer cells, to enhance helper T cells, and to influence cytokine production.

I recommend 1 to 3 milligrams of melatonin at bedtime. For troublesome insomnia, you can try 6 to 9 milligrams at night. Too much melatonin will make you sleepy, and some experts worry (I share their concern) that we do not fully understand the effects of megadoses of this hormone, especially over the long term. I usually tell my patients to take a break from melatonin for at least a couple of nights every so often, as frequently as every month or every few weeks.

Tea

It is believed that tea drinking originated in China almost five thousand years ago. There are three basic kinds of tea. They all come from the same plant, but the tea leaves are harvested and handled differently. The leaves of black tea are allowed to ferment (oxidize), the leaves of oolong tea are partially fermented, and the leaves of green tea are not fermented. When brewed, these different types of tea contain different polyphenols, but all types may be healthful.

Green tea may help prevent cardiovascular disease. Tea contains catechin, which is a potent antioxidant that helps to prevent lipid peroxidation, supports the liver, and works synergistically with other antioxidants. Tea has anticancer, antiviral, and antibacterial effects in humans; it has a beneficial effect on cholesterol levels; and it inhibits platelet aggregation.

Some studies have determined healthful effects from drinking more than 10 cups of green tea a day. This is a habit most Westerners don't have, so I recommend 100 to 300 milligrams of high-quality, decaffeinated green tea extract instead.

SPECIAL CIRCUMSTANCES

Different supplements can be helpful in particular situations. If any of the following circumstances apply to you, you may have an increased need for certain nutrients. Refer to the earlier discussion of each nutrient to determine the upper levels of safe dosages. Also, please remember that supplements are helpful, but they aren't everything. Don't forget to round out your healthful regimen with the rest of the Immune System Empowerment Program!

- **Stress.** Stress causes increased excretion of numerous vitamins and minerals, so if you are under stress (physical and/or emotional), take higher doses of magnesium, zinc, and the B vitamins (especially B_6). Also, to counteract adrenal fatigue, take additional vitamin C, vitamin B_5, and adrenal glandulars (see page 298).
- **Family history of cancer.** You can't change your family history, but you can take

higher doses of antioxidants, including selenium, vitamin C, vitamin E, and mixed carotenoids. Make a point of taking a broad array of the more potent antioxidants, including those in the flavonoid family (such as proanthocyanidins and quercetin), glutathione, CoQ10, and lipoic acid. I also recommend maintenance doses (not treatment doses) of immune-enhancing polysaccharides, including arabinogalactan and maitake mushroom.

- **Chemotherapy and/or radiation.** If you are currently undergoing chemotherapy and/or radiation for cancer, follow the anticancer antioxidant regimen above. There are also beneficial preparations of Chinese herbs (see Chapter 7) that are immunosupportive. In addition, take bovine cartilage and higher doses of alkylglycerols mentioned on page 191. (These treatments help protect normal cells from the toxicity of chemotherapy and radiation, but—contrary to popular myth—they are not protective of the tumor.) I also recommend some of the more advanced intravenous treatments, such as intravenous vitamin C and intravenous hydrogen peroxide (see Chapters 10 and 11).

- **Toxins.** If you are exposed to toxins where you live or work, follow the anticancer antioxidant regimen above. Also make a point of taking higher doses of NAC (N-acetylcysteine; mentioned on page 193) and a commercial liver support formula that includes glutathione, lipoic acid, silymarin, and dandelion root. (Liver support is discussed in depth in Chapter 9.)

- **Premenstrual syndrome.** I've had a lot of success treating PMS with supplements, (see including higher doses of magnesium on page 188), vitamin B$_6$ (page 179), and the essential fatty acids (particularly gamma-linolenic acid, which can be found in borage oil or evening primrose oil—see page 157). Take these supplements every day, and raise the levels a little further for the last 10 to 14 days of your monthly cycle. You may also wish to add natural progesterone to your regimen (see page 313).

- **Ten things you can do for a cold (or other viral illness).** Take:
1. Echinacea for 7 to 10 days
2. Goldenseal (an herb with antimicrobial and immune-stimulating effects) for 7 to 10 days
3. Frequent doses of vitamin C (1 gram every one to two hours, or 2 to 3 grams three or four times a day, or to bowel tolerance) as long as symptoms persist
4. 50,000 to 100,000 IU of vitamin A every day for five days (but no longer, as vitamin A has the potential of accumulating to toxic levels)
5. Zinc lozenges for one to three days
6. Garlic capsules in high numbers—fifteen to thirty a day for five to seven days (after seven days, go back to maintenance levels)
7. A homeopathic preparation (see page 223) until symptoms resolve
8. Immune-enhancing polysaccharides for seven to ten days, such as maitake mushroom and/or 1 teaspoon of arabinogalactan three times a day
9. A combination Chinese herbal preparation with antiviral herbs (such as Isatis Gold)
10. A thymus glandular preparation for one to two weeks

SUMMARY: IMMUNE SYSTEM BOOSTERS

I recommend that everyone take a comprehensive, high-potency, hypoallergenic, well-balanced multivitamin/mineral supplement every day, preferably in divided doses over the course of the day. Following are optimal daily (maintenance) doses of the immune-supportive nutrients discussed in this chapter. Doses may be higher in special circumstances, such as chronic or acute illness (see text).

Vitamin A	10,000 IU
Beta-carotene	15,000 to 50,000 IU
B vitamins	
Vitamin B_1	50 to 100 mg
Vitamin B_2	25 to 50 mg
Vitamin B_3	100 to 200 mg
Vitamin B_5	150 to 500 mg
Vitamin B_6	25 to 100 mg
Vitamin B_{12}	100 mcg
Folic acid	800 mcg
Biotin	300 mcg
Choline	50 to 150 mg
Inositol	25 to 100 mg
PABA	50 mg
Vitamin C	3,000 mg
Vitamin D	50 to 100 IU
Vitamin E (mixed natural tocopherols)	400 to 800 IU
Calcium	500 mg (with 500 mg magnesium)
Copper	2 to 3 mg (with 20 to 30 mg zinc)
Iron	None, unless for child or menstruating woman, or documented iron deficiency is present (adult maintenance dose 18 mg/day)
Magnesium	500 mg (with 500 mg calcium)
Selenium	200 mcg
Zinc	20 to 30 mg (with 2 to 3 mg copper)

Bioflavonoids (mixed)	200 to 1,500 mg
CoQ10	50 to 150 mg
Garlic	2 capsules (350 to 500 mg each) in divided doses
Glutathione	50 to 150 mg
Lipoic acid	100 to 300 mg

Following are daily doses of optional Immune System Boosters that may be beneficial for your particular symptoms or health situation. For serious illness, optimal doses may be even higher (see text). While the doses below are generally safe, consult a nutritionally oriented physician before taking treatment doses of any nutrient. All of the following nutrients should be taken in divided doses (except for melatonin).

Alkylglycerols	300 to 1,200 mg
Amino acids	
Arginine	1 to 6 g
Carnitine or acetyl L-carnitine	Up to 2,000 mg
N-acetylcysteine (NAC)	200 to 2,000 mg
Glutamine	500 mg to 12 g
Taurine	Up to 1,500 mg
Bioflavonoids	
Soy isoflavones	100 to 300 mg
Proanthocyanidins	50 to 300 mg
Quercetin	900 to 2,400 mg
Ginkgo biloba	120 to 240 mg
Cartilage	
Bovine cartilage	Up to 9 g
Shark cartilage	Up to ½ g per pound of body weight
Immune-enhancing polysaccharides	
Arabinogalactan	1 to 3 teaspoons
Modified citrus pectin	Up to 3 teaspoons
Echinacea	1 to 2 capsules or 20 drops, three to four times per day (dose may vary depending on product strength)
Maitake D-fraction	20 to 200 mg
Melatonin	1 to 9 mg
Tea (green tea extract)	100 to 300 mg

ᏝᏝᎧ DAVID'S STORY

I recommend supplements for nearly all my patients, usually as part of a larger regimen that includes other treatments as well. This makes it difficult to point to a case history that centers on supplements alone. However, David's story would have had a very different outcome if he had not received vitamin intervention.

When I first met David, he was nearly expressionless. He was severely depressed and totally lacking in energy. Formerly an accomplished writer, David had been unable to write for about a year and a half. He was profoundly upset about this, which was part of the reason he had driven six hours to see me in hopes of finding a cure. David said that he suffered from insomnia, panic attacks, persistent fatigue, and chronic constipation. It was hard to tell what kind of person he was, or what his likes and dislikes might have been. He seemed almost absent.

David was thirty-nine years old and married. There were no psychological problems in his family, and he'd had no noteworthy emotional problems until two and a half years earlier, when he had developed pneumonia and had been treated first with tetracycline and then with erythromycin. From that point on, David had developed emotional problems, and over time his anxiety and depression had worsened.

About a year before seeing me, David had consulted a well-known clinical ecologist who diagnosed candidiasis and treated David with nystatin. This was helpful, but it was not enough to stop David's descent into severe depression.

David got his local doctor to prescribe Ativan (an antianxiety agent) for him, but he had an adverse reaction to it. Next the doctor prescribed BuSpar (another antianxiety agent), but David couldn't tolerate that, either. Eventually he was admitted to a psychiatric hospital for several days, where he was treated with Mellaril (an antipsychotic medication) and released, but he had another adverse reaction. David was hospitalized again, and this time he was treated with still another antianxiety medication, Xanax, but it made him feel horrible. This is the point at which David came to see me.

It was clear that David suffered from anxiety and depression. What wasn't so clear to me was why. Were there physiological problems underlying his psychiatric problems? It seemed likely that David had chronic candidiasis, and I suspected underlying food allergies and nutritional deficiencies as well.

Intradermal skin testing revealed that David was allergic to corn, oats, pork, rice, and peas, and also to multiple molds. His blood work indicated abnormalities in his red blood cells that were suggestive of folic acid and/or vitamin B_{12} deficiency. A vitamin assay turned up equivocal vitamin B_{12} levels and a definite folic acid deficiency (the normal range is from

5 to 24 micrograms/liter; David tested at 3.6). A stool analysis indicated some abnormalities in his gastrointestinal flora.

To combat David's candidiasis, I prescribed natural antifungal agents as well as Diflucan (a stronger antifungal medicine than nystatin). I also started him on folic acid supplements, working up to 5 milligrams twice a day, which caused a noticeable improvement. After several months, David's folic acid levels reached normal, but I kept him on folic acid supplements because I suspected he had a biochemically unique increased need for this vitamin.

David's total regimen—in addition to the natural antifungal agents, Diflucan, and folic acid—included a multivitamin/mineral supplement, probiotics (such as acidophilus and bifidus), prebiotics (to support the probiotics), supplements for liver support (to offset any liver strain caused by the Diflucan), supplements for adrenal support, certain amino acids, flaxseed oil, buffered vitamin C, and natural gastrointestinal cleansers (for his constipation). David's psychiatrist prescribed Paxil (an antidepressant) and Klonopin (an antianxiety agent). David was able to tolerate these medications, but they did not relieve his depression.

David started to feel better, but he still was anxious, lacked self-confidence, and couldn't write. At this point his father died, and David's grief added to his difficulties.

Knowing that B vitamins are important for mental health, and suspecting that David had an increased need for these vitamins, I added niacinamide (a natural relaxant) to David's regimen, along with supplementary pantothenic acid and vitamin B_6. David found that this orthomolecular approach to his psychological problems was definitely helpful.

David's depression started to lift. He was sleeping better, and before long he reported to me that he'd had "twelve good days in a row." As the added nutrients began to take effect at the cellular level, David started to look like a different person. By the time one year had passed from the day of his first visit, David was looking like a different man. He started writing again, and soon was at work on a novel and some song lyrics. His appetite improved, he regained the sixteen pounds he'd lost when he wasn't feeling well, and he became energetic and animated.

David continued to wrestle with candidiasis. When he stopped taking the Diflucan, his yeast symptoms returned, so I started him on Sporanox (another prescription antifungal), which he also found helpful. I also initiated candida immunotherapy for David, and eventually he was able to get off the prescription antifungal medication while continuing to control his symptoms. David's psychiatrist began to taper off the psychiatric medications, and David felt better off the Klonopin than on it.

Over the course of two years, David was transformed from a depressed, nonfunctional person to an energized, productive, and prolific writer. Essentially he had rejoined the land of the living. High doses of certain supplements overcame David's functional insufficiencies and pushed his metabolism into a more functional state. Although psychiatric medications were a part of David's recovery, there is no doubt in my mind that they did not fully account for his recovery, and that he would not have responded as well to medications alone.

In David's file, I keep a copy of the chapter he sent to me after he started to feel better. To me it serves as a concrete example of the power of nutritional medicine, even to the point of turning around a life that was fairly rapidly ebbing away.

Chapter 7

ALTERNATIVE THERAPIES

> Science . . . must describe and accept "the way things are," the
> actual world as it is, understandable or not, meaningful or not,
> explainable or not.
>
> —ABRAHAM MASLOW

Conventional medicine has always looked askance at any therapies outside its parameters. While it is always important to be scientific, even skeptical, and to approach new
therapies objectively, it is not reasonable to believe that medical doctors know everything
worth knowing.

Here's a case in point. According to medical school legend, there was once a doctor in
the 1940s who lectured to a group of medical students about a new miracle drug. He showed
his research, presented case studies, and urged the students to take the drug seriously.

The chief of medicine, however, was scornful. If the drug were so miraculous, he argued, everyone would be using it—including their colleagues at such a renowned medical
school. It must be mere quackery.

The drug was penicillin.

The medical establishment is not known for being open-minded about new therapies,
or even about ancient therapies newly discovered. Because doctors won't try these therapies,
they have no way of knowing how effective they are. When they observe how effective
alternative therapies appear to be for other people, they chalk it up to the placebo effect—a
point of view that leaves their paradigm nicely intact. (The placebo effect itself is actually
nothing to scoff at—see page 236.)

Today more and more people are turning to alternative therapies. A 1991 poll by *Time*
magazine determined that 30 percent of respondents—nearly one in three—had tried some
form of alternative therapy.[1]

An article in *The New England Journal of Medicine* noted that, according to the results
of a survey conducted in 1991, "the frequency of use of unconventional therapy in the

211

United States is far higher than previously reported," and that in fact the number of visits to providers of unconventional therapies is greater than the number of visits to all U.S. primary care physicians. At an estimated cost of $13.7 billion per year, the economic impact of this trend is significant. The article also noted that 72 percent of survey respondents who used unconventional therapies did not inform their medical doctor that they had done so—even though unconventional therapies are most often used as adjuncts to conventional treatment.[2]

Some people consult alternative healers regularly; others do so only after an unpleasant experience with traditional medicine, or as a last resort for treating a chronic condition when conventional medicine has failed. Most alternative approaches are more holistic than allopathic medicine, with a greater emphasis on mind, body, and spirit. Alternative medicine also tends to be more preventive. When illness does develop, alternative healers usually focus on correcting underlying problems—a process that can be time-consuming—rather than simply making symptoms disappear.

Most traditional medical doctors view alternative therapies with deep suspicion. Many alternative treatments defy logic, and no one was clamoring for randomized double-blind placebo-controlled studies when ancient remedies like acupuncture were being developed. However, I *know* that certain kinds of alternative treatments work because I've read the literature about them (much of which, by the way, does not appear in the big-time medical journals), I've talked to like-minded holistic physicians about them, and I've documented successful results with my own patients, many of whom consulted many medical doctors and tried several courses of conventional treatments before coming to me.

Fortunately, attitudes *are* changing in medical circles. Recently there has been greater realization that ancient traditions of medicine from remote places actually may hold keys to treating some of our diseases, and more health care practitioners are seeing the relevance of the approaches of other cultures. Our challenge today is to bring these ancient methods and remedies to scientific scrutiny so they can be more widely understood and appreciated. The National Institutes of Health Office of Alternative Medicine is sponsoring research on alternative therapies, and as the results of these studies and others become known, alternative therapies may become more acceptable. Each tradition has its own way of viewing the human body, yet the human body itself has remained the same throughout the centuries. It stands to reason that some of the therapies that have withstood the test of time will still have relevance for us today.

WHAT IS AN ALTERNATIVE THERAPY?

Alternative therapies are, in the broadest sense, any medical treatments not embraced by traditional (allopathic) medicine and not taught at conventional medical schools. Some of these therapies go back thousands of years (for example, Ayurvedic medicine from India), some are new variations on ancient traditions (for example, the electrical stimulation of acupuncture points), and some are relatively new (for example, chelation therapy).

Many alternative practitioners see themselves as mainstream. Some chiropractors, for example, bristle at the idea that chiropractic could be considered unconventional medicine. Similarly, homeopaths practice a system of medicine that goes back two hundred years, and the remedies used by Chinese doctors go back thousands of years.

In this chapter I'll discuss three alternative systems of medicine that I incorporate into my own practice: acupuncture, Chinese herbs, and homeopathy. In other parts of this book you'll find additional information about other alternative treatments. For example, Chapter 8, Stress Management Techniques, includes information on biofeedback and other therapies that have been proven effective in handling stress. Chapter 10, Immune System Super Boosters, includes up-to-date treatments such as intravenous vitamin C, enzyme-potentiated desensitization (EPD), and hormone therapy, along with other approaches I use in certain circumstances for patients who are ill. In Chapter 11, Redox Medicine, I discuss oxidative therapies and ultraviolet blood irradiation.

It is not my purpose here to discuss every alternative therapy available. I do have patients who swear by aromatherapy, flower essences, and other forms of alternative therapies. If a particular treatment is not harmful and clearly has been helpful to one of my patients, I'll sometimes pass this information along to others. I don't try to offer every therapy that alternative healers are already offering. However, I do keep my eyes and ears open for new approaches that do no harm, appear sound, have been successfully tried and tested elsewhere, and yield quantifiable, reproducible results. Carefully I will build these treatments into my practice, observing what kind of results they bring.

Occasionally I hear about a new therapy that is supposed to be great, but the results that I see with my own patients are not as impressive as I'd hoped. Sometimes adjusting dosages or adding adjunctive therapies will help, but there are times when I decide that a particular approach is not worth pursuing. I do not chase after every alternative treatment I hear about, but I do suspend judgment about new therapies until I am able to gather evidence for or against them.

SEEKING ALTERNATIVE TREATMENTS

You may wish to try an alternative therapy to stay well or to get well. Either way, my advice to you is to proceed with care—but do proceed.

Some medical doctors offer alternative treatments, as I do, but the majority of alternative health care providers are not M.D.'s. Before consulting an alternative health care practitioner, inform yourself about his or her approach by tracking down as many resources as you can. Contact national organizations (you can start with the Resources list at the back of this book) and read whatever books, magazines, and journal articles you can find on the subject. The Internet has a wealth of information about alternative therapies. All of this detective work will help you understand what to expect, what you have to gain from a therapy, and how to judge the treatment you receive.

Choose your alternative healer with care. Find out what your state's licensing requirements are for the treatment you seek. Work the grapevine and talk to other people who have tried the therapy. Find the practitioner with the best reputation and the most experience with the condition you need to treat (if you know what it is). Where did he or she study? How long has this person been in practice? It is important that you feel comfortable with the healer who will be treating you, for if you genuinely trust him or her, this can enhance your progress.

Healing is very individual, so what works for someone else may not work for you (and vice versa). In any healing process, the road to recovery has bumps and turns. Sometimes it's hard to tell if you're getting anywhere. Many patients experience a "healing crisis," in which they feel worse before they feel better. Here you need to use common sense. If your condition steadily declines over weeks of treatment, your situation needs to be reassessed. My general rule of thumb is to try six treatments, provided all seems to be going well (for example, with acupuncture) and then evaluate your progress. No treatment should ever do you harm.

If you pursue treatment with an alternative healer, I hope you will simultaneously work with an open-minded primary care physician. As with any type of professional, alternative health care practitioners run the gamut from totally unselfish to greedy, and from brilliant to undiscerning. A physician who is truly interested in your health and well-being will remain open to and will help you evaluate the care you receive from other professionals.

CHINESE MEDICINE

Traditional Chinese medicine originated over five thousand years ago, when physicians relied on their five senses and their knowledge of nature to find effective methods of diagnosing and treating illness. The language of Chinese medicine is completely unfamiliar to Westerners, and a diagnosis from a Chinese doctor (for example, "exhausted fire of the middle burner, or deficient cold affecting the spleen") may sound more like poetry than a name for a particular illness. Chinese medicine is actually very systematic, but we lack the conceptual framework to fully appreciate this.

One of the first hurdles for us to overcome is that Chinese medicine uses the names of familiar organs in very unfamiliar ways. For example, according to ancient theory the spleen is associated with digestion. It is responsible for transforming the food we eat into usable energy, and for transporting that energy throughout the body. Our modern understanding of the spleen is that it filters and stores blood. So what a traditional Chinese doctor means by "spleen" (or "kidney," or "liver," or "heart," and so on) is something quite different from what we expect.

One important cause of disease in Chinese terms is the penetration of an external factor into the body. Usually the body's protective energy is strong enough to resist disease, but when we are in a weakened condition, we are vulnerable to wind, heat, cold, dampness, and dryness. If our protective energy is weak over a long period of time (i.e., our immune system is suppressed), we are susceptible to deeper forms of invasion, and more chronic illness can result.

One of the foundations of Chinese medicine is the concept of life energy, or Qi (pronounced "Chee"). This life force is constantly circulating throughout our bodies, nourishing our organs and guarding our health. According to the traditional Chinese point of view, our life energy can be weakened by any kind of overexertion, mental or physical. Other hazards include physical trauma (which can lead to local stagnation of Qi), exposure to poisons (or, in a modern update, to harmful microorganisms), and incorrect treatments (including excessive use of Western drugs such as antibiotics, painkillers, and psychotropic drugs).

On the other side of the balance sheet, we have two main sources of Qi: the food we eat and the air we breathe. A balanced diet of clean, unprocessed foods is essential for health, as are the consistent timing of meals and a peaceful environment in which to eat. Good exercise is also viewed as vital to maintaining health. Nothing unusual or alternative about that!

The Diagnosis

When a Doctor of Oriental Medicine makes a diagnosis, he (or she) first observes the patient's body language (for example, strong or frail, aggressive or timid, straight or collapsed). Then he looks in the patient's face for signs of internal imbalance. Different areas of the face correspond to different organs, and particular colors on the face all have certain implications. Deep lines on the face can also reveal imbalances in the body.

Another important part of the traditional Chinese medical diagnosis is examining the tongue. Different areas of the tongue correspond to different organs, so the color, surface (such as wet, dry, coated), and texture of the tongue all have certain meanings.

When the Chinese doctor takes a patient's pulse, he (or she) listens to not one but twelve separate pulses, six in each wrist (three superficial and three deep). He will listen not only for the pace of the pulse but for other characteristics as well. There are twenty-eight different pulse qualities described in Chinese texts (such as "slippery," "choppy," and "frail"). The pulses allow the doctor to hear if there is too much energy in one part of the body (upper, middle, or lower) at the expense of another part.

The doctor will also evaluate the patient's emotional state, again looking for imbalances, such as one emotion that is out of control or felt much more often than others. Interestingly,

Chinese doctors saw a connection between being excessively anxious to please (the "cancer personality" described in more detail in Chapter 8) and tumor growth centuries ago.

Then the Chinese doctor will ask all the usual questions that a physician would ask about the nature of the patient's problem, its duration, factors that make it worse or better (including the time of day or year), etc. The patient's tastes for certain foods can also be significant, as different tastes are believed to correspond to different organs. Cravings or aversions can indicate that a particular organ needs attention.

When the patient lies down, the doctor may check different areas of his or her body for dampness or dryness of the skin as well as for temperature variations (too hot may mean too much energy in a particular spot; too cold may indicate a deficiency). Different areas of the abdomen correspond to different organs and meridians, so feeling the abdomen can reveal imbalances as well. Taken into account are the level of tension or hypotonia (decreased muscle tone), pain or discomfort, and the quality of the patient's breathing.

Once the doctor has arrived at a diagnosis, he or she may administer acupuncture, Chinese herbs, or both.

Acupuncture

I have never learned how to do acupuncture myself, but I often refer my patients for acupuncture treatments. Over the years I have seen many patients improve their general state of health with acupuncture, and I've seen some remarkable recoveries as well.

One young woman was admitted to the hospital with an acute gallbladder attack. She was in extreme pain. In the hospital she was put on intravenous medications and fluids, and scheduled for surgery the next morning. Her parents, who were with her, were very uncomfortable about this and requested a second opinion from an acupuncturist friend of mine.

The acupuncturist came to the hospital and agreed that the young woman did indeed have an imbalance in her gallbladder energy (according to Chinese medicine diagnostics), but in her opinion the imbalance was not at such a level that surgery was required. She explained to the family that she would like to see if an acupuncture treatment could obviate the need for immediate surgery.

Once the needles were inserted into the appropriate acupuncture points, the patient began to relax and her pain began to dissipate. By the end of the treatment, the pain had completely disappeared and the young woman was feeling much better.

With the resolution of the patient's pain, the need for surgery became less urgent. The acupuncturist explained that if the pain returned, surgery might once again become an option. However, she could continue to give the young woman periodic treatments for her imbalance of gallbladder energy, with the hope and expectation of resolving her illness.

The pain did not return, and instead of having surgery the next morning, the young woman was discharged, smiling, from the hospital. The surgeon could see that she was much recovered, although he remained skeptical about the acupuncture, and even went so far as to suggest that the patient might be back someday.

This young woman never did have gallbladder surgery. The moral of this story is not that acupuncture can always prevent the need for surgery, nor that one treatment is usually as dramatically effective as it was in this case. This patient's experience does illustrate, however, the incredible potential of the healing power of acupuncture and the Chinese medical approach when applied by a skilled practitioner.

What Is Acupuncture?

Traditional Chinese medicine holds that the life force, Qi, flows through the body along various channels called *meridians,* which run along the surface of the body. There are twelve main meridians in the body, each named after an organ to which it corresponds (for example, the Spleen meridian, the Liver meridian, and so on). A blockage in a meridian is believed to cause ill health.

The word *acupuncture* is derived from the Latin roots *acus,* "needle," and *pungere,* "to pierce." Acupuncture is the process of inserting fine needles at certain points along the meridians—there are over a thousand specific acupuncture points that can be stimulated—to correct any imbalances (i.e., to bring energy into areas of deficiency and to draw energy away from areas of excess, such as an area of inflammation). The different meridians enable the surface of the body to connect with deep internal organs.

The needles used for acupuncture are hair-thin and made of stainless steel. They are available in different types and gauges. The number of needles inserted in one session varies,

---

೧~೨

COMMONLY ASKED QUESTION NO. 13:

I hate needles. Does acupuncture hurt?

Acupuncture does *not* feel the way it does when you stick yourself with a sewing needle! Acupuncture needles are thinner than a hair. Other than a kind of tug when the needles are inserted, you should not experience pain and should be able to relax. If you are uncomfortable during an acupuncture treatment, tell the practitioner immediately. Being able to fully relax is an important part of the treatment, for this allows energy to move through the body more easily.

೧~೨

but generally does not exceed twelve, and a treatment usually lasts from a half hour to an hour. In addition to the placement of the needle, the depth, angle, and direction are all important as well. Often a needle is turned after it is inserted. Sometimes an herb called moxa is burned on top.

Depending upon the severity of the problem, the patient usually receives acupuncture once or twice a week for several months. As he or she begins to feel better, treatments are spread further apart. Many acupuncture patients have a maintenance program of treatments every two months or so, or treatments at the beginning of each season. The change of seasons holds much significance in Chinese medicine.

Most of my patients have not experienced acupuncture, but I find it is helpful not only for pain relief (a common Western application of acupuncture) but also for numerous other conditions, including immune dysfunction, Lyme disease, digestive problems, allergies, chronic sinus problems, addictions, gynecological problems, and neurological disorders. Some practitioners believe acupuncture is also effective for acute medical problems, such as an asthma attack. Provided sterile, disposable needles are used (all reputable acupuncturists use a fresh set of needles for each patient), acupuncture does no harm, is relatively painless, and has no side effects—yet it is powerful enough to be used in China as a local anesthetic during major surgery, including brain surgery.

How Does Acupuncture Work?

Acupuncture is based on Chinese philosophy, which holds that the opposites *yin* (restraint, darkness, passivity) and *yang* (vigor, brightness, activity) are always present together in the universe. Acupuncture is used to bring yin and yang back into balance in the body. These and other Chinese concepts are unfamiliar to Westerners, who have a hard time explaining the effectiveness of acupuncture using standard medical terms.

Acupuncture causes the release of natural painkillers called *endorphins*, and the needles stimulate peripheral nerves. (A Swedish study notes that acupuncture stimulates the same nerve receptors that are activated by strong muscle contractions, giving an effect similar to that of protracted exercise.[3]) Also, as you'll see in the next chapter, chemical messengers generated by the nervous system in response to acupuncture can be received and acted upon by cells of the immune system. It has also been found that many acupuncture points have significantly decreased electrical resistance compared to that of the surrounding skin.[4] Even so, there appears to be more to acupuncture than we can adequately express in terms of current medical dogma.

One study tried to determine if the effects of acupuncture are due to a placebo response by comparing the results of "real" and "fake" acupuncture in patients who had just had molars surgically extracted. Those who received the genuine acupuncture experienced less pain than the other group.[5] It is believed that stimulating false acupuncture points fails to release the same kind of neurotransmitters.

In another study, a French researcher, interested in proving whether or not meridians really exist, injected radioactive isotopes into the acupuncture points of humans and tracked their movement with a special gamma imaging camera. The isotopes could be seen to travel along the meridians. When the same isotopes were injected into blood vessels at random areas of the body, they did not travel in the same manner. This study supports the theory that the meridians are a system of pathways separate from the vascular and lymphatic systems.[6]

Chinese Herbs

For many centuries, herbal medicine was the most common form of medical treatment. Just because herbs are naturally occurring doesn't mean they don't present powerful treatment options. In fact, a survey back in 1975 showed that 74 percent of all prescription drugs were directly derived from plants.[7]

I give Chinese herbal preparations for infections that don't require antibiotics (for example, a viral infection), to obviate the need for antibiotics, and for chronic conditions that require immune system strengthening (including recurrent infections, chronic fatigue immune dysfunction syndrome, and cancer). Chinese herbs are frequently used in conjunction with acupuncture. They are also used as an adjunctive therapy to minimize the side effects of conventional treatments like chemotherapy and radiation.

Chinese herbs are described by their taste (bitter, sweet, sour, salty, and acrid), and different tastes are associated with different effects. Herbs are also said to be warm, neutral, cool, or cold, and have an affinity for certain organs or meridians. They also can be classified according to the five elements of traditional Chinese medicine: fire, earth, metal, water, and wood. *Tonics* are herbs that nourish the body. *Toxin-clearing* herbs cleanse the body, while *blood-activating* herbs maintain the free motion of blood.

Chinese herbs are often dried, powdered, and then prepared in a water decoction. Alcohol extracts are generally not used, as alcohol extraction changes the properties of the herbs.

Combining Herbs

Fu zhen (or *fuzheng*), which means "to restore normalcy and balance to the body," is an important Chinese herbal treatment. Fu zhen uses Chinese herbs in combination to normalize the physiology and to enhance immunity. It relies upon herbs that act as adaptogens—substances that enhance host resistance and help the patient adapt to external influences, including surgery, radiation, chemotherapy, and viral activity. The purpose of fu zhen is not to attack a specific pathogen, or to stimulate just one aspect of the immune system, but instead to provide general strengthening and immune rehabilitation. Fu zhen is generally used to treat patients who have been severely weakened, either by disease or by the side effects of the conventional medical therapies they have received.

Back in 1982, clinicians at the Department of Medical Oncology at Beijing Cancer Institute reported significant increases in the survival rates of patients who received fu zhen herbs in addition to conventional therapy. There was a notable drop in the immunosuppressive effects of radiation and chemotherapy (which are both destructive therapies) when fu zhen herbs were added to the protocol.[8]

In another study, seventy-six patients with second-stage liver cancer were divided into four groups: radiation therapy only, chemotherapy only, radiation plus fu zhen, and chemo plus fu zhen. At the end of one year, six of the thirty patients who had received only conventional treatment were still alive, but twenty-nine of the forty-six who had received fu zhen therapy in addition to conventional treatments were still alive. At the end of three years, all of the survivors from the conventional therapy groups were dead, but ten of the fu zhen patients survived for three years.[9]

As Chinese herbs become more popular, there are more reputable companies producing these herbs and herbal combinations. I have recently begun to use two specific combination herbal formulas that were designed for adjunctive use with chemotherapy and radiation therapy. These products—appropriately entitled Chemo-Support and Radio-Support—function as adaptogens and are given to cancer patients during treatment. Chemo-Support is made up of sixteen different Chinese herbs, while Radio-Support contains thirteen herbs in a different combination.

The major herbs used in fu zhen therapy are astragalus, atractylodes, codonopsis, ganoderma, ginseng, and ligustrum (see below). Recent studies—many involving laboratory animals, and most (but not all) conducted in China or Japan—have demonstrated that each herb has specific effects on the immune system, and that combinations of herbs can stimulate the immune system in different ways. Herbs can enhance the production of interferon and the production of antibodies; they can have anti-inflammatory and antimicrobial effects; they can enhance T cell maturation and stimulate the production of either red blood cells or white blood cells. Combination herbal therapies have multiple effects that have been, and continue to be, scientifically validated.

I use different commercially prepared herbal formulas for immune system support, including RESIST and several formulations of the Astra series. Usually I recommend RESIST for patients with recurrent or chronic viral illness, and Astra 8 or Astra Essence for patients who are in serious need of immune strengthening, including cancer patients. RESIST is currently undergoing testing with AIDS patients in San Francisco.

RESIST consists of:

Astragalus	Sand root	Chinese yam root
Ganoderma	Schisandra	Balloon flower root
Codonopsis	Ginger	Ligustrum
Atractylodes	Jujube fruit	Peony root
Licorice	Millettia root	Tangerine peel
Rehmannia	Dodder seeds	

Astra 8 was formulated by Subhuti Dharmananda, Ph.D., an expert on Chinese herbs and director of the Institute for Traditional Medicine and Preventive Health Care. This formula consists of eight Chinese herbs: astragalus, atractylodes, codonopsis, ganoderma, licorice, ligustrum, schisandra, and Siberian ginseng. Dr. Dharmananda's writings describe in detail the effects and importance of Chinese herbs.[10]

Some of the more important Chinese herbs are the following:

• **Astragalus** *(Huang Qi)* is the main ingredient of RESIST and is one of the most studied Chinese herbs. It's an important part of all Chinese strengthening formulas and was traditionally used to give vitality to the weakened patient and to increase resistance to disease. In animal studies, astragalus has been shown to increase the number of macrophages, enhance T cell maturation, increase phagocytosis, and promote the production of interferon. In human clinical trials, astragalus improved the survival rates of cancer patients receiving radiation or chemotherapy. In the treatment of people susceptible to the common cold, astragalus increased the number of antibodies in the blood.

A study published in the *Journal of Clinical and Laboratory Immunology* concluded that different fractions derived from *Astragalus membranaceus* were capable of "fully correcting *in vitro* T cell function deficiency found in cancer patients."[11] This study found that astragalus completely restored T cell function *in vitro* to a level that equaled that of cells derived from healthy subjects. A follow-up study by the same authors, published in the same journal, proved the efficacy of *Astragalus membranaceus* with an *in vivo* experiment that involved laboratory rats.[12] In these experiments, as well as others, astragalus proved to be a powerful biological response modifier.

• **Berberis** *(Sankezhen)*, prepared from a root, contains berberine and other active ingredients that significantly increase the number of white blood cells. Berberis also has antimicrobial effects (antifungal, antiprotozoan, etc.) and has been shown to have antitumor effects in rats.[13]

• **Codonopsis** *(Dang Shen)*, which today is commercially cultivated, is cheaper than ginseng but has similar effects. The root of the codonopsis herb stimulates the growth of red blood cells (but not white blood cells), enhances T cell maturation, and stimulates phagocytosis.

• **Ganoderma** *(Ling Zhi)*, a fungus that grows on trees, is now commercially cultivated. In Japan, ganoderma is known as *reishi* mushroom. Ganoderma was found in laboratory studies to increase T cell activity and macrophage activity. Known as an immune system stimulant, ganoderma stimulates phagocytosis by reticuloendothelial cells, enhances cell-mediated immunity, and increases the number of white blood cells in peripheral vessels. It is also used to counteract the effects of stress and to lower cholesterol.

• **Gentiana** *(Long Dan)* promotes phagocytic function and has antibacterial effects, but it is also known to protect the liver from chemical damage. Gentiana increases bile flow and urine excretion and reduces inflammation and blood pressure. I also use gentiana, alone at times, in patients with imbalances in their intestinal flora when a pathogenic organism that is sensitive to gentiana is found (using a comprehensive stool analysis).

• **Ginseng** *(Ren Shen).* The original, true ginseng *(Panax ginseng)* is a rare and venerable Chinese herb. Research on this plant has shown it to be a strong adaptogen. *Panax ginseng* owes its beneficial effects to a group of compounds called *ginsenosides* that are not found in any other genus.[14]

• **Siberian Ginseng** *(Ci Wu Jia).* Today many formulas substitute Siberian ginseng *(Eleuthero ginseng),* which is actually from another plant family but has similar effects. (There is also a third variety, American ginseng *[Panax quinquefolius],* which is considered less stimulating.) Siberian ginseng also is an adaptogen. Its root and leaves are used to prevent colds, flu, and bronchitis; to treat cardiovascular disease; to speed postoperative recovery; to counteract the effects of stress; and to moderate the destructive effects of radiation therapy. According to Dr. Dharmananda, cancer patients undergoing radiation therapy who receive ginseng have higher recovery rates and report a greater sense of well-being than patients who receive radiation alone.

• **Ho Shou Wu.** The name of this tonic herb means "Mr. Ho has black hair." Traditionally used for longevity, this herb promotes lymphocyte transformation, increases the number of leukocytes, and enhances phagocytosis.

• **Licorice** *(Gan Cao).* The root and lower stem of licorice *(Glycyrrhiza glabra* or *Glycyrrhiza uralensis)* are widely used in Chinese medicine. One of its active ingredients, glycyrrhizin, has antiviral properties and is effective in treating acute and chronic viral hepatitis. Licorice has antibacterial effects and it also activates the body's interferon mechanism.[15] In addition, licorice is anti-inflammatory, which can be helpful for patients with allergies or autoimmune problems. Licorice is considered a "harmonizer" for the other herbs that are present in a combination formula.

I use a commercial licorice extract formulation that contains glycyrrhizin in my intravenous treatments when appropriate. I've found it to be helpful for detoxification as well as for treating allergic and autoimmune disorders, inflammatory diseases, and viral illnesses (especially hepatitis).

• **Ligustrum** *(Nu Zhen Zi)* is derived from the fruit of an evergreen shrub that grows in China. Ligustrum is a diuretic and cardiac stimulant. It also has antibacterial effects and has been shown to raise the white blood cell counts of patients undergoing cancer therapies. Traditionally ligustrum has been used as a tonic herb when there is rapid deterioration of the body. Although ligustrum does not attack tumors directly, it does have anticancer properties due to its immune-enhancing effects.

• **Shiitake Mushrooms,** which are now widely available either fresh or dried, have a long history of use in China as an immune stimulant. This mushroom stimulates the release of interferon, enhances phagocytosis, and enhances T cell maturation.

• **Rehmannia** *(Shu Di Huang)* strengthens the immune system by increasing phagocytic activity, promoting lymphocyte transformation, and increasing the production of immunoglobulin. Rehmannia also is protective of the liver.

- **Schisandra** *(Wu Wei Zi)*. Preparations derived from the ripe fruit of schisandra, a woody vine native to northern China, stimulate the nervous system. Schisandra helps to counteract the effects of stress and fatigue by enhancing body energy and mental activity. This herb also protects the liver and is used to treat hepatitis. In addition, schisandra is used to treat acute gastrointestinal infections. In lab animals, schisandra was shown to enhance lymphocyte transformation.

- **White Atractylodes** *(Bai Zhu)*. The dried root of this herb, which is not commercially cultivated, enhances the phagocytic functions of white blood cells and also increases their number. It also acts as a diuretic, reduces platelet aggregation (which helps to explain its effectiveness in cardiovascular conditions), and protects the liver against toxins.

HOMEOPATHY

Back in the 1800s there were several medical schools that trained physicians in homeopathy. The first homeopathic medical school in the United States was founded in 1835, and the American Institute of Homeopathy—the first national medical association in the United States—was formed in 1844. By 1847, the American Medical Association was formed, and it moved quickly to denounce homeopathy. In fact, at that time, physicians who practiced homeopathy were not allowed to be members of the AMA.

With the arrival of "miracle" drugs (and the subsequent rise in influence of the pharmaceutical industry), homeopathy became less and less utilized. However, with the advent of new enthusiasm regarding alternative medicine, homeopathy is experiencing a surge in interest, utilization, and inquiry in the United States. Homeopathy is more accepted in Europe. In France, pharmacies are required to carry homeopathic remedies along with conventional drugs. In England, homeopathic hospitals and clinics are part of the national health system.[16]

Homeopathic Remedies

Homeopathic preparations are derived from plant, animal, or mineral substances and are greatly diluted in pure water or alcohol. Classical homeopathy consists of finding one precisely correct remedy, used in the minimum dose. We have found much success with the newer protocols that use combination therapies. These do not require the inordinate time and attention to minute details that are necessary in monotherapy.

Very strict homeopaths do not believe in the use of antibiotics. Having seen patients who were treated homeopathically for a bacterial illness, such as Lyme disease, but whose condition worsened, I cannot fully endorse this viewpoint. However, I do know respected homeopaths who feel they can effectively treat bacterial illness with homeopathic remedies.

COMMONLY ASKED QUESTION NO. 14:

What is homeopathy?

The term *homeopathy* is derived from the Greek words *homoios,* or "similar," and *pathos,* or "suffering." Homeopathy follows three principles set forth by Samuel Hahnemann, the German physician who originated homeopathy in the late 1700s:

1. Like cures like (the Law of Similars).
2. The further a remedy is diluted, the greater its potency (the Law of the Infinitesimal Dose).
3. Each illness is specific to the individual.

In homeopathy, a substance that causes a certain set of symptoms in a healthy person is made into a preparation (through a process called *dilution and succussion*) to give relief to someone who is sick with the same symptoms. For example, someone who has diarrhea would be treated with a minute amount of laxative. In this way, homeopathy resembles modern "allergy shots" (in which allergic people are injected with ever-increasing doses of allergens until they are fully desensitized). In fact, homeopaths were using pollen extracts to treat hay fever at least twenty years before immunotherapy injections were introduced in 1911.[17]

In the case of an infection that I don't deem to be severe, I may first give the patient a trial of homeopathic treatment. If the response is inadequate, I may move on to an antibiotic. In those situations when I must put a patient on antibiotics, I may also recommend homeopathy as an adjunctive or follow-up treatment.

I also know of one strict homeopath who refused to use conventional medical diagnoses. A child with measles, for example, was simply said to have a rash, which was treated homeopathically. In my practice, I prefer to ascertain a diagnosis (to the extent possible) and then consider options and alternatives using this information.

In my experience, I have found that combination homeopathic remedies follow the $\frac{1}{3}$, $\frac{1}{3}$, $\frac{1}{3}$ rule I learned in medical school: they work extremely well in approximately one-third of patients, moderately well in another third of patients, and have little or no effect in the final third of patients. I always tell patients before recommending these remedies that this is my experience. Being nontoxic, inexpensive, and potentially very effective, homeopathic treatments are certainly worth a try.

Some of the combination remedies I have found effective include Husteel (used for colds, bronchitis, and coughs), Drosera Homacord (used for bronchitis, bronchial asthma, and bronchial cough), and Euphorbium nasal spray (used for nasal and sinus problems). These preparations can be effective for sinus and respiratory infections when taken together or singly. At the first sign of a cold or upper respiratory infection, I sometimes advise patients to take a very helpful remedy called Oscillococcinum. I also use Lymphomyosot (to promote lymph drainage during infections) and Gallium-Heel (to help with the Herxheimer, or die-off, reactions we sometimes see during recovery from Lyme disease and chronic candidiasis). For relaxation, I recommend Valerianaheel and Calming (which can also be helpful for insomnia).

When patients take a combination homeopathic remedy for an acute illness, they need to take it only as long as they have symptoms. This is in contrast to antibiotics, which must be taken for at least ten days, even if the problem—for example, a sore throat—becomes asymptomatic in two or three days.

Does Homeopathy Really Work?

It's difficult to prove the viability of homeopathy using conventionally constructed studies. For one thing, homeopathic treatments usually are highly individualized—that is, ten people with the same medical diagnosis could receive ten separate homeopathic preparations. In addition, homeopathic treatments can have long-lasting effects, making crossover studies (in which groups of patients switch treatments) problematic.

However, even with these inherent problems, many convincing studies on the efficacy of homeopathy have been done. One study determined that homeopathic treatment resulted in a statistically significant decrease in the duration of acute diarrhea in children in Nicaragua. (Acute diarrhea is the leading cause of pediatric illness and death worldwide.)[18] In another tightly controlled study that was reported in the *Lancet*, twenty-eight patients with asthma were randomly assigned to two groups. One group received a homeopathic treatment, while the other received a placebo (a biologically inert substance). All of the patients continued with their conventional medical therapies. The homeopathically treated group showed greater improvement in respiratory function tests within one week, and the beneficial effects of the homeopathic treatment lasted for up to eight weeks. The authors conclude their article (entitled "Is Evidence for Homeopathy Reproducible?") with a challenge to the medical community: Either homeopathy works, or the clinical trial model does not.[19]

Many studies have been done about homeopathy—if it were an orthodox system of medicine, it probably would have been incorporated into conventional treatment protocols by now. However, homeopathy is not an orthodox approach, and it is impossible to explain its effectiveness using conventional medical concepts.

Homeopathy does at first seem to defy logic. Victor Herbert, M.D., an outspoken critic of alternative therapies, has said, "It is obviously fraudulent when bottles of homeopathic remedies 'potentized' by having been diluted past Avogadro's number—so that there is one molecule or less of active agent per ten bottles—are sold with representations of potency against dysfunction and disease."[20]

Because conventional medications are dose-dependent, homeopathic remedies do not fit the paradigm of Western pharmacology. However, as we saw in Chapter 4, the nature of an immune response is harmonic. (Some people call this the "oscillating response curve.") When we position immune responses along a sine curve (remember the sea monster on page 98?), it becomes clear that we do not need large quantities of a treatment to effect a response—all we need is just the right treatment dose. Viewed this way, homeopathy makes more sense. (Keep this principle in mind, for we will be returning to it when we discuss oral tolerance immunotherapy in Chapter 10, Immune System Super Boosters.)

Another study published in the *Lancet* ("Is Homeopathy a Placebo Response?") compared the effects of a homeopathic treatment for hay fever (a preparation of mixed grass pollens) with a placebo in 144 patients with active hay fever. The homeopathically treated patients experienced a significant reduction of symptoms, as assessed by both doctors and the patients themselves. The other group did not show any improvement. The article concludes, "The drug we used was potentised *[sic]* to the point where, in theory, none of the original material remained. Yet these results and those of the pilot study offer no support for the suggestion that the observed effects were wholly due to placebo responses."[21]

So how do we explain the effectiveness of homeopathic remedies that have been diluted to the point where even a single molecule of the original substance is no longer present? The answer seems to lie in the process of succussing, or vigorously shaking successive dilutions of a remedy. Some researchers have theorized that succussion causes some kind of electrochemical patterning of the original substance in each dilution. A physicist has suggested that succussion produces energy storage in the bonds of the dilution in the infrared spectrum which "downloads" when it comes in contact with water in the body. Somehow biological information is encoded in the remedy and "read" by living cells. Here the discussion clearly veers away from the biochemical and into the bioenergetic. (For more information on energetic medicine, see page 331.)

It may be many years before we can explain homeopathy to the satisfaction of the American Medical Association. In the meantime, I know that I can help certain patients with homeopathic treatments that are both safe and effective.

OTHER KINDS OF DOCTORS

I'm a medical doctor, or M.D. I earned a medical school degree, I'm licensed to practice medicine in the state of New York, board certified in family practice, and I periodically have to take exams in order to maintain my family practice board certification. In terms of alternative credentials, I am board certified in chelation therapy and oxidative medicine.

Other doctors use different systems of medicine. Their credentials look like this:

- **M.D. (China)** or **O.M.D.** is a degree from medical school in China. A foreign medical degree is not automatically recognized as equivalent to a U.S. medical degree (and consulting a Chinese doctor may not be recognized as a legitimate medical expense by your health insurance company).

- **M.D. (Ayurvedic)** is a degree from an Ayurvedic medical school. Ayurvedic medicine, recently popularized in several books by medical doctor Deepak Chopra, has been practiced in India for five thousand years. Ayurvedic medicine places equal emphasis on the patient's body, mind, and spirit and is based on three basic *doshas,* or metabolic body types: *vata* (changeable, quick, and thin), *pitta* (predictable, methodical, and of medium build), and *kapha* (relaxed, slow, and heavyset). Each *dosha* is associated with certain innate tendencies. All of us are a mixture of all three, with one dominant *dosha.* Ayurvedic medicine combines many therapies, including herbal preparations, fasting, chanting, yoga exercises, breathing techniques, meditation, diet, exercise, and massage.

- **N.D. (Doctor of Naturopathy)** is a degree from a school of naturopathic medicine. The term *naturopath* dates from the turn of the century, when naturopathy became popular. A naturopathic doctor may not write prescriptions or perform major surgery—but then again, he or she probably doesn't want to. Naturopaths believe that the key to health is natural living (avoiding anything artificial, unnatural, or toxic), and that our bodies contain everything we need to overcome disease. Naturopaths use different therapeutic methods to restore health, including fasting and detoxification, dietary manipulation, nutrients, herbal preparations, homeopathy, acupuncture, physical therapy, and counseling.

- **D.O. (Doctor of Osteopathy)** is a degree from osteopathic medical school. Osteopathy dates from the late 1800s, and the first school of osteopathic medicine was established in 1892. Osteopaths attend medical school and do rotations just as medical doctors do, and they are fully licensed physicians who may prescribe medications and practice in all branches of medicine and surgery. Unlike medical doctors, osteopaths receive additional training in osteopathic medicine, which emphasizes the importance of the musculoskeletal system. Osteopaths believe that any mechanical restriction in the body—which may be traced to any number of causes, from an old injury to emotional tensions—can influence the healthy functioning of our organs and bodily processes. (One osteopath compared this disruption to cutting a triangle out of a sweater. You can sew up the hole, but the entire sweater will be affected.) By using manipulative treatments, osteopaths correct the body's mechanical structure and thereby normalize body functions, including breathing. *Cranial osteopathy* involves making subtle adjustments to increase the mobility of the cranial (head) bones. This technique is controversial, as conventional medicine holds that the bones of the skull eventually fuse together.

Probably due to pressure from medical doctors, or possibly feeling that they want to be recognized as medical doctors, many osteopaths have given up this valuable skill of manipulation and have moved into the arena of prescription-based medicine. In the hands of a skilled practitioner, this cranial-sacral manipulation can be extremely effective for a multitude of problems, ranging from headaches and back pain to recurrent ear infections in children.

• D.C. (Doctor of Chiropractic) is a degree from a chiropractic school. Chiropractic evolved at about the same time as osteopathy, but chiropractors may not prescribe drugs or perform surgery. Chiropractors emphasize the relationship between the musculoskeletal system, particularly the spine, and the nervous system. They view disease as a lack of normal nerve function due to some irregularity in the spine. Health is restored by manipulating the vertebrae. Chiropractors generally believe that continual adjustments are needed to maintain optimal health, with the frequency of treatment depending upon the circumstances.

Would You Believe . . . Progressive Medical Doctor (P.M.D.)?

In my view, no one system of medicine—allopathic, Ayurvedic, or Chinese; chiropractic, homeopathy, naturopathy, or osteopathy—is a complete health care system. As I said earlier, progressive medicine combines the best of traditional (allopathic) medicine with the best of alternative medicine to give patients a complete program for health and healing.

Progressive medicine is hard work. It's like a journey that is never done—or, as a friend joked, it has a "learning curve" that looks like a straight trajectory into outer space. Many doctors aren't interested in alternative therapies, and others are unwilling to reeducate themselves.

When my colleagues and I completed our residencies, we all had been trained to do a certain job, and to do it well. Most of my fellow residents were eager to put into practice right away what they had learned. Going back to square one and starting a new learning process just wasn't appealing to most of them. Why would they want to take on something so difficult when they could go out and be successful right away?

All good doctors make every effort to keep abreast of new developments in medicine, but I find it's even more challenging and rewarding to chase down reliable, valid, clinically applicable alternative therapies. This interest of mine is what caused me to take a different path after completing my residency and that path has led to progressive medicine—what I believe is the medicine for the next millennium.

ᕱᕇᕲ EDIE'S STORY

To illustrate the enormous potential of alternative therapies, I have borrowed a striking case history from my brother, Steve. In this case, acupuncture caused a dramatic turnaround in a patient's condition and obviated the need for major surgery.

When Edie first visited Steve, she was fifty-one years old and had been diagnosed with a uterine fibroid tumor bigger than a grapefruit. She had consulted two gynecologists, both of whom had recommended that Edie have a hysterectomy. Edie had been given an outside limit of three to six months to seek other solutions. She was not familiar with progressive medicine, but she was willing to give it a try if it meant possibly avoiding surgery.

Edie's tumor was not cancerous, but it was causing problems. She had abdominal discomfort—as you can imagine—and was experiencing heavy menstrual bleeding. On examination, Edie's uterus could be palpated 1 inch below her navel, indicating that it was greatly enlarged. Edie had constant nasal congestion and sinus trouble, persistent fatigue, and gastrointestinal bloating and constipation. She also almost always felt cold. All of these symptoms have particular significance in Chinese medicine.

Steve immediately placed Edie on nutritional supplements, probiotics (such as acidophilus and bifidus), and Chinese herbs. Because Edie was a recovering alcoholic, Steve also started her on a liver detoxification program to help correct any damaging effects alcohol had had on her liver. It's possible that Edie's tumor was estrogen-related, and that her overstressed liver had not been able to efficiently process estrogen as it was produced by her body, leading to complications from improper hormone balance.

In Chinese medicine, a fibroid is a sign of blood and Qi stagnation. Qi moves through the body in a cyclical (not linear) manner; areas of stagnation need to be unblocked if the Qi is to keep moving. Steve administered acupuncture to Edie to stimulate her spleen (in the Chinese sense) and to eliminate the stagnation in her menstrual system by correcting her liver energy (also in the Chinese sense—in Chinese medicine, the liver is responsible for a woman's monthly cycle). Edie had never tried acupuncture before, but she was game.

After her first acupuncture treatment, which involved the placing of needles in her hands and feet to stimulate the movement of her Qi, Edie felt better. It was too soon for tissue changes to be apparent, but it was clear that on a functional level, changes were already occurring.

By October of that year, Edie's uterus could be palpated 3 inches below her navel. The fibroid was shrinking. Edie had less discomfort and was feeling better overall. Her sinuses had cleared, and she was now a convert regarding acupuncture.

By the following March, ultrasound showed that Edie's tumor was the size of an orange. It appeared that Edie's bodily systems were rebalancing themselves. She'd lost weight, and she had more energy. Surgery was clearly no longer necessary, although it would take more time for the fibroid to actually melt away.

Two years later, Edie's tumor was reduced to the size of a lemon. She no longer had pelvic pain or excessive menstrual bleeding. After a dozen treatments in all, acupuncture was stopped. Edie kept taking her nutritional supplements, but she no longer needed to take the Chinese herbs.

Today Edie comes into the office about once a year, and her fibroid tumor is no longer a concern. By expanding her horizons and embracing alternative therapies, Edie was able to keep her uterus and avoid almost certain surgery. I sometimes wonder how many other hysterectomies could be avoided if more patients—and more doctors—took these options as seriously as they deserve to be taken.

Chapter 8

❧❦❧

STRESS MANAGEMENT TECHNIQUES

The greatest discovery of any generation is that human beings can alter their lives by altering the attitudes of their minds.
—ALBERT SCHWEITZER

Stress often is the "last straw" that puts us over the top of our Immune System Kettle. Even a small stress can put us over our immune threshold when it is imposed upon a huge immune burden. Alternatively, an intense stress can tip the scales toward immune dysfunction even when our immune load is relatively low. There are two ways to restore immune balance: lower the overall load in the kettle and reduce the amount of stress. Sometimes we can remove sources of stress from our lives altogether, but even if that's not possible, we can certainly learn and use stress management techniques that have verifiable physical benefits.

My patient Hannah was shocked when she was diagnosed with thyroid cancer. "This is so unfair!" she objected. "How come *I'm* the one who got cancer?"

Hannah did everything "right." She was a vegetarian, she rarely ate sugary or fatty foods, and she took a variety of supplements to replenish and rejuvenate her immune system. Hannah had two beautiful children, delivered by natural childbirth, for whom she made organic baby food from scratch and knitted homemade sweaters of natural wool. When Hannah wasn't driving the children to their classes—including swimming lessons, music appreciation, gym time, and introduction to computers—she could usually be found either working out at the club or cross-training on her bike. She also was a gifted hostess and was known for her beautiful floral arrangements.

Hannah had surgery to remove her cancerous thyroid. While she was hospitalized, she gave her husband lists of things to do and planned a family trip to Normandy. The day Hannah was released from the hospital, her parents came to visit from Florida; that evening she was at the stove cooking homemade tomato sauce with fresh tomatoes from her garden.

With thyroid medication, Hannah was quickly back to her usual schedule, and the trip to Normandy went off as planned. People were universally admiring of how indomitable

Hannah was. However, all did not go smoothly. Two years later, Hannah's parents were killed in a car accident, and a year after that Hannah felt a lump in one breast.

Tests revealed that the lump was malignant. Hannah went back into the hospital. By this time the children were in different schools and on different schedules, so Hannah had to rely on friends to get them where they needed to be and to look after them in the afternoons. Although she found it difficult asking for help, she discovered that no one else minded in the least.

As Hannah lay in her hospital bed one long night, wondering how much the cancer had spread in her body and what her surgery the next day would reveal, she suddenly realized how very tired she was. For the first time, she considered the possibility of dying. She started to reflect on the things that were truly important in her life. Flower arranging was nice, but it wasn't one of them. By dawn, Hannah had decided that if she was lucky enough to live much longer, she'd make fewer lists and spend more time with her family. What she really wanted to do was go for a walk with her husband and children. This resolution sustained her as she was prepared for surgery, and it was her last thought before the general anesthetic took effect.

Fortunately, Hannah's breast cancer was not far advanced. As soon as she got home, she took that walk with her family, and appreciated it in a way she never had before. After follow-up chemotherapy, she was pronounced clear and clean of cancer.

Today Hannah is a noticeably different woman. She told me that whenever one of the kids chooses a polyester superhero T-shirt at the store or puts on mismatched socks, she just smiles and enjoys the moment. In fact, she appreciates each moment in ways she'd never imagined possible. She has slowed down and no longer has to be the perfect, accomplished superwoman. Hannah also has a new rule: When her "to do" list gets overwhelming, she deliberately crosses off three items. The world hasn't ended yet, her family is doing fine—and she's still cancer-free.

STRESS: THE UNIVERSAL RISK FACTOR

There's no question that lung cancer is associated with smoking. The majority of people who develop lung cancer have a history of smoking. On the other hand, most cigarette smokers do not get lung cancer. How do we account for this?

A study evaluating the psychosocial risk factors for lung cancer revealed that the single most important predictor of cancer was a significant loss experience within the previous five years. Other factors—such as depression and an inability to express emotions—were also associated with the development of cancer. The bottom line: psychosocial factors were one to two times as important as smoking history in predicting lung cancer.[1]

Whether or not we get sick—with cancer or with something less scary—depends in part on factors over which we have no control (for example, our genetic makeup), factors over which we have little control (such as global pollution), and factors we can control if we make the effort. Stress is a risk factor for illness that *can* be controlled.

What Is Stress, Anyway?

Actually, stress is difficult to define, particularly because it means different things to different people. For example, discovering that your shirt has been buttoned wrong all morning could be horrifying or amusing, depending upon your outlook. Similarly, a new job turning around a Fortune 500 company could be an exhilarating challenge or a frightening experience.

Picture Joanne and Celia approaching a stoplight in their identical cars. Joanne is very tense, in a rush. She drives rapidly up to the light, hoping to get through but having to stop short when it turns red. She waits anxiously, fidgeting, gripping the steering wheel, impatient for the light to turn green. For her, this stoplight is stressful. Celia approaches the stoplight, sees it turn yellow, slowly puts on the brakes, stops, and waits calmly for the light to turn green, realizing she has no control over the light and there is nothing she can do to change the situation.

These two women may be going to the same meeting and may be on the same schedule, but Celia is not stressed by the delay. The stoplight—the objective phenomenon—is a subjective stress for Joanne, but not for Celia. Clearly, how we interpret events is more important than the events themselves. Even an event that is not stressful to us in one set of circumstances may be in another.

Hans Selye first defined biological stress as the "nonspecific response of the body to any demands put upon it." In other words, stress isn't the traffic light, or your boss, or your divorce. Stress is your response.

A certain amount of stress is an inevitable part of life. Some stresses are actually pleasurable or exciting. What really matters is our outlook, whether we see something as a catastrophe or a challenge, and whether or not we can learn to relax in spite of it. Too much stress—either chronic, low-level stress; unpredictable bursts of stress; or sudden, devastating stress—can lead to distress, which has a negative impact on the immune system.

As I mentioned in Chapter 2, up to 90 percent of trips to the doctor are stress related. Stress plays a part in chronic problems such as high blood pressure, cardiovascular disease, headaches, backaches, depression, allergies, asthma, arthritis, cancer, and AIDS. Stress also has been linked to anxiety, insomnia, ulcers, panic attacks, alcoholism and substance abuse, and immunosuppression.[2]

One study found that the more stressed people are, the more likely they are to catch a cold. When the study subjects were systematically exposed to a cold virus, just 27 percent of the low-stress individuals got sick, whereas 47 percent of those with the most stressful lives caught colds.[3]

Modern life is stressful, and this stress is making us sick. Why?

STRESS RESPONSES

While people don't necessarily agree about stressors, we all show our stressful feelings in one of three ways: an upregulated response, a downregulated response, or a coping response.

The Upregulated Stress Response: Fight or Flight

It's 3:00 A.M. and something awakens you from a deep sleep. You hear a sound downstairs. Footsteps? There it is again! An intruder? You freeze, totally alert. Your heart jumps, your mouth goes dry, your muscles tense, and you scarcely dare to breathe. Time seems to slow down while your mind races.

Under maximum stress, everyone responds the same way. The body releases a flood of hormones that quicken the heartbeat and breathing rate, widen the airways, and dilate blood vessels in the muscles while simultaneously constricting those in the skin and abdominal organs. Glucose is released into the bloodstream for quick energy and blood pressure goes up. As a result of these changes, oxygen and nutrients are redirected to the central nervous system and to stressed body sites, and energy is directed away from the reproductive and digestive systems.

During this "fight or flight" response, the brain goes into high gear. Our attention is totally focused. This adaptive mechanism no doubt helped our cavemen ancestors when they were being menaced by saber-toothed tigers and noticing the smallest sound could mean the difference between life and death.

Researchers have now determined that stress hormones actually help what is known as "emotional learning" (learning that takes place when intense emotions have been aroused, including pain or fear). In fact, one study determined that human subjects who were given beta-blockers (medication that blocks the effects of stress hormones) had considerably poorer recall of a disturbing slide show about a young boy's terrible accident than participants who did not take beta-blockers.[4] Evidently, the same stress hormones that cause our heart to race also help imprint information deep within our brains.

The upregulated stress response is still useful today when we are in danger and need a burst of energy. However, these days we are menaced by ongoing stressors such as job pressures, family problems, financial worries, chronic illness, and other troubles of modern-day life. These threats bring on the upregulated hormonal surge, but are not resolved through either fight or flight.

Being constantly in a hyperresponsive state is not good for us. Chronic stress suppresses the immune system (more about this in a moment). Excess stress hormones take a toll on the body, and while we're stressed, energy is diverted away from processes like eating, digesting, growing, and reproducing. Stress has been linked to anorexia and weight loss, and prolonged stress leads to the suppression of growth hormone secretion. In some people stress appears to interfere with fertility as well. Severe trauma that lasts for months or even years on end—experienced, for example, by soldiers or abused children—may damage the hippocampus (a part of the brain that is crucial for short-term verbal memory).[5]

The Downregulated Stress Response: Hopelessness and Helplessness

You've been out of work since last November. You sent out copies of your résumé, but got a poor response. You figure probably nobody wants to hire somebody so close to retirement. Now it's July, and most companies just aren't hiring. You've been running through your savings—something you hate to do, but you don't see any alternative. At this point it's getting harder and harder to face each day.

The downregulated stress response slows us down instead of speeding us up. People in a hyporesponsive state feel helpless and hopeless when confronted with adversity. They see no way out of their situation, so they tune out and give up.

You have no doubt heard that a fighting spirit can make a difference in recovering from illness. People who have a lot to live for sometimes extend their lives as if by the force of sheer willpower. On the other hand, patients who wish to die usually do so. A downregulated stress response sends a "give up" message to the body. Not surprisingly, it is associated with fatigue, hypersomnia (excessive sleep), weight gain, and depression.

The Coping Response: "I Can Handle This"

Your home caught fire and sustained a lot of smoke and water damage. Fortunately, everybody got out safely. You were planning to take a cruise this winter, but obviously there's no money for a cruise now. You'll have to rebuild the house and buy a lot of new furniture. You still cry when you think of the family photographs and other irreplaceable belongings you lost, but then you figure it could have been a lot worse. This is difficult, to be sure, but everyone is being really helpful and already you've got a contractor lined up.

The individual with a "stress-hardy personality" feels in control and is actively engaged in finding solutions to problems. Effective copers experience just as many stressors as the rest of us, but they seem to have a knack for staying optimistic and focusing on the present, rather than agitating over "what if" or "what could have been." Worrying uses up a lot of energy, in essence wasting one of our most valuable resources.

In his book *The Health of Nations*, Leonard A. Sagan, M.D., discusses what he considers to be the main psychological characteristics of the healthy person. You can read the full text in his book, but I've taken the liberty of condensing them as follows:

1. Healthy people have a high level of self-esteem, and they believe that their personal decisions can make a difference.

2. They are committed to goals other than their own personal welfare and have a strong sense of community.

3. They place a high value on health and survival.

4. They are future oriented and well-informed.

5. They are trusting, affectionate, and capable of commitment.

6. They relish companionship but also value solitude and contemplation.

7. They pursue knowledge and find meaning in life events.[6]

Later in this chapter you'll find a rundown of stress management techniques anyone can use to help get a handle on stress and to become a healthier, stress-hardier person.

THE MIND/BODY CONNECTION

It's a little silly that we have to reunite mind and body at all, but we're still dealing with the aftereffects of the deal Descartes made with the Roman Catholic Church back in the seventeenth century. He pursued the study of science as we now know it, but left the mind, soul, and consciousness to the Church. Now that we're putting the whole picture back together again, we're starting to see just how intricate the puzzle is.

The Power of Suggestion

A simple example of the mind/body connection is blushing. When we feel embarrassed, the blood vessels in our face dilate and we turn pink. It stands to reason that other kinds of feelings can have other kinds of effects, including more serious ones. Mind and body communicate with each other in profound ways that can propel us toward either healing or death. Once we realize how powerful these messages are, we can begin to try to influence them in positive ways.

Take the placebo effect, for example. It is well known that people will respond positively to substances they believe are curative, even if these remedies are in fact inert or even harmful. In one remarkable and often-cited study from 1950, women with morning sickness were given syrup of ipecac (which is used to induce vomiting) and were told it was a powerful antinausea medicine. Astonishingly, they stopped throwing up. The power of their belief overrode any nausea they might otherwise have felt.

The placebo effect has successfully been used in healing on many occasions (more about this in Chapter 13, Healing Begins with Acceptance), and in fact may have far more to do with the history of medicine than most physicians care to admit. In medical school, I learned that 30 to 40 percent of patients who are given an inert substance will experience a positive (placebo) effect. In his book *The Psychobiology of Mind-Body Healing,* Ernest Lawrence Rossi, Ph.D., notes that there may be a 55 percent placebo response in many, if not all, healing procedures.[7] This is placing a great deal of power in the mind of the patient.

Just as belief can heal, it also can kill. There are well-documented cases in which individuals have lain down and died because curses were cast upon them and they believed their time was up. These "voodoo deaths" are not caused by heart attacks or other disease. In this culture, a doctor's prognosis can be equally powerful. Patients given three months to live sometimes believe they are not entitled to live any longer and die on schedule.

We humans are more suggestible in some states than in others. For example, if a hypnotized person is touched with a cold coin, but told he is being burned with a hot iron, a blister can actually appear on the skin. One woman was asked during hypnotherapy to imagine she was on a sunny beach, whereupon she cried out in pain and developed a "sunless sunburn" on her face, shoulders, and upper arms that lasted eighteen hours.[8] Bernie Siegel, M.D., who is well known for his best-selling books and lectures on the mind/body connection, routinely asks anesthetized patients to correct their pulse rate or to stop excessive bleeding during surgery—and they oblige.[9] Similarly, there are many stories of comatose patients being fully aware of conversations held at their bedside. In all these states, information is received, understood, and transmitted to the body without the benefit of conscious thought. In fact, removing the mind's interference seems to enable us to unconsciously transform thought into physical reality.

Conditioning the Immune System

In a groundbreaking study with mice, Robert Ader, Ph.D., showed that mice could be given a drug to suppress their immune system, and then be conditioned to continue suppressing their immune system even after the drug was taken away. Dr. Ader put saccharin—a distinctive flavor—in the animals' drinking water, and paired this with an injection of an immunosuppressant drug. One of the many fascinating aspects of this experiment is that the mice "understood" that the immunosuppressant was bad for them. When the mice were reexposed to the saccharin-flavored water, they did not receive any immunosuppressant— but some of them dropped dead anyway! Dr. Ader noted that the mice who died were those who had consumed the most saccharin.

The human immune system can be conditioned as well. In one case, a boy who was severely allergic to roses was observed to have an allergic reaction to *plastic* roses. His immune system was so overzealous that in effect it became a gun turned against the self. Another boy who suffered from multiple personality disorder was allergic to orange juice in all but one of his personalities. If he drank orange juice in this personality, but switched to another too soon, he would break out in a rash.[10]

Wondering if she could use immune system conditioning to advantage, pediatrician Karen Olness, M.D., tried a variation of Dr. Ader's experiment with a girl named Marette who was suffering from lupus. Marette's life was in danger, and her doctors felt it was necessary to put her on an immunosuppressant drug that was known to cause severe side effects. (In this case, the immunosuppressant drug was life-saving, not life-threatening.) After getting all the necessary consents, Dr. Olness gave Marette the drug, but paired it with the strong taste of cod liver oil and the pungent smell of rose perfume. Taste and smell are most easily conditioned, so the idea was to double the chance of successful conditioning by using both. With each treatment, Marette would sip cod liver oil and smell the perfume. Over time, her doses of immunosuppressant drug were reduced, but Marette did as well as children who received the full amount. Marette came to absolutely detest the taste of cod liver oil, but by that time her immune system had already responded to the cues it had received.[11]

Why do our perceptions play such a strong role in our immune responses? Because various systems of the body work together to coordinate one integrated response, as we'll now see.

PSYCHONEUROIMMUNOLOGY (PNI)

Psychoneuroimmunology, the study of mind/body medicine that was once on the fringe of reputable inquiry, has become mainstream medicine. PNI holds that our thoughts, feelings, and personality are expressed through our brain and nervous system, influencing our immune responses and therefore our health. We now know that our nervous, immune, and and endocrine systems are interrelated, and that the best way to understand our health is not to tease these systems apart, but to observe them together.

As I mentioned back in Chapter 3, the different systems of the body communicate by means of biochemical messengers. If cells, tissues, and organs are our "hardware," then these messengers are the "software" that tell the hardware what to do.

The Autonomic Nervous System

The *autonomic nervous system* is the part of the central nervous system that controls involuntary bodily activities such as heartbeat and breathing. *Neurotransmitters* are chemicals that carry messages between nerve cells or from nerve cells to muscle cells. Some neurotransmitters act locally, while others are released into the bloodstream so they can initiate a response at a distance.

The autonomic nervous system comprises two parts that act together and balance each other: the *sympathetic nervous system* and the *parasympathetic nervous system*. The sympathetic nervous system generally has stimulating effects and is dominant during stress or excitement. It secretes *epinephrine* (also known as *adrenaline*) and *norepinephrine* (also called *noradrenaline*), which are responsible for the upregulated, high-anxiety response described earlier. The parasympathetic nervous system generally has relaxing effects and is dominant during sleep. It secretes *acetylcholine,* which (among other effects) slows the heart and speeds digestion.

The Endocrine System

The *endocrine system* is made up of different glands (including the pancreas and the thyroid, pituitary, and adrenal glands) that are involved with growth, metabolism, and sexual development and functioning. The endocrine system secretes many different *hormones,* which are chemical messengers that are necessary for normal body functioning.

The *hypothalamus,* located in the brain, is the control center that tells the pituitary which gland-stimulating hormone to produce. Under stress, the adrenal glands secrete epinephrine and norepinephrine as well as corticosteroid hormones such as *cortisol.* This is why chronic stress can deplete the adrenals. (For information on adrenal support, see Chapter 10, Immune System Super Boosters.)

The Immune System

As we saw in Chapter 3, the immune system is made up of the thymus, spleen, lymphoid tissue, bone marrow, and various types of white blood cells. The immune system secretes chemical messengers called cytokines that include lymphokines, monokines, interleukins, interferons, tumor necrosis factor, and others. These substances have a multitude of effects, and their influence is not limited to the immune system.

Look Who's Talking

We used to believe that each of these systems spoke a different language. If the nervous system spoke French, then the endocrine system spoke German and the immune system spoke Spanish. This point of view turned the human body into a sort of United Nations, with different conversations going on in different languages.

We now know that this is an outmoded way of viewing the human body. The nervous system, endocrine system, and immune system communicate back and forth in a language that is received and understood by all three systems. It's true that each system issues its own particular chemical messengers, but even here there may be some overlap. For example, the pituitary gland is usually credited with turning out adrenocorticotropic hormone, or ACTH, but it is now known that lymphocytes can produce an ACTH-like peptide, too.[12] Because of the intense level of communication that goes back and forth among the nervous, endocrine, and immune systems, it makes sense to view their different biochemical messengers more as different dialects of a common language.

ᑐᗢᎮ

COMMONLY ASKED QUESTION NO. 15:

What is a psychosomatic illness?

Medicine has long recognized that bona fide physical disorders can be caused by, or worsened by, psychological factors. A psychosomatic illness is one that has a psychological connection. If you feel nauseated every time you set foot in a hospital, it's possible that something about hospitals makes you so anxious that you get a stomachache. Other psychosomatic illnesses can be much more subtle.

When traditional doctors cannot confirm a diagnosis, they sometimes tell patients that their problem is all in their head. I have seen virtually hundreds of patients who were told by other doctors that their illness was psychosomatic. In the vast majority of cases, *it was not.*

Physical factors can underlie psychiatric disorders just as often as the reverse occurs. Somatopsychic problems are far more common than most physicians recognize. Nutrient deficiencies have contributed to memory loss; food allergies can cause behavioral problems; Lyme disease can cause depression; candida overgrowth can lead to fuzzy thinking. Sometimes it is extremely difficult to tell whether a psychological problem is being expressed in the body, or a physical problem is being expressed in the mind.

ᑐᗢᎮ

When David Felton, M.D., was looking through a microscope at sections of immune tissue, guess what he discovered? Bunches of nerve fibers. What were nerve cells doing in the middle of immune tissue? Eventually he and others discovered that nerve fibers are "hard-wired" to virtually every organ of the immune system.[13]

Immune cells have dozens of receptors on their surface, not only for cytokines, but also for neurotransmitters and hormones. This explains how chemical messengers from the nervous system and endocrine system can have immunomodulatory effects. This information was a real eye-opener for me when it first became known in medical circles in the 1980s. Finally I had an explanation for the immunomodulatory effects of acupuncture and of stress management techniques that I had already observed in my patients.

Signals generated by the immune system are also received and acted upon by the nervous and endocrine systems. This explains why the activation of the immune system can be accompanied by neurological and psychiatric effects. For example, an immune response can influence eating and sleeping patterns, mood states, movement, and other behavior.

The bidirectional nature of these communications is one of the things that makes psychoneuroimmunology so interesting. Not only do we now have a framework for understanding immunologically based changes in behavior, but we also have the basis for understanding behaviorally induced changes in immune function.

HOW THOUGHTS MODULATE CELLULAR ACTIVITY

We've always known that it's possible to die of a broken heart. Now we know why. Psychosocial factors and emotional states influence cellular activity, including the initiation and progression of disease. Here's how this works:

Step 1: Brain activity. In response to our environment (which includes both stressful and relaxing life experiences), the cortex, or higher part of the brain, forms certain perceptions and makes interpretations. Thoughts and images are generated by means of electrical impulses in the brain.

Step 2: Neurotransmitters. The electrical impulses from the cortex are filtered through the lower parts of the brain and are transduced into different kinds of neurotransmitters. In this way, feelings and impressions become biochemical substances. Candace Pert, Ph.D., a leader in the field of PNI, refers to these messenger molecules as the "biochemical units of emotion."[14]

Step 3: Responses by the autonomic nervous system. Neurotransmitters initiate the production of hormones like epinephrine (stimulating) and acetylcholine (relaxing). The immune system picks up the thread of conversation when immune cells are exposed to neurotransmitters and hormones.

Step 4: Cellular activity. Surface receptors on individual cells are stimulated by the neurotransmitters, hormones, and immune system messengers that have now been produced. When the surface receptors are activated, the interior machinery of the cell is turned on, including the cell's genetic machinery. The genes within each cell are the ultimate blueprint for how that cell will be constructed, organized, and regulated, and ultimately determine just what that cell will do.

This process helps us see how beliefs and attitudes can translate into either sickness or health. Because of this mind/body connection, our state of mind can have an effect on both our susceptibility to and recovery from disease. I happen to believe that our attitudes, thoughts, and feelings originate at higher energy levels and are laid down in our bodies. Level by level, our attitudes resonate with our organs, tissues, and cells. As Bernie Siegel, M.D., says in his book *Peace, Love and Healing,* "Body and mind are different expressions of the same information."[15]

Attitude and Health

The Type A personality—aggressive, competitive, hard-driving, fierce, often hostile—consistently churns out high levels of stress hormones. Type A people race their engine constantly and experience more maintenance problems more quickly than steadier folks who go through life at a lower idle. Type A people have changes in their serum cholesterol, triglycerides, and blood sugar that put them at an increased risk of coronary heart disease and heart attack, even in the absence of other risk factors like genetic predisposition, smoking, obesity, high blood pressure, lack of exercise, and a fatty diet.

A cancer personality has also been proposed. This personality—mild, polite, unemotional, compliant, uncomplaining, easily victimized—seems to correspond to a downregulated immune system. Rather than taking out their hostility on the world, such people are thought to "sacrifice" themselves by growing tumors.

I don't particularly like stereotypes, but I do see correlations in my patients between outlook, life experiences, and health. For example, one of my patients who was sexually molested as a young girl developed a hypervigilant attitude toward life. Understandably, she grew up to be a wary adult, always sensitive to any perceived invasion of her personal boundaries. Not surprisingly, she has developed an autoimmune disorder, the result of an overzealous immune system. Another young patient who is extremely sensitive to sights, sounds, and other stimuli also has extensive allergies, as if he were physically trying to ward off the world. Similarly, I have had many depressed patients with underactive immune systems who were susceptible to recurrent infections and chronic diseases. Successfully treating their depression was an important part of rehabilitating their immune system.

It really shouldn't be so surprising that the mind and the immune system are so clearly linked. Both have the responsibility of defining and remembering who we are. Most cells of the body turn over, but brain cells and certain immune cells do not. These cells are part of our permanent self and hold long-lasting information about our experiences. In addition, both the brain and the immune system are in the business of patrolling boundaries—cognitive, spiritual, and psychological boundaries as well as the physical boundaries of self and not-self.

Dr. Sagan, who proposed those characteristics of psychologically healthy people, takes issue with the ideal of good health that is being marketed these days. Physical fitness, he argues, is not the same as good health. Health is "largely cognitive and emotional," he notes. "It is the brain that is the true health provider."[16]

STRESS AND THE IMMUNE SYSTEM

So we know the immune system does not work in a vacuum. It responds in a neuroendocrine environment that is affected by our thoughts, beliefs, and responses to life events.

Chronic or severe stress has a debilitating effect on the immune system that can be measured and quantified. How much the immune system is disrupted depends upon many factors, including the type of stressor we experience, its duration, our personal coping abilities, how healthy our environment and lifestyle are, and "host factors" such as our age, sex, and genetic predisposition.

Excess stress hormones have been shown to suppress immune system activity. Although the corticosteroids are anti-inflammatory and are important in helping the body recover from stress, an overabundance of corticosteroids inhibits the function of macrophages and lymphocytes and interferes with the ability of lymphocytes to divide. In fact, corticosteroids are used as immune-suppressing drugs in the treatment of allergies, arthritis, and other ailments associated with an upregulated immune system.

Epinephrine gives the body the kick it needs to respond to a stressful situation. However, too much epinephrine inhibits white blood cell function, lowers the number of helper T cells, raises the number of suppressor T cells, and causes important lymphoid tissue to wither.

Stressful experiences are associated with decreased production of cytokines, increased susceptibility to infection and tumors, and the reactivation of latent viruses (viruses like the Epstein-Barr virus) that are commonly present in our bodies but are kept under control by the immune system. When we're stressed, a normally inconsequential exposure to a pathogen is more likely to lead to disease.

As we saw earlier, thoughts are transformed into chemicals that ultimately can affect our cells. Stress is associated with dysfunctions on the molecular level, and it has been found that the repair of DNA—the genetic material in the nucleus of cells—is defective in people subjected to psychological stress.[17]

Few life events are as stressful as losing a loved one, which helps explain why bereaved spouses are more likely to die within eighteen months of their loss. A bereavement study showed that widowers had unchanged T cell and B cell counts, but their lymphocyte function was suppressed.[18] This is another example of functional rather than structural or numerical changes. In this case, a routine white blood cell count would not indicate immunosuppression, even though it is present.

Another study of stressed individuals involved medical students. This study compared certain biochemical and cellular markers one month before the students' exams and on the last day of exams. The stress of exams caused the students to have decreased NK cell activity (particularly the lonelier students), decreased numbers of helper T cells, and decreased interferon production. The students also had increased antibody titers to Epstein-Barr virus, herpes simplex virus, and cytomegalovirus, indicating their cellular immune systems were doing a poorer job of controlling latent viruses. All told, the stress of exams translated into increased susceptibility to infection.[19]

While very stressful situations have been shown to modulate immune activity, it's also true that ordinary daily hassles have an effect on the immune system. One study of the secretory IgA in saliva—one of our first lines of defense—showed that daily fluctuations in mood and minor stresses are associated with immunological changes. On a good day, our secretory IgA levels are high. On a bad day, they drop—which gives invading microorganisms easier access to the body.[20]

As I mentioned above, depression can go hand in hand with immune system changes. Researchers have determined that depressed people can have a decreased number of NK cells, reduced NK cell activity, and decreased numbers of T cells and B cells, including fewer helper T cells and fewer cytotoxic T cells.[21] Their psychological vulnerability is mirrored by physical vulnerability in the form of immunosuppression.

STRESS MANAGEMENT

Now that we know all this information, what do we do with it? There's really only one conclusion to reach: stress-relieving techniques maximize our defense against disease and promote healing. By altering our state of mind, we can alter our state of health.

Conveniently—at least in this situation—the mind doesn't make judgments about what is "real." Imagine tasting a ripe, summer peach and you'll start to salivate. If you imagine a peaceful walk along a deserted beach, your body will relax—even though you're stuck in traffic. This kind of "mind game" can be very helpful to our health.

In his book *Healing and the Mind*, Bill Moyers tells the story of being connected to a biofeedback machine by Dr. Karen Olness—the pediatrician mentioned earlier—and being instructed to think of a very relaxing, comfortable place. He closed his eyes and imagined standing on a favorite mountain peak with a gorgeous 360-degree view of the Rockies, a place he had visited only once before. His heart rate, indicated by a white line on the biofeedback machine, became nice and steady, and Dr. Olness was pleased.

"I'll have to go back one day," Bill Moyers said.

"You just did," Dr. Olness replied.[22]

The Relaxation Response

Herbert Benson, M.D., author of *The Relaxation Response*, found that when we deliberately relax, we can achieve a state that is the opposite of the "fight or flight" response. Our heart rate and respiration slow down, our blood pressure normalizes, our muscles relax, and our breathing becomes deeper and more regular. Alpha waves in the brain, which are associated with feeling fully relaxed, increase. While we're in this state, the effects of stress-related hormones diminish, and our body consumes less oxygen and uses less energy. By periodically conserving energy with the relaxation response, we can compensate for the furious rate at which we use energy during our other waking moments. With practice, we can even create an overdraft on our energy bank account.

The health benefits of stress-reducing activities are significant. According to a 1996 *Time* magazine article, studies have shown that routinely eliciting the relaxation response caused 75 percent of insomniacs to start sleeping normally, 35 percent of infertile women to become pregnant, and 34 percent of sufferers of chronic pain to reduce their use of painkillers.[23]

Remember those stressed-out medical students who were preparing for exams? Half of them were randomly assigned to a relaxation group. The relaxers' blood showed better immune function than the control group's—and the more often they took time out to relax, the higher were their ratios of helper T cells to suppressor T cells.[24]

Another study divided elderly subjects into three groups: one that met three times a week for one month for training in progressive relaxation, another that met just as frequently to socialize, and the third, a control group that did neither. The health benefits for the relaxers included greater NK cell activity and lower antibody levels to herpes simplex virus (meaning the virus was successfully kept in check). They also reported feeling less distress. The other two groups had no significant changes.[25]

STRESS MANAGEMENT TECHNIQUES

To get started on your stress reduction program, read the descriptions of the stress management techniques that follow. Reducing stress can be as simple as taking a walk with a friend. If you're interested in learning a new skill (for example, yoga or biofeedback), consider getting advice from an expert. In our health centers, we have someone on staff to give patients short-term instruction on stress management techniques that they can then use on their own. My patients frequently resist this, perhaps because of the investment of time and money, or perhaps because they envision a long-term process like psychotherapy. After they finally avail themselves of these tools, they invariably tell me that they can't believe they waited so long.

Change can be difficult, particularly when it involves taking a hard look at our own fears and ingrained behaviors. Most people need a crisis—for example, an illness—to motivate them to start changing their attitudes. I urge you not to wait until a crisis gives you an incentive to take stress management seriously.

Whatever you do, pick activities you enjoy. Your stress reduction program is not supposed to be stressful! In addition to taking stress breaks every day, try to maintain a regular schedule of eating and sleeping. It amazes me how often I have to tell my patients to pay attention to their body's needs for food and rest. Rest is not something to be cavalier about. For patients recovering from viral illnesses such as Epstein-Barr (mononucleosis) or hepatitis, rest is an integral part of their treatment program. Even for day-to-day health maintenance, appropriate rest is essential. Many of us persist past the point of hunger or exhaustion and get out of the habit of heeding the messages our bodies are trying to send us.

To complete your stress reduction program, look for ways to reduce stress in your daily life. Can you free up some of your time? Get help with an obligation that is a real burden? Eliminate a source of argument at home? You might need to make some long-term changes, too, such as getting out of an unhealthy relationship or switching jobs. I can't count how many of my patients have needed to make such significant changes. After they mustered the courage to do what they needed to do, the subsequent improvement in their immune health was well worth the effort. One of my patients gave up a lucrative marketing job that required extensive travel and ninety-hour workweeks for a less prestigious job at a local newspaper. Her health has greatly improved, as has her quality of life.

Allow yourself to take a vacation, to take a leisurely bath, to go for a walk on the beach, or to play your favorite music. You'll ease your mind as well as your body. Remember to be present in every moment. As the saying goes, life is not a dress rehearsal.

Attitude Adjustment

Stress is a subjective response to an objective phenomenon. Knowing this empowers us to reframe or to modify our reactions. There's no question that life can be hard, but we often make it harder by using outdated or counterproductive thought patterns. This has been compared to building a jail and then volunteering to live in it.[26]

Remember the sixties saying, "Be Here Now"? Many stress-reducing activities come down to accepting the present moment—no more and no less. Maybe it's a tribute to our complexity as human beings, but most of us have a lot of trouble staying in the present, without replaying tapes from the past or borrowing trouble from the future. This is why a conversation about laundry detergent can escalate into "Mom always loved you best," or "You just don't understand my needs!" Laundry detergent is not, in and of itself, particularly stressful, but—being human—we can create huge amounts of stress over any issue at a moment's notice.

I've observed many mental traps over the years, both in my patients and in myself. I've also had the help of some very wise advisers in different courses I've taken about spiritual healing. Following are some recommendations for reducing stress and anxiety through attitude adjustment.

• **Recognize that nothing is 100 percent.** People generally see things in a strictly dualistic fashion. We are either happy or sad, right or wrong; situations are either good or bad; experiences are either positive or negative. We believe we have to be "perfect," or else we will be completely "imperfect," and in some irrational way this will mean we are worthless. Talk about stress! Having to pick and defend one position (because the opposite seems unacceptable) is like constantly being embroiled in a wartime effort. Just as it is draining for the immune system to be fighting numerous border skirmishes, so does constantly defending extreme positions drain energy from more constructive and reparative purposes, including immune repair. It's hard to relax when you feel so threatened by other points of view. This kind of thinking is very prevalent in our society and in our world, whether we recognize it or not.

Either/or thinking is simplistic and unforgiving. It took a professional training course for me to realize that "100/100" thinking (i.e., 100 percent this *or* 100 percent that) is artificial and unrealistic. A much more accepting attitude is 50/50 (i.e., 50 percent this *and* 50 percent that). Actually, 50/50 symbolizes an attitude or consciousness toward life rather than a specific equation. Situations need not be split down the middle. More important than percentages is the concept of "bothness," or this *and* that. This allows the coexistence of opposites. People can be both weak and strong, selfish and selfless, tired and exhilarated; situations can be both good and bad, and experiences can be both positive and negative.

Once we free ourselves of 100/100 thinking, we are liberated from taking and defending extreme positions. This frees up a tremendous amount of energy that can be put toward constructive purposes elsewhere. Years ago I was unable to accept weakness within myself because of my unwitting adherence to the 100/100 rule, which held that if I was weak in any way, I could not also be strong. When I finally grasped the 50/50 concept on a deep level, I realized that I could experience weakness or vulnerability, and still be strong. This allowed me to be more open to and accepting of my own feelings, and more sensitive to the feelings of my patients. The 50/50 point of view has enabled me to help my patients recognize and accept their internal conflicts. Just as the balance of opposing forces is the key to immune system health, so is this balance of thoughts, feelings, and beliefs essential to our emotional and spiritual health.

• **Recognize that there is no absolute reality.** We all have a tendency to believe that "our" reality is the only one. Total breakdowns in communication can occur when two people make assumptions about each other's perspective. For example, my wife and I once attended a movie with another couple. We loved it; they hated it. We thought it was funny; they thought it was boring. I remember standing on the sidewalk outside the movie theater with my jaw hanging open. How could they have missed the humor? Had we even been to the same movie? Well, not really. The movie each of us saw had been filtered through our individual personalities—yielding four different movies.

In this case, we laughed at our differences of opinion. Basically it didn't matter if we agreed or not. Nobody got entrenched in trying to persuade the others that they were wrong. In more serious circumstances, however, our differences of opinion might have escalated into a stressful battle of wills. Just as a healthy immune system recognizes but tolerates certain foreign substances, such as dust or pollen, so must we learn to acknowledge foreign perspectives without feeling the need to defend ourselves.

• **"Cook" your feelings, rather than serving them up raw.** Denying or repressing feelings uses up energy and leads to internal distress. I don't mean to suggest, however, that it's healthy to just let our emotions rip. One of our greatest gifts is the ability to be self-aware.

All kinds of impulses bubble up from our unconscious. The idea is not to push them back down again, but to bring them to the forefront of our consciousness.

There is a great Zen concept called "hold your seat" that refers to bringing these kinds of impulses to awareness and working through them without actually acting upon them. Again, we are talking about balance—in this case, "holding our seat" between the overexpression and underexpression of our impulses. Overexpression of our aggressive impulses correlates with Type A behavior, while underexpression corresponds with the cancer personality. Dark, destructive impulses from our "shadow self" are very powerful. Accessing this aggression in a positive, constructive way can redirect our internal destructive energy toward healing and understanding.

- **Dig up what you've been hiding from yourself.** When very young children play hide-and-seek, they put their hands over their eyes to make themselves disappear. Even though we're all grown up now, we sometimes still believe that what we don't see doesn't exist. We all have experiences and suspicions we back away from, and uncomfortable or unkind feelings we'd rather deny exist. It can be a huge stress reliever to come to terms with deeply hidden concerns (with professional help, if necessary). If our innermost fears are not allowed entrance into our consciousness, they may instead find expression in the body as chronic illness.

- **Don't get trapped in unhappiness.** So many people live lives full of stress and unhappiness. In essence, they are hemorrhaging energy. Parts of themselves and their spirit are dying on an everyday basis. Often we regard the way out of our stress-filled life as more frightening than just keeping going the way we are. Sometimes the alternative can seem so overwhelming and so fearful that we continue to live in misery. In this situation, the only escape is illness.

One of my seriously ill patients finally found the strength to deal with her unhappy marriage when she developed cancer. "I see now that on some level, I believed that getting sick was the only way out," she explained to me. "Now I can't believe I was willing to die rather than help myself."

W. H. Auden wrote, "We would rather be ruined than changed." Obviously it is more beneficial to change our point of view so that alternatives, although difficult, are no longer so frightening, and we don't slip into severe emotional or physical illness to escape.

- **Drop outdated behavior.** Suppose you were scratched by a cat when you were little. You would immediately learn a valuable lesson: cats can be dangerous. However, you might go on to be afraid of all cats in all situations for the rest of your life. You might even teach your children (knowingly or unwittingly) to fear cats, too. You might avoid visiting friends with cats, and make a point of crossing to the other side of the street when you see a cat in someone's yard. Old fears and resentments can imbue the most ordinary events with high anxiety and make life unnecessarily stressful.

• **Don't borrow trouble.** It's distressing, and very tiring, to keep imagining the worst that could happen. Because the list of dreadful possibilities is endless, you can never reach a constructive conclusion. You just have to make yourself stop, for to continue is a tremendous strain on your whole system, including your immune and hormonal systems. As a doctor, I sometimes have to present patients with a best- and a worst-case scenario, but I always carefully reassure each patient that whatever happens, we'll deal with it. This also holds true for any event in life. Dealing with whatever is in front of us is very much in tune with healthful living. Being consumed with a list of dreadful or potential negative outcomes—living in dread, living in fear—prevents us from living in the present, and not experiencing the present is the equivalent of not really living.

• **Avoid woulda/coulda/shoulda.** Life is full of regrets and miscalculations, great and small. It bears repeating: Everybody makes mistakes. That's one way we learn. Accepting mistakes as a natural and integral part of being human allows us to avoid the trap of woulda/coulda/shoulda. It also allows us to forgive ourselves as well as others when things don't turn out exactly as we had hoped or planned. In my experience, forgiveness is one of the healthiest states for emotional as well as immune system balance.

• **Avoid the "if only" trap.** We've all had times when we were sure things would be different if only we had more money, or if only we lost ten pounds, or if only we found the right boyfriend/girlfriend. It's healthy to have goals, but it's stressful to be perpetually dissatisfied with life as it is.

We've all met people who have very much in their lives and yet are unhappy and dissatisfied, seemingly always wanting more. The other side of this endless wanting is endless "not wanting," or giving up wanting. This response is not the real solution to endless wanting and, when taken to the extreme, can result in depression. The true solution to this 100/100 duality is being grateful—a state of 50/50 acceptance. This state of being grateful for what we have allows us to appreciate life on its own terms, including all those little things we tend to overlook, such as being in the presence of a loving relative or friend.

Picture a spoiled child at a birthday party who gets so many presents he just rips through them, never stopping to appreciate any of them, always wanting more. Another child may receive much less, but totally and completely love and be grateful for what he has. All of us have moments when we act like spoiled children, forgetting to be grateful for everything that is right and joyous about our lives. Contentment is healthy for us emotionally and healthy for our immune system.

• **Let your anger dissipate.** Holding on to anger is sometimes compared to holding a hot coal: you're the one who gets burned. If you are really entrenched in being angry about something, remember that no one is ever 100 percent right. Chances are your emotions are based on some kind of misconception, and only by delving beneath the anger and turning your awareness inward to expose your misconception(s) will you allow your anger to dissipate, thereby releasing the hot coal and relieving the burn.

Anger is a health hazard. One researcher found that those physicians who scored highest on a test of hostility while still in medical school were *seven times* as likely to have died by the age of fifty as their colleagues with low hostility scores.[27] This makes being prone to anger a stronger predictor of dying young than smoking, high blood pressure, or high cholesterol.

If you naturally have a hot temper, try taking the proverbial three deep breaths (they'll counteract the surge of stress hormones you're experiencing) and saying to yourself with each breath, "I am not my anger" or "I will let go of this anger." Another way to defuse your anger is to look deeper into the fear that underlies this anger and to ask yourself a question: What are you afraid of that is making you so angry? Some people hold on to their anger because they believe it will protect them from being taken advantage of again and again. If this sounds like you, recognize that there are more constructive ways to protect yourself.

In certain extreme situations, anger is appropriate and can even be lifesaving. For the long haul, however, forgiveness is much easier on and healthier for the immune system than persisting rage, anger, or resentment.

• **Avoid blaming yourself or others.** Ours is a culture in love with blame. We like to blame more than we like to accept responsibility. Remember the story about the woman who scalded herself with hot coffee and sued McDonald's? Blame is a two-edged sword: blaming others helps us save face, but it also makes us the victim. As we've seen, feeling powerless sends the wrong message to our immune system. Don't make others responsible for your happiness/unhappiness or your success/failure.

• **Recognize your idealized self-image.** We spend tremendous amounts of energy hiding who we really are and preparing our face—our mask—to meet the world. The more false our presentation, the more energy we use keeping it up. In fact, it's quite possible (and not that unusual) to maintain a superficial self that is quite at odds with the inner self. These exhausting efforts at concealment deplete our cellular energy. This depletion of energy can result in mitochondrial problems (mitochondria, you'll recall, are the powerhouses of our cells) and cellular fatigue, and subsequently can lead to chronic fatigue, neurological diseases, and chronic illness. Being totally who we are allows us to interact directly with others and to use our emotional energy for truly constructive purposes, such as healing.

• **Look for solutions.** The stress-hardy person takes action when possible. As we've already seen, hopelessness and helplessness suppress the immune system. Sometimes, however, the appropriate action is that of surrender or letting go. When no further action is possible, surrender *is* the solution. By letting go—becoming an empty vessel, if you will—we open ourselves to help, guidance, and new points of view. I am reminded of the prayer that goes something like, "God give me the strength to change the things I can, the courage to bear the things I can't, and the wisdom to know the difference!"

Frequently I tell patients that the best way to reduce stress is to sit quietly, accepting that our life is unfolding exactly as it is meant to—or, as Deepak Chopra, M.D., has said, that each moment is "as it should be." On a global level, certainly our lives are unfolding the way they should be. On the more day-to-day level of human interaction, it's not always easy to maintain that perspective. For example, it's not easy for me to look a Holocaust survivor in the eye and tell her that her life unfolded just the way it should, any more than I can look a newly diagnosed advanced cancer patient in the eye and tell him that his life is "unfolding as it should." At that moment, it certainly doesn't seem like it is. And yet, if we stay the course, and stay connected to our feelings, we can frequently transform this initially shocking and painful experience into a much different one. If we can go through the initial shock, denial, anger, grief, etc.—those feelings that are associated with dire circumstances—we may be transformed. It never ceases to amaze me how many of my patients can open up to parts of themselves that they were not in touch with, discovering not only inner strength and inner peace but also a sense of relatedness and connectedness to other people and to the world that they had never known before. Through this whole process there is a deep sense of acceptance—an acceptance of things as they are, and an even deeper acceptance that life is indeed giving us what we need and giving us the opportunity for deep inner growth. Acceptance allows us to see difficulties and obstacles as gifts and as vehicles for this transformation.

Biofeedback

Biofeedback is a technique that helps us harness the mind's influence on the body for the purposes of stress reduction or healing. Over the years biofeedback has gained more acceptance, probably due to its use of technology—a sensitive machine that monitors and measures physical responses (including skin temperature, muscle tension, or brain waves) in an easily recognizable way.

In the most common form of biofeedback, the patient is taught to increase the blood flow to his or her hands by relaxing the autonomic nerves that regulate this blood flow. (Stress constricts the blood vessels to the hands and feet, causing our extremities to become cooler.) As the patient thinks about raising the temperature of his or her fingers, the biofeedback equipment converts the actual temperature of the fingers into a sound or a display that presents "feedback," in real time, about how the patient is doing. With practice, the patient can be taught to increase blood flow to the fingers and thereby raise their temperature, thus regulating a process we formerly thought was beyond the mind's influence (a so-called involuntary reflex).

Because of the direct connection between the nervous system and the immune system, self-regulation techniques learned through the use of biofeedback have the potential of giving us some voluntary control over processes that affect the immune system. It's possible that biofeedback will enable us to bring consciousness to every organ, tissue, and cell of the body, including the cells of the immune system.

Although you can self-regulate without biofeedback equipment, in my experience people like having concrete evidence that they are undeniably controlling certain physiological changes. Eventually, after they have mastered self-regulation techniques with the help of an expert, they can continue using the techniques at home without any biofeedback equipment or with an inexpensive unit. This takes away the dependence on another person and empowers patients to take responsibility for their own healing.

Biofeedback can be used to reverse some of the immune system's learned responses, such as allergies. It's also useful for any stress-related disorder, including asthma, hypertension, irritable bowel syndrome, chronic pain, migraines, immune disorders, and more.

Breathing Exercises

In many ways, breath is the essence of life, for our bodies cannot function without taking in oxygen. In fact, all of us are born knowing how to breathe properly, but somewhere along the line we forget how. Stress and anxiety make our muscles tense and our breathing fast and shallow. This chest-breathing does not provide an optimal air exchange, and it is tiring because it uses up a lot of energy. Proper breathing—abdominal breathing—uses less energy and supplies our body with more oxygen.

Deep breathing helps to calm us down. It also helps to oxygenate the brain and to cleanse the lungs. In addition, taking deep breaths helps pump our lymphatic fluid through the lymphatic channels, sweeping waste products like dead cells, bacteria, and virus particles out of our lymph nodes.

A full abdominal breath moves eight to ten times as much air as a chest breath.[28] Every deep breath is an opportunity to feed the brain and to let go of tension. In the absence of abdominal breathing, the body will use sighs and yawns to get a deep air exchange and to relieve tension.

Since breathing is something we do all day, we have plenty of opportunities to try to get it right. Try to remember to take deep breaths from time to time all day. For the full effect, take a few minutes to concentrate just on your breathing.

1. Start with one or two full exhalations, breathing in through the nose and out through the mouth (like a sigh of relief). Remember to squeeze out the last bit of air at the end of each exhalation. This will enable you to take in more air when you subsequently inhale.

2. Take several deep, abdominal breaths. Some people imagine a balloon in their belly slowly filling up with air. After about ten breaths you should feel both more alert and more calm.

There are more complicated breathing exercises—for example, the *pranayama* techniques associated with yoga—but you can do deep breathing anywhere, anytime, with no assistance from anyone. If you combine abdominal breathing with meditating or deep relaxation, soon you will condition your nervous system to slow down quickly with just a few deep breaths. Deep breathing is always good for relieving tension, but it is even more effective when your body associates it with total physical relaxation and emotional calm.

Deep Relaxation

Deep relaxation is often combined with other stress-relieving techniques, such as deep breathing or meditation. The purpose of deep relaxation is to eliminate tension from your body. While you want to stay alert and focused while meditating, you may wish to use deep relaxation just to calm down or even to fall asleep. Some people combine deep relaxation with positive or healing affirmations (more about healing visualization is included in Chapter 13).

Progressive relaxation is simply a systematic way of relaxing all your muscles from head to toe—or, more correctly, from toe to head. Here's what to do:

1. Pick a comfortable place to lie on your back (on the floor or in bed). Lie with your feet apart and your arms out flat, palms up.

2. Start with five deep breaths, imagining that you are sinking farther into the floor (or bed) with each exhalation.

3. Now, systematically tense and relax your muscles, one muscle group at a time, starting with your feet and working your way up to your shoulders, neck, head, and finally face. (If you've never tried this before, you'll be amazed at how much tension is carried in your facial muscles alone.)

4. If you wish, imagine that you are someplace pleasant—on a cloud, at the beach, whatever works for you.

5. Finish with ten more deep breaths.

Many of us get so keyed up during the day that we're not even aware how physically tense we are. Maintaining all that tension in our muscles uses up energy and perpetuates an upregulated stress response. As we've already seen, the "relaxation response" has the opposite effect and helps to undo all the damage caused by an excess of stress hormones.

Emotional Support

What keeps us going when things get tough? How do we recharge our emotional batteries? To whom do we turn when we're in trouble?

Many people are sustained by their religious faith. Some individuals have an intimate relationship with God or another religious figure, while others feel a more generalized spiritual connection to a higher power or to the universe. There is no question that faith is sustaining, and there is evidence that faith is curative as well. One survey of heart surgery patients revealed that those who did not have religious faith had a death rate more than three times greater than those who did. Another study of patients recovering from hip fractures found that those who regarded God as a source of strength and comfort were able to walk farther when discharged and had lower rates of depression than those with little faith.[29]

Religious faith is often accompanied by social support in the form of a congregation or church group. Several studies indicate that churchgoers have lower blood pressure, lower suicide rates, less depression, and half the risk of dying from coronary artery disease as people who rarely go to church.[30] Although churchgoing may be associated with clean living, there is evidence that it's the emotional support, not the lifestyle, that makes the difference.

The town of Roseto, Pennsylvania, had an unusually low incidence of heart disease. The folks in Roseto had a sedentary lifestyle and consumed plenty of calories, including meat and fat, and many of them smoked—but they still had few heart attacks. When researchers descended on Roseto to determine why, they discovered a remarkably close-knit community made up of large extended families. The social network in Roseto acted as a buffer against stress and stress-related diseases. Social support turned out to be a more important predictor of heart disease than health habits.

Further evidence that emotional support can counteract the unhealthy effects of stress comes from a study of Swedish men. Seven hundred and fifty-two men were given free medical exams. When they were contacted again seven years later, 41 had died. Men who had originally reported being extremely stressed had a death rate three times greater than those who reported placid lives. However, among men who had dependable emotional support, there was *no relationship whatever* between high stress levels and death. Social support proved to be an antidote to stress.[31]

I believe that human beings are not meant to "go it alone." (This helps explain why solitary confinement is one of our society's harshest punishments.) Time and again I see my hospital patients brighten when visitors stop by, and I've had patients rally against unbelievable odds because they knew they had to get well for an important social event such as a wedding, christening, birthday, bar mitzvah, or graduation. People who are socially active—who love and are loved—are more resistant to disease and death than people who are isolated, embittered, or distrustful. Connected people are hardier; lonely people are sicker.

Research has shown that breast cancer patients who receive group social support may live twice as long as those who do not.[32] Evidence is increasing that support groups, behavior therapy, and stress management can improve the survival rate of heart attack patients by as much as 25 percent—which is comparable to the effect of beta-blockers.[33]

Modern life moves us toward isolation rather than connectedness. We may attend five schools in three years, or change jobs repeatedly, or live thousands of miles away from our parents and our children. Just as social connectedness protects us from stress, isolation leaves us vulnerable to distress. Part of stress management, then, is encouraging supportive relationships. It is possible to seek and receive emotional support from a spouse, family members, friends, a support group, or even a pet. The time that you put into these relationships is not frivolous; it's an investment in your health.

Exercise

Everybody knows exercise is good for you. It has cardiovascular benefits (such as low-ered cholesterol levels and lowered blood pressure), it helps protect bone density, it helps with weight control, it increases blood flow to the brain (which can improve mental health and cognitive function), and it relieves stress. Aerobic exercise enhances oxygenation throughout the body and improves metabolic processes. Moderate exercise is immune en-hancing, but studies yield different results on this subject because there are so many variables involved, including the type of exercise, the methods used to measure immunological com-petence, the fitness of the individual, and the timing of the observation (some immune effects are transient). There is growing evidence that regular moderate exercise may be pro-tective against cancer. If you don't already exercise regularly, please start.

If you have been seriously ill, you may need to start with physical therapy to relieve discomfort and to promote flexibility. Hot packs, range-of-motion exercises, and other body work may be helpful, including massage therapy, gentle chiropractic adjustments, and acu-puncture. From here you can move on to stretching and strengthening exercises. Do not attempt a program that is too vigorous or you may set back your recovery. Slowly introduce a gradual advancement of well-tolerated aerobic exercise as you feel stronger.

If you've been physically inactive, there are many ways to get started on an exercise program. One of my older patients started by jogging to her mailbox and back. Eventually she was jogging several miles a week—something she never imagined she'd be able to accom-plish.

If you have a health condition, talk to your physician about an exercise regimen that would be appropriate for you. Once you get started, don't judge yourself harshly, and defi-nitely don't compare yourself to the aerobics instructors in leotards on television. Instead of thinking "that was nothing," tell yourself: "I did it!" Acknowledge yourself for whatever you achieved, even the little things.

Try to exercise for at least half an hour at a time, preferably several days a week. It takes a half hour of exercise to improve the circulation to the deeper organs of your body (such as your spleen, liver, kidneys, and bone marrow) and to circulate the lymphatic fluid and flush out your lymph nodes. In addition, it takes about thirty minutes of aerobic exercise to awaken the dormant white blood cells that have been parked on the inside walls of your blood vessels and to sweep them back into circulation, where they can do their job most effectively.

Overexertion is not healthy. In addition to the risk of muscle damage, overexertion can cause an "open window" while the immune system is temporarily suppressed. After pro-longed and excessive exercise, the number of lymphocytes in the blood is reduced and NK cell function is depressed, which can leave the body more vulnerable to infection.[34] This is not a problem, however, with moderate exercise—and by far most exercise can be considered moderate—which is immune enhancing.

Hypnosis and Self-Hypnosis

In his book *Discovering the Power of Self-Hypnosis,* Stanley Fisher, Ph.D., notes that all hypnosis is really self-hypnosis. Dr. Fisher compares self-hypnosis to a pathway to a special room within ourselves where we can restructure our thoughts, beliefs, feelings, and responses.[35]

COMMONLY ASKED QUESTION NO. 16:

Will I lose control if I let someone hypnotize me?

Hypnosis is poorly understood. In the past, it was associated with kooks and quacks and with overdramatic situations in which people were put into a trance and made to do outrageous things. I can see the fear in some of my patients when I refer them for hypnotherapy with the certified hypnotherapist who works in my office.

In truth, hypnosis is simply a state of focused concentration. During hypnosis, you're mentally alert but physically at rest. You're not asleep, and you do not lose control, although hypnotized subjects may be more receptive to input from other people. People who are hypnotized are able to set aside distractions—sounds, feelings, or sensations—and to fix their attention upon certain thoughts or images. We're actually in a hypnotic trance whenever we're thoroughly preoccupied—for example, when we're so involved with an activity that we don't hear the phone ring, or we're so lost in thought that we drive right past the highway exit we had planned to take.

During hypnosis, the background fades, and we can communicate clearly with all aspects of the self—both body and mind. If we imagine a hot summer day, we can see the scene, feel the warmth of the sun, and re-create the experience. In this state, we can use the power of suggestion to modify bodily functions that are usually considered involuntary and beyond the reach of conscious thought.

Hypnosis can cause powerful changes within the body and is used in mind/body healing to influence the action of the immune cells. Medical literature gives many examples of patients who were cured of skin disorders and other problems while hypnotized. Self-hypnosis is also useful for behavior modification (for example, helping people to stop smoking or to stop overeating) and surgery (to make the surgery less stressful for the body and to make recovery more rapid). It is also used for pain control (the hypnotized person is aware of the pain, but is able to ignore it) and stress reduction. During hypnosis, patients can face a stressful problem without having their body switch into an upregulated stress response. After they focus on the problem, they can set it aside instead of continuing to agitate over it.

A trained hypnotherapist can give you self-hypnosis exercises to practice at home. Although self-hypnosis is described in different books, I recommend seeking the advice of a professional who can get you started on the right track.

Meditation

Meditation is mindful relaxation. During meditation we can bring about the "relaxation response" that counteracts the effects of stress and distress. Our heart and breathing rates slow down, our blood pressure normalizes, our muscles relax, and we stop churning out stress hormones. Meditation is so effective at reducing stress that in 1984 the National Institutes of Health recommended meditation over prescription drugs as the first treatment for mild hypertension.[36]

To meditate, all you need is yourself, a quiet space, and maybe a chair or pillow.

1. Pick a quiet spot—someplace restful, with no distractions. Turn off the phone, and let people know it's not okay to interrupt you. If you meditate regularly in the same location within your home, that spot will soon become associated with peaceful contemplation. Just sitting there, or even passing by, will be calming.

2. Pick a good time—not after eating (you'll fall asleep). Many people meditate before breakfast and/or before dinner. Try to meditate for ten to twenty minutes, preferably twice a day. If you have only five minutes, then take five. Maybe it will turn into ten.

3. Get comfortable, but don't lie down (that's *too* comfortable). You can sit in a chair or on a pillow on the floor. Put your hands in your lap or on your legs. You want to be able to relax, but you also need to stay awake.

4. Close your eyes.

5. Start with some deep breaths. Focus on abdominal breathing for a few minutes to get centered.

6. Deeply relax from your feet to your head. Let go of tension with each exhalation.

7. As you sit quietly, breathing slowly, focus on a word or phrase with each exhalation. Some people use a prayer or a fragment of a prayer; others have a special mantra; some use the word *one;* others simply count from one to ten over and over. In her book *Minding the Body, Mending the Mind,* Joan Borysenko, Ph.D., refers to this as "dropping the anchor of attention."[37]

8. Your mind will definitely wander. Observe your thoughts, but let them go. This process is sometimes compared to watching a stream go by. Don't force, stop, or judge your thoughts—and do not write memos to yourself! Refocus after you get distracted. The idea is to get beyond your conscious thoughts to a place where it is quiet. Gradually you will peel

off layers of stress and move deeper and deeper into a state of relaxed awareness in which you are completely present in the moment.

9. Avoid performance anxiety. Whatever you're doing is just fine. It's important to maintain a passive attitude. Don't worry about your success or about whether you're meditating correctly.

10. When your time is up (it's okay to look at your watch), sit quietly for a couple of minutes before getting up.

Sometimes disconcerting or distressing thoughts emerge during meditation. If your mind has been wrapped around a problem for a long time, it may choose to reveal this problem while you are peacefully meditating. Dr. Borysenko compares this process to the body rejecting a splinter.[38] It is a healthful process. Try to meditate through it.

Meditating gets easier with practice. Jon Kabat-Zinn, Ph.D., founder of the Stress Reduction Clinic at the University of Massachusetts Medical Center, compares meditating to weaving a parachute. Meditation is a way of being. "You don't want to start weaving the parachute when you're about to jump out of the plane," he explains. You have to weave it day in and day out ahead of time so that when you need it, it will hold you.[39]

Yoga

The word *yoga* means "yoke" or "union." Yoga combines physical, mental, and spiritual energies to enhance health and well-being. It also is meant to help us realize that the individual is one with the universe.

The earliest descriptions of yoga date from the second century B.C. in India. Since that time—and probably since before that time—people have been using the physical postures, breathing exercises, and meditation practices of yoga to reduce stress and to help regulate bodily processes that are usually carried out unconsciously. People tend to enjoy yoga because it gives the body something to do while meditating. It combines full-body strengthening and conditioning with mindful relaxation.

Yoga has many different aspects. A common form is hatha yoga, which combines physical postures with mental awareness. Each position creates a balance between movement and stillness, and different positions increase circulation in different parts of the body. *Pranayama* focuses on the regulation of breathing. When the mind is calm and attentive, the breathing is steady and rhythmic. When the mind is restless, the breathing will be jagged.

Yoga is associated with vitality and peace of mind—both physical and mental limberness. Yoga can be used to reduce anxiety, control pain, and alleviate a wide variety of stress-related disorders.

⌒ MEG'S STORY

When Meg, a fifty-five-year-old divorcée, first came to see me, her main symptoms were persistent fatigue and depression. She didn't have the entire constellation of signs and symptoms required for the diagnosis of chronic fatigue immune dysfunction syndrome, but simple activities like housework or yardwork exhausted her, and she told me that at her job she sometimes fell asleep sitting in her chair.

Meg had assorted other complaints, including multiple food allergies (because of these, she ate little), many chemical sensitivities (to perfume, fresh paint, and gas, among others), and drug allergies as well. She had chronic rhinitis, recurrent yeast infections, and frequent sore throats. Meg also reported that she felt shaky and light-headed if she didn't eat or if meals were delayed. In addition, Meg's temperature was lower than normal (her resting axillary temperature was 96.8 degrees, as opposed to a normal reading of 97.8 to 98.2 degrees).

I talked with Meg about her lifestyle and learned that she had been under terrific stress for several years. A couple of years before, a dog had bitten both her hands, which plunged Meg into a deep depression because she needed her hands to produce her artwork. In addition, one of Meg's brothers had died of lung cancer, and the other had received a heart transplant. Her nephew had serious asthma, and her niece had cancer. Meg currently worked long hours as an office manager, a job that was extremely stressful. She had also gone back to college, but she could barely get through her classes. Although her depression sometimes lifted, her energy level never improved.

After I learned all of this, the pieces of Meg's puzzle started to fit into place. On her chart I wrote, "Check labs. Rest. Stress management." I suspected that Meg's chronic stress overload had caused low adrenal function (stress taxes the adrenal glands). I also felt Meg probably had an underactive thyroid, allergic asthma, allergic rhinitis, reactive hypoglycemia, and possibly an underlying fungal hypersensitivity.

Meg's test results basically confirmed my suspicions. She had severe reactive hypoglycemia (her fasting blood sugar level was 105, but three hours into a glucose tolerance test it measured just 32), low adrenal function, and borderline functional hypothyroidism.

I started Meg on an immune-empowering regimen that ultimately included natural desiccated thyroid, a high-potency multivitamin/mineral supplement especially formulated for patients with chronic fatigue, a homeopathic remedy for allergies, supplements for adrenal support, buffered vitamin C powder, probiotics (such as acidophilus and bifidus), prebiotics (to support the probiotics), CoQ10, borage oil, chromium picolinate, quercetin, dry vitamin E, and a preparation of Chinese ginseng. Meg also started taking intravenous vitamin C with nutrients. Meg's gynecologist had placed her on estrogen replacement therapy, and I recommended a "Women's Formula" calcium and magnesium supplement to help prevent osteoporosis.

I referred Meg to our nutritionist, with whom she worked out a hypoglycemic, hypoallergenic, yeast-free Immune Empowering Diet. I also referred Meg for stress management, but this did not appeal to her. We talked about the importance of rest and lifestyle modification at Meg's first visit and at every visit thereafter, but she did not immediately take this as seriously as I hoped she would.

Meg began to feel better, but for me the most exciting part of her recovery was her recognition of the involvement of stress in her illness. When she finally made this connection in a heartfelt manner, it made a huge difference in the way that she saw things and in the way events affected her. She started practicing yoga and made important attitude adjustments toward her family, boss, and colleagues. Over time, Meg worked on becoming less reactive to stressors. She learned to shrug it off when her boss yelled at her. As she started feeling less overwhelmed, she began to take more interest in her life.

I raised the level of Meg's thyroid medication and also added DHEA to her regimen. Overall Meg was feeling so much better that she never pursued allergy testing. She now had increased energy, increased learning ability, increased powers of concentration, and increased tolerance for activity. She mentioned that she had days when she could be in motion all day long without collapsing.

About two years after her initial visit, Meg had finally become accepting of the need to make some major lifestyle changes. She found a new job that paid more, which helped alleviate some of her financial stress. "I have changed my whole attitude," she told me. Meg really felt that she was now able to control her stress, instead of the other way around. As an extra bonus, she found that as long as she was handling her stress well, she seldom needed to use her asthma medications. Meg learned to set boundaries and to say no, and was more accepting of her limitations. If she got a sore throat, that was a sign for her to cut back.

Meg continued with her intravenous vitamin C treatments and felt she definitely benefited from them. Unfortunately, her insurance company stopped covering them because vitamin C is a nutritionally based therapy. Meg kept up with her other supplements, although we had to modify her regimen somewhat because realistically she couldn't work in taking supplements three times a day.

At her last visit, Meg was cheerful and serene. She still had problems in her life—who doesn't?—and suffered an occasional sleepless night, but she was no longer the fatigued, depressed woman she had been when we'd first met. With attitude adjustment, stress management, and an immune-empowering regimen—and without antidepressants—Meg had returned not only to a more functional life, but to a much happier and healthier one as well.

Chapter 9

❧

GUT AND LIVER FUNCTION: WHAT'S THE STORY?

> If it be true that precocious old age is due to poisoning of the
> tissues, it is clear that agents which arrest intestinal
> putrefaction must at the same time postpone and ameliorate
> the conditions of old age.
>
> —ELIE METCHNIKOFF (1845–1916)

When Elie Metchnikoff—deputy director of the Pasteur Institute, originator of the theory of phagocytosis, and winner of a Nobel prize in 1908 for his work in immunity—suggested that humans should consume milk fermented with lactobacilli (i.e., yogurt) for good health and longevity, people were skeptical. Metchnikoff believed that beneficial lactobacilli could displace less favorable organisms in the gut, some of which were known even during his time to produce toxins. Metchnikoff also believed that the status of a patient's intestinal flora could affect the outcome of an infection.

Although we lack sufficient double-blind placebo-controlled studies to satisfy all members of the medical community that fermented milk products contribute to a healthy old age, it is unquestionably true that Metchnikoff was on the right track. We may never have irrefutable scientific proof about his theory, in part due to the limitations inherent in conducting experiments with living, breathing human beings. However, we do have clinical evidence in abundance, along with plenty of supporting studies, indicating that gut health is far more important than most people (including physicians) realize.

DETOXIFICATION: THE MISSING LINK

As I've mentioned before, we are constantly bombarded with poisonous substances from outside the body (exotoxins) as well as inside our body (endotoxins). These poisons are processed primarily by the liver, which alters the chemical composition of toxins so they can be excreted as waste products. If the liver is already overwhelmed—and it has plenty to do, even under the best of circumstances—then toxins may accumulate in the tissues of the liver or elsewhere in the body. This bioaccumulation of toxins can adversely affect the immune system and other bodily systems as well. It's amazing to realize that what starts as toxic overload can end up as any number of illnesses, from chronic fatigue to autoimmune problems to immunosuppression. There is even some evidence linking toxins to autism and certain behavioral problems.

Reducing our exposure to toxins has been discussed elsewhere in this book. In addition to limiting our exposure to harmful chemicals, we also can alleviate our toxic burden by making changes on the inside. By making sure the gastrointestinal tract is healthy, by clearing the body's detoxification pathways, and by improving the liver's detoxifying capabilities, we can revitalize our ability to handle toxins efficiently.

Under the congestion model of disease, most chronic diseases are traced to poor elimination of waste products from the bowel or to poor detoxification processes. The buildup of waste products and toxins leads to cellular "suffocation," and from there, to disease. If the immune system is constantly diverting nutrients and energy to detoxification, it can't keep up with its defense and repair duties. When cells throughout the body do not take in the nutrients they need, or get rid of toxins promptly, this can result in increased oxidant stress (free radical damage as well as mitochondrial problems) and subsequent immunosuppression (which may show up as recurrent or chronic infections). When the bioaccumulation of toxins causes disease, detoxification becomes the missing link between sickness and health.

Because microorganisms in the gastrointestinal tract generate toxins that must be processed by the liver, a good place to begin any detoxification program is with the bowel. Making sure the intestinal tract contains the correct balance of microorganisms and digestive enzymes is called *gastrointestinal detoxification*.

Decreasing the amount of toxins that originate in the gut decreases, in turn, the burden placed on the liver. We also can help the liver detoxify these poisons more efficiently by providing it with generous quantities of the nutrients and cofactors it needs to function effectively, as well as with plenty of antioxidants to protect it from the free radical damage that can occur during the biotransformation of toxins. Rehabilitating the liver's ability to process toxins is known as *liver detoxification*.

As you can see, *detoxification* refers to two different processes: the act of breaking down toxins so they can be excreted, and the process of clearing the body of excess toxins. Some people refer to gastrointestinal and liver detoxification as "cleansing" to avoid any confusion, but detoxification is really the more accurate term.

Detoxification (cleansing) isn't the answer to everything, but it does have a place in any program designed to combat chronic illness. Someone who has a mild overgrowth of yeast in the digestive tract will require less intervention than someone who has been living for years with a toxic bowel, but in either case, detoxification treats underlying problems that undermine good health.

Detoxification is like wiping the slate clean and starting anew. It's a process of restoration, like rebuilding an old house that has acquired layers of aluminum siding, old paint, peeling wallpaper, and cracked linoleum. First you strip away the damaged parts in order to expose the strong and stable parts of the home; then you carefully rehabilitate the original structure until it looks (and functions) like new.

I've found that I keep returning to this concept of the "clean slate" in my practice. For me to fully appreciate each new patient's problems, I have to wipe my own mental blackboard clean. For patients to get well, they often have to drop their preconceptions and expectations about what they think is happening and assume a more open attitude.

You may have heard the ancient Chinese legend about the wise man and the scholar. The scholar, who knows a great deal, goes to visit the wise man, about whom he has heard much. The wise man offers the scholar tea, and proceeds to fill his cup. The tea wells up and over the rim of the cup, and still the wise man keeps pouring. The scholar jumps up, indignant, and demands to know what the wise man thinks he is doing. Unfazed, the wise man replies that in order to learn, one must become an empty vessel, for it is impossible to add to a cup that is already full. Just as the scholar needed to set aside his knowledge in order to really hear the wise man, so does the body (including the bowel) benefit from being "emptied" and then restored and rebalanced when it has acquired functional problems.

Detoxification: A Concept Whose Time Has Come

I didn't always take gastrointestinal and liver detoxification as seriously as I do today. When I was first practicing medicine, it seemed like most of the people who favored detoxification were into coffee enemas, colonics (colon cleansing), and other procedures or potions that just didn't strike me as very scientific. Detoxification was something you'd encounter in a fringe practice, and coffee enemas were sure to obscure my efforts to establish a respectable practice based on progressive medicine.

On the other side of the issue were the traditional allopathic doctors and the heavy-duty medical journals, which recognized the existence of localized bowel and liver diseases, but paid little (if any) attention to the importance of gut and liver support, or to the effects of toxins on the body. The traditional medical model is to treat symptoms with medications, not to worry about xenobiotics (chemical compounds that are not-self) or nutritional intervention. Even today the importance of detoxification is highly underrecognized by the medical profession.

I would like to acknowledge the brilliant work of my colleague Jeff Bland, whom I've referred to before but must mention again in this context. He has been greatly instrumental in increasing awareness of the importance of liver detoxification, and has helped to scientifically support its transit from the fringes of medical care toward the mainstream. Times definitely are changing. I was happy to see a 1996 article in *The Journal of the American Medical Association (JAMA)* entitled "Biotherapeutic Agents: A Neglected Modality for the Treatment and Prevention of Selected Intestinal and Vaginal Infections." This article concludes that the administration of selected organisms—including lactobacilli—can be beneficial in the treatment of certain types of diarrhea and possibly vaginal infections as well.[1] Metchnikoff would be pleased.

Biochemical Individuality (Again)

Remember Mr. Benedi, who consumed Tylenol and ended up with a liver transplant? And Mr. Latimer, who went out to mow his (chemically treated) lawn and was never the same again? Both of these men were poisoned when their detoxification pathways became overwhelmed.

These stories are striking because neither Mr. Benedi nor Mr. Latimer did anything all that unusual, but they suffered permanent physical damage. These are yet more illustrations of biochemical individuality. Each of us handles toxins—which include acetaminophen and pesticides, as well as innumerable other substances—in a unique way.

Here's another illustration. A standard anticancer drug, 5-fluorouracil, is utilized by some people, completely ineffectual for others, and toxic for the rest. Why? Because of genetic differences in detoxification. A person with normal amounts of the enzyme DPD will clear a dose of 5-fluorouracil in 8 to 10 minutes. However, someone with superfast DPD enzymes will clear the drug in seconds and get little or no therapeutic effect. Another individual with abnormally low amounts of DPD may require 159 minutes to clear the drug, a situation which can prove fatal. Researchers have observed hundredfold differences in enzyme activity, and also have found that slow detoxifiers are more likely to get cancer.[2]

Factors That Affect Our Detoxification Capabilities

Whether or not you are an efficient detoxifier depends on many factors, some of which you can control and some of which you can't. The list includes:

• **Age.** Younger people are generally at an advantage when it comes to detoxification, in part because they have accumulated less cellular wear and tear. Also, enzyme activity and nutrient resources tend to decline with age.

• **Nutritional status.** The detoxification process requires different nutrient cofactors. If these cofactors aren't available in sufficient amounts, toxins will not be efficiently processed.

• **Hormone levels.** Hormones—including estrogen, testosterone, insulin, cortisol, and adrenaline, among others—are released and metabolized according to the body's needs.

Birth control pills and steroids contribute to the body's hormone burden, and hormones are processed by the liver.

- **Genetic predisposition.** Some people are born with sluggish detoxification pathways due to insufficient enzyme activity. This is the luck of the draw, but we now know that we can partially offset genetic predispositions with the appropriate nutritional intervention.

- **Immunological competence.** A flagging immune system is less able to control the proliferation of unfavorable microorganisms, and it is less efficient at filtering antigen/antibody complexes from the blood and lymph. As we've already seen, disruptions in immune balance tend to spiral into more serious conditions as energy and nutrients are diverted away from cellular defense and repair. Toxins can build up, and chronic illness can develop. Detoxification is one way to break this vicious cycle.

- **Lifestyle and habits.** Smoking, antibiotics and other prescription medications, nonsteroidal anti-inflammatory drugs (NSAIDs such as Advil), food additives, and environmental pollutants all place toxic burdens on the body. If your body is already busy trying to handle all these demands, it will have a limited capacity to deal with additional detoxification needs.

- **Gastrointestinal health.** As Metchnikoff knew way back in the early 1900s, organisms in the gut can release toxins that are absorbed into the bloodstream. Imbalances in the gastrointestinal tract can cause excessive amounts of toxins to reach the liver, which can contribute to a backlog in detoxification pathways.

- **Liver disease.** A liver that is diseased (for example, with hepatitis, which causes inflammation, or cirrhosis, which causes scarring) is less able to keep up with its detoxification duties.

HOW DIGESTION IS SUPPOSED TO WORK

Our digestive tract breaks our food down into usable particles, which are then absorbed into the bloodstream. Because we take in undesirable microorganisms along with our food, nature has provided the gastrointestinal tract with plenty of immune support to prevent antigens from taking hold in the body.

It has been estimated that there are more bacteria in and on one person at any time than there are people on this earth. The intestines alone are inhabited by 100 trillion bacteria.[3] In fact, the total weight of bacteria in the gut is thought to equal the weight of the liver (around 3½ pounds)!

Intestinal flora influence our nutritional status, response to medications, aging processes, handling of toxins, development of cancer, and resistance to infection. Our intestinal ecology has a profound effect on our well-being in general, and on our immune system in particular. Following is a quick tour of the digestive tract to show why this is true.

The Mouth

Other chapters have already addressed the importance of what goes into our mouth. Your body will thank you for eating a high-fiber, nutrient-dense diet with plenty of pure water, a reasonable amount of protein, and a minimum of sugar, chemicals, and contaminants.

The process of breaking down food begins with chewing. Actually, most of us don't chew enough. I got into the habit of eating fast when I was young—probably for survival, having an older brother who was one of the fastest eaters in the East—and since then I've had to learn to slow down. Chewing grinds up food into small pieces and mixes them with saliva, which contains enzymes that start digesting food. Each bite spends less than a minute in the mouth before beginning its long journey through the rest of the digestive tract.

The entire gastrointestinal tract, including the mouth, is lined with mucosal tissue that secretes the protective antibodies known as secretory IgA. As I've mentioned elsewhere, secretory IgA is an important part of our immune defenses. It inhibits the penetration of antigens into the body and also helps to neutralize toxins. High levels of secretory IgA protect us from bacteria, viruses, parasites, yeast, and toxins. We can easily assess the status of a patient's secretory IgA by measuring its level in saliva.

The Stomach

Digestion continues in the stomach, which churns food for two to four hours, mixing it with hydrochloric acid and digestive enzymes secreted by the stomach lining. Many Americans are afraid of "stomach acid" because of the intense amount of advertising put out by the manufacturers of antacids, but in truth the highly acidic environment of the stomach is a key part of the digestive process. In fact, low stomach acid (hypochlorhydria) is more common than most people, including doctors, realize, and can greatly impede proper digestion and cause bloating and gas. The stomach provides the perfect surroundings in which pepsin (an enzyme that works on proteins) can do its job, and also kills off many antigens. Only the most durable microorganisms survive the passage through an optimally acidified stomach.

The Small Intestine

From the stomach, food passes into the duodenum, the first part of the small intestine. Here digestive enzymes from the liver, gallbladder, and pancreas are added to the partially digested food. The liver and gallbladder both secrete bile (when it leaves the liver, bile is somewhat diluted, but when it leaves the gallbladder, bile is concentrated). Bile works on fats and helps with the absorption of essential fatty acids and fat-soluble vitamins. Pancreatic enzymes—including chymotrypsin, trypsin, amylase, and lipase—help digest food further. Because pancreatic and intestinal enzymes need a more alkaline environment in which to work (less acidic than the stomach), the pancreas also releases bicarbonate to help establish the correct pH level in the intestines.

Food spends from one to four hours in the small intestine, which generally is about 25 feet long. Glands in the lining of the small intestine secrete more digestive enzymes. Food that has been sufficiently digested at this point is absorbed into the small blood vessels in the lining of the intestine. This absorption process is selective. When the small intestine is functioning properly, beneficial nutrients are absorbed through its mucosal lining, but toxins and antigens are not. This explains why the integrity of the mucosal lining is so vital to our good health.

All those billions of intestinal microorganisms I mentioned earlier maintain a complex and somewhat precarious balance with their human host. A symbiotic relationship—one that benefits both sides—exists as long as the correct balance of beneficial bacteria and yeast is maintained. We provide a warm and secure environment and a steady supply of nutrients to the intestinal flora, and they, in return, provide many beneficial services for us (see below).

Peristalsis

Food progresses through the digestive tract by means of *peristalsis,* the rhythmic contraction of muscles that squeezes undigested food along. Fiber helps to keep the inside of the gastrointestinal tract clean by picking up waste products and transporting them out of the body.

Beneficial (and not so beneficial) microorganisms adhere to the mucosal lining of the intestinal tract to keep from being swept away. The ability of a microorganism to adhere to the epithelial cells of a particular host will determine whether or not it can successfully colonize that species. Different strains compete for space and, just to make things more interesting, various types of epithelial cells at different sites have striking differences in how suitable they are for the adherence of individual kinds of bacteria.[4] This helps explain why different bacteria colonize different parts of the GI tract.

The Large Intestine (Colon)

Although most nutrients have already been absorbed by this point, the remaining food spends about ten hours winding its way through the large intestine. At about 5 feet long, the large intestine isn't nearly as long as the small intestine, but it is over twice as wide (about 2½ inches).

Like the small intestine, the large intestine is colonized by microorganisms. There are at least fifty genera of bacteria in the large intestine, and several hundred species.[5] Most of the microorganisms in the human large intestine are anaerobes, meaning they do not require oxygen to complete their metabolic processes.

The large intestine primarily digests fiber and absorbs water. Toxins and waste products accumulate in the large intestine and are excreted as fecal matter. Ideally, the contents of the large intestine should not linger too long. A healthy gastrointestinal tract with an adequate supply of fiber usually produces at least one ample, effortless bowel movement a day.

The Portal Vein

The portal vein gathers nutrient-rich blood from the network of blood vessels in and around the stomach and intestines and transports it to the liver for further processing. This is a little like emptying a full net's catch onto the deck of a fishing boat. In addition to a variety of fish you might also find sharks, weeds, jellyfish, mermaids, or anything else from the deep sea. The liver sorts out the amino acids, fatty acids, sugars, vitamins, and minerals from the toxins, antigens, cellular debris, and other substances that have been absorbed from the gut. (Liver function is discussed in more detail later in this chapter.)

The portal vein and liver are not considered parts of the digestive tract. However, the body could not get nourishment and energy without them. Also, the welfare of the liver depends in part upon how well the digestive tract is working, which in turn depends upon who is living there.

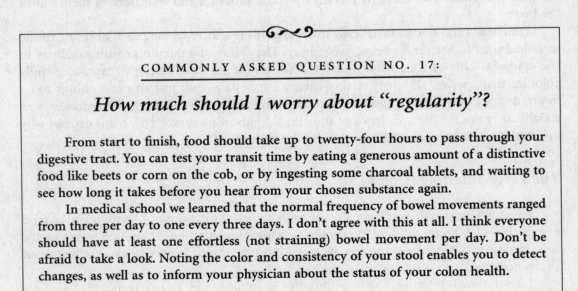

ᏨᎨᎧ

COMMONLY ASKED QUESTION NO. 17:

How much should I worry about "regularity"?

From start to finish, food should take up to twenty-four hours to pass through your digestive tract. You can test your transit time by eating a generous amount of a distinctive food like beets or corn on the cob, or by ingesting some charcoal tablets, and waiting to see how long it takes before you hear from your chosen substance again.

In medical school we learned that the normal frequency of bowel movements ranged from three per day to one every three days. I don't agree with this at all. I think everyone should have at least one effortless (not straining) bowel movement per day. Don't be afraid to take a look. Noting the color and consistency of your stool enables you to detect changes, as well as to inform your physician about the status of your colon health.

ᏨᎨᎧ

The Digestive Tract

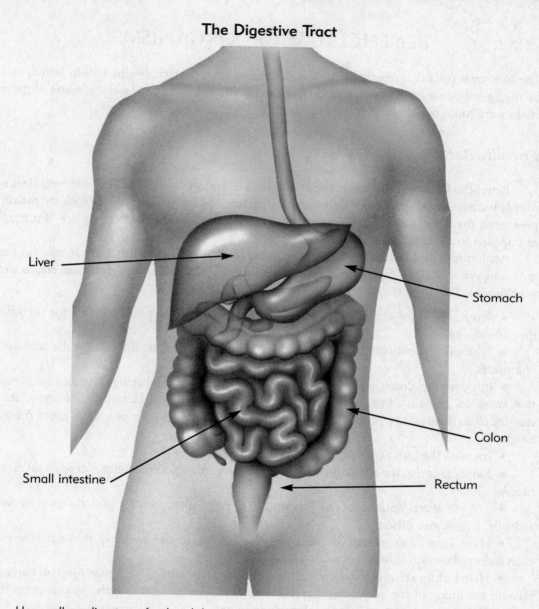

Liver

Stomach

Colon

Small intestine

Rectum

How well we digest our food and the general state of health of our digestive tract have a profound influence on our health. It is now known that many systemic disorders originate in the gut.

Illustration by Gary Carlson

BENEFICIAL MICROORGANISMS

The intestinal tract is sterile at birth. The colonization of bacteria begins within hours, and by the age of one month, newborns have characteristic adult flora.[6] However, some of these critters are more beneficial than others.

Friendly Bacteria

Beneficial bacteria that live in the gut include *Lactobacillus acidophilus* (different strains of this bacterium live primarily in the small intestine) and *Bifidobacterium bifidum* (mainly present in the large intestine). These organisms are known as *probiotics* (they are "for life," as opposed to antibiotics, which are "against life").

Acidophilus and bifidus have many beneficial effects on our health, both locally (in the gut) and systemically. They do not function in exactly the same way, but their effects are very similar. Together, they:

• Synthesize short-chain fatty acids (such as butyrate), the preferred fuel for the cells that line the colon.

• Synthesize significant amounts of the B complex vitamins, including folic acid and vitamin B_{12}.

• Improve our digestion and absorption of nutrients by producing proteases (enzymes that work on protein), lipases (enzymes that work on fat), and lactase (the enzyme that enables us to digest dairy products). More efficient digestion in turn promotes more robust health.

• Increase the bioavailability of vitamins and minerals.

• Biodegrade bacterial toxins, detoxify carcinogens, and metabolize drugs and hormones.

• Act as natural antimicrobials (helping to prevent infections by bacteria such as *Salmonella, E. coli*, and others).

• Have anticancer effects (by reducing the activity of the enzymes that catalyze the conversion of certain substances into carcinogens).[7]

• Help reduce serum cholesterol. (It is speculated that acidophilus may bind up cholesterol in the lining of the intestines, thereby reducing its absorption into the bloodstream.[8])

• Help prevent parasites from colonizing the gut.

• Decrease the amount of ammonia produced by bacteria in the gut. (This reduces the burden on the liver, which detoxifies the ammonia.)

• Inhibit the growth of undesirable microorganisms, including candida, by helping to keep the environment within the intestines optimally acidic. (This helps prevent secondary problems associated with yeast overgrowth, which can be severe.)

• Strengthen the immune system by stimulating macrophages and lymphocytes. (This, in turn, causes increased resistance to infection.)

• Indirectly stimulate the production of gamma interferon by regulating the release of certain cytokines. (This leads to increased T cell activity.)

Both healthy and unwell people can benefit from taking in large amounts of acidophilus and bifidus. These friendly bacteria are severely affected by antibiotics and can also be disrupted by many other factors, including diet, stress, diabetes, viral infections, and even space travel! Our levels of acidophilus and bifidus naturally decline with age, but this is easily corrected by eating yogurt. Some people attribute the long lives of many people in the Balkans to their ingestion of large quantities of fermented dairy products such as yogurt and kefir.

Researchers have found that germ-free animals (grown in a laboratory) have mild to moderate defects in immune function, including lower levels of natural antibodies, less responsive macrophages and neutrophils, and defective cytokine production. This suggests that the absence of gut bacteria allows the immune system to get sleepy—or, more correctly, that the beneficial endogenous intestinal flora are immune stimulating. However, nothing about the immune system is simple, so I should note that while germ-free animals are at increased risk of certain kinds of infections (for example, intracellular parasites), they fare better than control animals in other situations (for example, diseases in which the immune response is the primary cause of pathology).[9]

Friendly Yeast

Throughout this book I've issued repeated warnings about *Candida albicans,* a type of yeast that can overpopulate the human body. However, there is a beneficial yeast for the gut—no relation to *Candida albicans*—called *Saccharomyces boulardii,* which, like acidophilus and bifidus, is considered a probiotic.

S. boulardii has several beneficial effects:

• It ferments carbohydrates.

• It produces lactase, which helps us digest dairy products.

• It acidifies its environment (most yeast prefer a more alkaline environment) and strengthens mucosal tissue.

• It is antagonistic against several bacterial pathogens and against candida.

• It increases the enzyme activity of the intestinal mucosa.

• It stimulates the secretion of intestinal secretory IgA as well as other immunoglobulins.

• It increases the number of white blood cells and cells of the reticuloendothelial system, as well as complement proteins.

S. boulardii is known to prevent antibiotic-associated diarrhea (AAD)[10] and is used commonly in Europe for this purpose. Several different mechanisms could account for this, although one study points to *S. boulardii*'s ability to stimulate secretory IgA.[11]

PROBLEMS IN THE DIGESTIVE TRACT

So far we've been looking at digestion under ideal circumstances. However, as a physician I commonly see patients with bowel complaints. Problems elsewhere in the body can affect the gastrointestinal tract, and problems in the GI tract can affect other tissues and systems of the body. Like the chicken/egg dilemma, sometimes it's difficult to tell which came first, the systemic problem or the intestinal problem—but the intestinal problem comes first more often than many people realize.

The flora in the digestive tract are part of a complex ecosystem that is regulated by many factors. This important balance can be thrown off by:

- Poor diet (not enough fiber, too few nutrients, too much protein, too much sugar, etc.)
- Diarrhea, constipation, or impaired peristalsis (which can be caused by conditions such as diabetes, scleroderma, or intestinal obstructions)
- Toxins, chemical pollutants, heavy metals
- Chronic inflammation or irritation in the gut
- Stress
- Travel, exposure to new microorganisms
- Medications, antibiotics
- Hormonal fluctuations, birth control pills, steroids
- Alcohol
- Gastric surgery
- Chemotherapy, radiation
- Intestinal infections (bacterial, viral, fungal, parasitic)
- Low stomach acid, overuse of antacids
- Insufficient bile
- Inadequate amounts of pancreatic enzymes
- Decreased acidity of intestinal environment
- Advancing age
- Bacterial interactions (including competition for nutrients, production of growth inhibitors or growth promoters, and direct antibiotic effects)
- Low secretory IgA. Immunosuppression in the digestive tract will obviously affect microbial colonization, allowing pathogenic bacteria and yeast a better chance of survival. IgA deficiency is the most common immunodeficiency, affecting from 1 in 200 to 1 in 1,000

people.[12] Low levels of secretory IgA in the intestinal mucosa cause impaired resistance to harmful microorganisms, which in turn can cause more antigens to be absorbed through the walls of the intestine, placing a larger burden on the liver and other parts of the immune system.

Dysbiosis

It would be nice if intestinal flora could live in happy harmony forever, but any of the factors above can throw off the delicate balance in the gut and allow unfriendly microorganisms to flourish. A state of imbalance in gut ecology that results in disease is called *dysbiosis*.

When the wrong kinds of microorganisms colonize in the intestines, they can wreak havoc in many ways.

- Gut flora can produce toxins that enter the bloodstream, burden the liver, and poison tissues at a distance from the digestive tract.
- Bacterial overgrowth can cause fat malabsorption (because the bacteria break down bile acids, which are needed for fat digestion) as well as hypoproteinemia, a low level of protein in the blood (because the bacteria use up the protein before the host can take advantage of it).
- Intestinal flora can cause vitamin B_{12} deficiency by using the vitamin themselves and making it unavailable to the host.
- Unfriendly microorganisms can disturb the normal pH of the intestines, creating an environment more favorable for themselves and other pathogens.
- Certain bacteria can ferment carbohydrates to ethanol (alcohol), which is then absorbed into the blood. There have even been reports of "drunken" behavior associated with this abnormal gut fermentation. One of my patients was arrested for DWI. As it turned out, he had not been drinking, but his gut flora had turned him into a walking distillery.
- Pathogenic bacteria and yeast can cause the lining of the intestinal tract to become inflamed, leading to chronic bowel diseases and to the malabsorption of nutrients. Undernutrition contributes to any number of problems, from deficiency-related diseases like anemia and osteoporosis to fatigue and lowered immune competence.
- When they attach themselves to the inside of the intestines, unfriendly microorganisms can break the immune barrier. Candida yeast actually extends roots into the mucosal lining, breaching the body's first line of defense and weakening the barrier between the gut and the bloodstream.
- Intestinal flora themselves can be absorbed into the bloodstream, a feat called *translocation*. Bacterial translocation is most likely to occur when the normal ecologic balance of the intestinal flora has been disturbed, when the host's immune defenses are impaired, and/or when the mucosal barrier in the gut has been physically disrupted. Bacteria that have

translocated can invade the organs and bloodstream. Interestingly, this translocation process can induce systemic nonspecific cell-mediated immune suppression.[13] This phenomenon seems to be related to *oral tolerance,* which is the body's ability to accept foreign matter in the gut without mounting an immune defense. Oral tolerance is presently being researched for its usefulness in treating autoimmune disorders such as rheumatoid arthritis and multiple sclerosis.

• Surface proteins released by the gut flora (both friendly and unfriendly) can be absorbed into the bloodstream, where they may be recognized and attacked by the immune system. This sets the stage for immune cross-reactions and autoimmune problems. It appears that the level of exposure is more important in setting off a response than whether a particular microorganism is "good" or "bad."[14] However, once the immune system is sensitized, it will recognize more and more antigens—first new epitopes (peptide sequences) on the original antigen, then epitopes on new antigens. This phenomenon, known as *epitope spreading,* helps explain why exposure to foreign antigens that mimic self epitopes may ultimately lead to immune responses to a wide range of antigens.

• Some microorganisms set off immune reactions that persist only as long as the antigen continues to provoke an immune response. In a true autoimmune disease, the immune system consistently attacks the self and can't be persuaded to stop. Some inflammatory diseases that are autoimmune in nature don't quite fit this profile because they seem to depend upon the presence of a microbial antigen (not necessarily the live organism, but at least some particle thereof). For example, one man's arthritic symptoms went into complete remission when he was treated for the *Giardia* parasite. When he picked up another intestinal "bug," this time an ameba during a trip to Egypt, his symptoms returned. When he was treated for amebiasis, he went into remission again.[15] This kind of situation blurs the line between autoimmune and infectious diseases. Some syndromes that we regard as autoimmune diseases may actually be more correctly viewed as chronic infections with autoimmune side effects. This certainly has very important implications for treatment.

• There is evidence that a persistent immune response to a particular antigen (for example, an intestinal bacteria) can continue even in the absence of viable organisms. Microbial products that linger in the body and are not completely cleared—sometimes called *persistent microbial antigens*—have been detected weeks, months, and even years after the original intestinal infection. Some experiments have identified immunoreactive antigens and particles without finding any cellular DNA.[16] This means an intestinal infection that has come and gone can continue to cause symptoms elsewhere in the body.

Pathogenic intestinal microorganisms are especially dangerous for people who are already immunocompromised, such as AIDS patients. The intestines are a portal of entry for bacteria, viruses, fungi, and parasites that can cause life-threatening infections. Also, as we just saw, translocation from the gut can depress systemic immunity.

GI and Liver Health:
The Big Picture

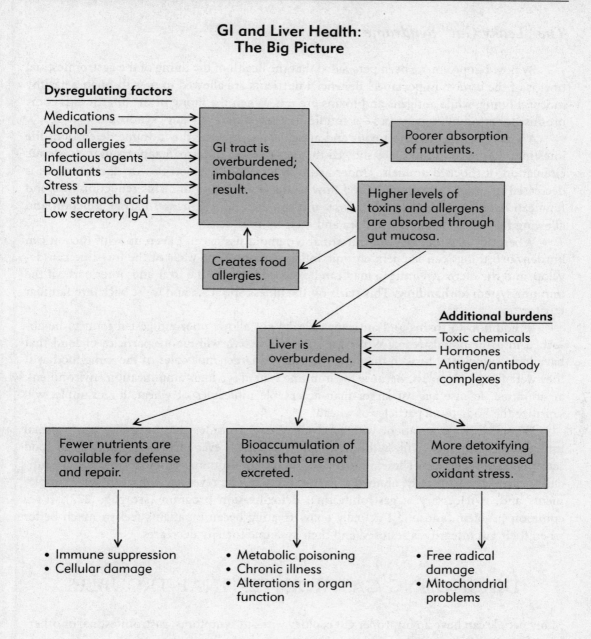

Dysregulating factors

Medications →
Alcohol →
Food allergies →
Infectious agents →
Pollutants →
Stress →
Low stomach acid →
Low secretory IgA →

GI tract is overburdened; imbalances result.

→ Poorer absorption of nutrients.

→ Higher levels of toxins and allergens are absorbed through gut mucosa.

Creates food allergies.

Liver is overburdened.

Additional burdens
← Toxic chemicals
← Hormones
← Antigen/antibody complexes

Fewer nutrients are available for defense and repair.

Bioaccumulation of toxins that are not excreted.

More detoxifying creates increased oxidant stress.

- Immune suppression
- Cellular damage

- Metabolic poisoning
- Chronic illness
- Alterations in organ function

- Free radical damage
- Mitochondrial problems

The "Leaky Gut" Syndrome

By now I hope you've been persuaded that the health of the lining of the gastrointestinal tract is of the utmost importance. Beneficial nutrients are allowed to pass through a healthy mucosal lining, while antigens and toxins are not. When the lining of the intestines is compromised, permeability increases—a condition known as "leaky gut" syndrome.

A leaky gut allows more toxins and antigens to penetrate the immune defenses of the intestines. Research in the 1960s showed that gut-derived endotoxin appears in the systemic circulation of shocked animals. Under acute stress (shock), blood flow to the intestines is decreased in order to maintain blood flow to the heart and brain. This reduction in blood flow can damage the intestinal mucosa, thereby disrupting mucosal barrier function and allowing the translocation of gut flora and their by-products.[17]

When the secretory IgA and intestinal lymphoid tissue can't keep up with the antigen burden, two things can happen: chronic inflammation of the walls of the intestine can develop, and the increased antigen load can be passed along to the liver and other parts of the immune system for handling. This starts off the Illness Spiral . . . and we're back into familiar territory.

In addition to toxins and antigens, a leaky gut allows poorly digested food to be absorbed into the bloodstream. While the immune system will ignore particles of food that have been sufficiently broken down, it will react to larger molecules of the same food as if they were foreign invaders. Because the immune system is a high-amplification environment, an immune defense against larger-than-acceptable molecules of wheat, for example, will sensitize the body to *all* particles of wheat.

Whenever I see a patient with food allergies, I consider the possibility of abnormal intestinal permeability. Unless the leaky gut is repaired, ever-increasing numbers of food sensitivities will develop. These, in turn, can set off autoimmune problems that can be difficult to correct. Fortunately, abnormal permeability can be reversed with nutritional supplements and, if necessary, a gastrointestinal detoxification program (see page 277). It's a common problem, and one I actually enjoy treating because patients feel so much better when their gut integrity is restored and their systemic toxicity decreases.

DIAGNOSING GASTROINTESTINAL TROUBLES

Many people can have an improper gut ecology without symptoms, gastrointestinal or otherwise. Others may experience all kinds of symptoms, including:

- Fatigue
- Bloating, gas
- Diarrhea, constipation

- Unintentional weight gain (or loss)
- Food allergies, chemical sensitivities
- Behavioral changes
- Asthma
- Eczema
- Inflammatory disorders (such as arthritis)
- Immunosuppression
- Autoimmune problems (such as lupus)
- Malnutrition
- Migraines

Whether or not someone is symptomatic depends in part upon the nature of the dysbiosis and in part upon genetically determined factors.

One of the time-honored ways of finding out what is happening in your gut is to send a stool sample for testing. We send a stool for Comprehensive Digestive Stool Analysis (CDSA) by Great Smokies Diagnostic Laboratory and get a great deal of useful information regarding gut dysbiosis, digestive enzymes, yeast overgrowth, and malabsorption.

Also valuable is the lactulose/mannitol challenge test. Lactulose is a nonabsorbable disaccharide; mannitol is a nonmetabolized disaccharide. After fasting, you drink the lactulose/mannitol beverage, and urine is collected for six hours afterward. Lactulose should be minimally absorbed, so a high level in the urine suggests abnormal permeability. Mannitol should be absorbed, so a low level in the urine suggests abnormal metabolic processes in the gut. We also look at the ratio of lactulose to mannitol because an increased ratio suggests abnormal intestinal permeability.

GASTROINTESTINAL DETOXIFICATION

To detoxify the gut, you first clear away what shouldn't be there, then fortify what should. This process is very individual. For some of my patients it is relatively quick and simple; others need to proceed more slowly and combine several approaches.

The first step is to remove allergens, toxins, chemicals, sugar, antacids, processed foods, and toxic fats (margarine, fried foods, refined vegetable oils) from the diet, and to adopt the Immune Empowering Diet, including added fiber (psyllium) and pure water. Some people find it helpful to adopt a limited diet of foods that very rarely provoke allergic responses (the elimination diet, or a modified elimination diet—see page 288). Others benefit from going on a liquid diet that consists of a hypoallergenic, predigested formula that contains many nutrients, cofactors, and antioxidants, plus beneficial proteins. People who are very ill may need to get their nourishment intravenously if their intestines are simply incapable of absorbing nutrients. (This is referred to as *intravenous hyperalimentation*.)

Before going any further, it's important to treat any problems such as parasitic infections or yeast overgrowth. Depending upon the severity of the problem, this can be achieved either with herbs (such as paramicocidin, artemisia, garlic, and black walnut) or medications (such as Flagyl or Yodoxin).

Some people use natural bowel purgatives. I frequently start patients on a 3- to 4-week herbal GI detoxification program to help them begin with a "clean slate." Aloe is an effective natural laxative that soothes inflammation in the gastrointestinal tract.

It may be necessary to replace hydrochloric acid in the stomach or pancreatic enzymes in the intestines. Each of these can be assessed by an appropriate test. There are natural substances that help restore optimal digestion, such as chamomile and ginger root. Restoring proper levels of stomach acid and digestive enzymes allows the body to make the most of beneficial nutrients.

I have my detox patients take specific nutrients that are beneficial both for detoxification processes and for the gastrointestinal tract, including:

- Antioxidants (zinc, selenium, vitamin C, vitamin E, beta-carotene)
- Pantothenic acid (vitamin B_5)
- Essential fatty acids
- Butyric acid (to provide energy to the epithelial cells of the colon)
- Clay (bentonite) or herbal detoxification formulas to bind with toxins and remove them from the body
- Glutathione, N-acetylcysteine, and cysteine (to boost glutathione levels in the liver)
- Glutamine (a preferred food of the intestinal cells that enhances cellular repair)

Probiotic Supplements

A very important part of gastrointestinal detoxification is restoring the ecologic balance of the microorganisms in the gut. I give my patients high levels of *Lactobacillus acidophilus*, bifidobacteria, and *S. boulardii* to help repopulate their intestines with beneficial flora. When using these kinds of supplements, it's important to choose high-quality products that live up to their claims (see the Resources section at the back of this book for details). Some products have been found to contain far fewer microorganisms than they advertise. Others contain the wrong bacteria, or the right bacteria—but the wrong strain. The correct flora must be able to:

- Survive the acidic environment of the stomach
- Tolerate bile
- Adhere to the host's mucosal lining (different strains are better adapted to different hosts)
- Multiply in sufficient numbers to make a difference to the host

It is necessary to ingest high numbers of beneficial microorganisms because the cards are basically stacked against them. First, they have to survive their journey through the stomach, followed by a bath of bile. Once they make it to the intestines, they have to compete with other microorganisms for space on the mucosal lining of the GI tract, even as they are being pushed along the intestines with waste products that are being swept out of the body. Many beneficial microorganisms will fall by the wayside, but the hardy survivors will soon bring about beneficial changes.

Recently more attention has been paid to the importance of *prebiotics,* or foods that nourish the probiotics. The right substances—including fructo-oligosaccharides (FOS) and inulin—can selectively enhance the growth and activity of beneficial flora. Prebiotics are an important part of gastrointestinal detoxification.

ANTIBIOTICS AND GUT HEALTH

I have mixed feelings about antibiotics. I understand and value their utility in certain situations (such as Lyme disease and strep throat), and at the same time I am cognizant of and unhappy with the side effects that frequently can accompany their use—especially their overuse. Unlike naturopaths, I will prescribe an antibiotic when I feel it is called for, although I certainly try to avoid using them as much as possible. I am very much opposed to the medical practice of giving antibiotic after antibiotic, such as for children with recurrent ear infections, or adults with recurrent bronchitis. Generally, depending on the situation, such as when an infection is not severe, I have a patient try natural antimicrobial agents first. If these are not enough to help the patient's immune system conquer an infection, then we may need to move on to antibiotics.

As I've already mentioned, antibiotics can wreak havoc with gut ecology, particularly when taken in high doses or for a long period. They kill off the friendly bacteria in your gut right when you need them most, and in the absence of these beneficial bacteria, pathogenic bacteria and yeast may overpopulate your intestines. The result? Diarrhea, inflammation, and increased permeability, which can lead to all the secondary disorders discussed earlier in this chapter, including bacterial translocation.[18]

Antibiotic-associated diarrhea (AAD) is no joke. It is the most common adverse effect of antimicrobial therapy, occurring in up to 29 percent of all hospital patients and associated with a threefold risk of increased mortality.[19]

Unlike most physicians, I will not prescribe an antibiotic without giving my patients probiotics, prebiotics, and herbs to offset the dysregulating effects antibiotics have on the body. I ask my patients to take *S. boulardii, Lactobacillus acidophilus,* and bifidobacteria *before* they develop any symptoms of intestinal upset, and to keep taking probiotics for at least one and up to two weeks after they have finished their course of antibiotics. (For ease of administration, I have combined these three probiotics into one formula that I call Co-

Biotic.) Natural antifungal agents can help reduce the risk of yeast overgrowth, and prescription antifungals can be used if necessary (although having to process yet another medication further strains the liver). I also recommend immune system boosters (supplements) for all my patients on antibiotics, and sometimes will add Immune System Super Boosters (such as intravenous vitamin C) as well. When a patient is taking an antibiotic that I know is metabolized by the liver, I will also recommend supplements specifically for liver support (see page 287).

There is no question that physicians today overprescribe antibiotics. Often they are pressured by the patient to do so ("Doctor, you have to give me something!"), sometimes doctors want to help but know of nothing else they can offer, and sometimes, unfortunately, antibiotics are just the quickest and easiest option. Half of all antibiotics are thought to be prescribed inappropriately or unnecessarily—for example, to treat a viral infection (antibiotics are not effective against viruses). The overuse of antibiotics in this culture is leading to robust, antibiotic-resistant forms of bacteria. Bacteria multiply so rapidly that they can evolve many generations in just hours, changing their chemistry and genes so that a particular antibiotic no longer has any effect. In response, doctors prescribe larger and larger doses, or newer and newer drugs. Some experts have proposed a grim future that includes wards for patients with untreatable conditions.

The shortcomings of antibiotics are forcing many of us to reexamine techniques that were in use *before* penicillin was introduced in 1942. I am quite excited about the possibilities of many of these immune-stimulating modalities (see Chapter 10, Immune System Super Boosters).

The 1996 JAMA article I cited earlier in this chapter sounded a clarion call to physicians to develop new strategies for the treatment and prevention of infectious diseases. Ideally, beneficial microorganisms like probiotics—referred to in this article as *biotherapeutic agents*—do no harm to the host, act against pathogens by means of several different mechanisms (thus minimizing the risk of the development of resistance), stimulate the host's defenses to destroy an invading pathogen, act promptly (unlike, for example, a vaccine), and aren't too expensive.

Antibiotics can be lifesaving, but they also upset natural bodily processes. With the correct adjunctive treatments, it is possible to maximize their effectiveness while minimizing the damage they cause.

CANDIDIASIS

A very common consequence of antibiotic therapy is the overgrowth of *Candida albicans* in the gut. Candida organisms are normally present in the body in limited numbers and are considered *commensal* (i.e., they are neither beneficial nor harmful). However, they always hold the potential for overgrowth (a condition called candidiasis or yeast infection). *Candida* is one of the oldest surviving life-forms and it has had eons to perfect its adaptability.

As we've already seen, candida organisms compete with acidophilus and bifidobacteria for attachment sites along the intestinal walls. When antibiotics kill off its competitors, candida will seize this opportunity to take the upper hand. Other factors that encourage the candida overgrowth include sugar in the diet (sugar not only feeds the candida, but also suppresses the immune system), a high intake of carbohydrates (which are broken down into simple sugars), hormonal changes (including those brought about by oral contraceptives and pregnancy), the use of antacids and H2 blockers (which decrease the acidity of the digestive tract, promoting maximal attachment of candida), and immune suppression (due to steroids, chemotherapy, or illness).

When they are present in large numbers, candida organisms can:

• Sensitize the host to yeast and molds (leading to allergic responses, including asthma, hives, eczema, and food sensitivities).

• Colonize the gastrointestinal tract by attaching themselves to the mucosa and putting out roots (thereby compromising the barrier between the gastrointestinal tract and the bloodstream).

• Release toxic by-products (mycotoxins) that are absorbed into the bloodstream and can disturb organs and tissues in other more distant bodily systems.

• Release immunosuppressive factors that in low doses specifically inhibit lymphocyte response to candida (and possibly, in high doses, have broader immune suppressive effects).

• Have an amplifying effect on the virulence of other pathogens, such as staphylococcal bacteria. It is even suspected that the immunosuppressive effects of candida sensitivity in women with recurrent vaginal candidiasis may help promote viral infection of the uterine cervix.[20]

Candida overgrowth is not a rare disorder, characterized by few symptoms in immunosuppressed hosts, as the medical establishment maintains. On the contrary, I have found it to be quite common and associated with many symptoms, from mild to debilitating. Candida overgrowth can be a multisymptom, multisystem disorder that greatly complicates a patient's clinical picture.

Signs and symptoms of candidiasis include:

• Fatigue
• Depression
• Insomnia
• Poor memory
• "Brain fog"
• Muscle aches
• Joint pain or swelling
• Impotence
• Gastrointestinal complaints, bloating, nausea
• Chronic stuffy nose

- White tongue, white patches in mouth
- Recurrent fungal infections of the fingernails/toenails
- Recurrent vaginal infections
- Headaches
- Rashes and other skin problems
- Cravings for sweets
- Premenstrual syndrome
- Sensitivity to yeast/mold
- Chemical sensitivities, food intolerances
- Autoimmune problems
- Puffiness, water retention
- Nausea (can lead to unintentional weight loss)
- Weight gain, difficulty losing weight

Many of my patients have had such a severe yeast problem that their quality of life suffered greatly. However, they have made dramatic turnarounds after taking steps to control the candida overgrowth. Treatment for candidiasis depends upon the severity of the symptoms and can include:

- **Dietary modifications.** Eliminate sugar; avoid fruit and fruit juices; avoid dairy products; eliminate yeast-containing foods (including bread); avoid fermented foods, such as vinegar; eliminate alcohol; eliminate processed foods; and eliminate any foods to which you are sensitive. Follow the low-carbohydrate Immune Empowering Diet on page 135.

- **Natural antifungal agents.** I give my patients paramicocidin (derived from grapefruit seeds), caprylic acid (derived from coconut), garlic, and berberine.

- **Prescription antifungal medications.** Nystatin is a widely prescribed antifungal that is not absorbed, so systemic side effects are few. In fact, it is one of the few drugs that are not problematic during pregnancy. However, yeast die-off can be greater with nystatin. We use a gradually increasing dose protocol that minimizes the risk of die-off reactions. Stronger systemic antifungals, including fluconazole (Diflucan), itraconazole (Sporanox), and ketoconazole (Nizoral) can be even more effective in certain circumstances. However, liver function must be monitored with these medications, especially with Nizoral, as they can adversely affect the liver. My experience with many, many hundreds of patients is that the occurrence of liver problems with the newer medications (Diflucan and Sporanox) are infrequent and fully reversible upon discontinuation of the drug. I routinely add liver-protective nutrients and herbs (see pages 286–87) whenever I use stronger systemic antifungals.

- **Probiotics and prebiotics.** It's important to restock the GI tract with friendly microorganisms, which, as you now know, have many beneficial effects (and no known side effects). One study published in the *Annals of Internal Medicine* concluded that "daily ingestion of 8 ounces of yogurt containing *Lactobacillus acidophilus* decreased both candidal colonization and infection."[21] That's certainly an easy regimen to follow!

COMMONLY ASKED QUESTION NO. 18:

What is yeast die-off?

As antifungal measures take effect, it is possible to experience symptoms related to yeast die-off. This is one of those situations in which patients feel worse before they feel better. A die-off reaction (similar to the Herxheimer reaction, which is an intensification of symptoms due to a bacterial die-off, first observed in association with the treatment of syphilis with penicillin) usually occurs early in the treatment (not, for example, three months later). Symptoms last a few days to a week (rarely, up to three weeks) and usually subside if you continue taking your medications and probiotics. In certain severe die-off reactions, the medication may need to be stopped temporarily, then restarted at a much lower dose and increased very slowly.

When my patient Lacey first came to see me, she already suspected she might have candidiasis. Her manicurist had just finished being treated for candida overgrowth and was telling everyone who came into her shop how much better she was feeling.

Lacey's medical history presented an almost classic case of candidiasis. She'd had recurrent urinary tract infections plus respiratory and ear infections, all of which had been treated with repeated courses of antibiotics. When she was younger, she'd had recurrent strep throat and tonsillitis, which were also treated with antibiotics. Now, at age twenty-eight, Lacey had what she described as a "more or less permanent" vaginal yeast infection, gastrointestinal symptoms (including abdominal bloating and chronic constipation), and chemical sensitivities and food allergies. Lacey said she was chronically fatigued and drowsy, to the point where her family had started teasing her about falling asleep all the time.

Lacey admitted that she loved pizza and occasionally went overboard with sugar, particularly around the time of her menses. She drank 6 cups of coffee a day and also ate bread daily.

Lacey adopted a yeast-free diet and also started on nystatin. She felt much better, but was still troubled by vaginal symptoms. Lacey's severe, chronic vaginitis turned out to be tough to beat. A vaginal culture indicated bacterial vaginosis, so we put Lacey on antibiotics again—which always complicates the picture for someone who already has candidiasis. However, this needed to be treated, as coexisting infections can be synergistic in their negative effect on health. We were able to minimize any ill effects from the antibiotic by giving Lacey immune system boosters, probiotics, and prebiotics.

I believe that Lacey's intractable yeast overgrowth had led to immune dysfunction. The yeast overgrowth itself was probably in part due to some inherent immune defect that prevented her from being able to effectively control yeast. Her body was simply not able to resolve her chronic infections. Oxidative therapy (an Immune System Super Booster) helped greatly with this. (Lacey also told me that the oxidative treatments helped with her "mental fuzziness.") Enzyme-potentiated desensitization (EPD) helped Lacey with her chemical sensitivities and food allergies, and specific immunotherapy to candida helped her immune system to better control this troublesome yeast as well.

Lacey still has a recurrence of symptoms from time to time, probably due to this ongoing impairment in her ability to effectively control yeast in her body. She has intermittent treatment with antifungal agents (both oral and vaginal) when necessary, and also has regular oxidative and EPD treatments to keep her yeast symptoms under control.

Today Lacey is much happier, brighter, and more energetic than she was when I first met her. In spite of the fact that she continues to need periodic treatments, she feels that her anticandida regimen has been extremely successful, and she continues to have far fewer symptoms than she ever thought possible.

WHAT THE LIVER DOES

Just as we can't live without a heart, we cannot survive without a liver. The largest organ in the body, the liver is incredibly responsive to the body's changing needs and has a fascinating ability to regenerate. Approximately 1½ quarts of blood flow through the liver *each minute* as it performs its many varied functions.

Although it is not part of the digestive tract, the liver has an all-important role in processing nutrients. It processes fat, carbohydrates, and protein, turning nutrient building blocks into many different substances, from cholesterol to immune system complement proteins. It also metabolizes nutrients (producing glutathione, for example, and turning beta-carotene into vitamin A), and regulates the blood's level of amino acids and glucose.

In addition, the liver synthesizes and secretes bile (many toxic substances are eliminated via bile), and acts as a storehouse for blood, iron, glycogen, and vitamins (such as vitamins A, D, and B_{12}). The liver converts glycogen to glucose when necessary, and does the reverse as well.

Most important for our discussion here, the liver filters from the blood toxins, bacteria, and antigen/antibody complexes that are absorbed from the gut. It also detoxifies pollutants, hormones, mycotoxins (toxic substances produced by fungi), histamines, and ammonia in the blood.

We've all had the experience of being asked to do just one more thing, and wondering where we would get the energy to do it. I am reminded of the feeling I get when I have to squeeze another patient into my already packed schedule. The liver, too, has times when it is asked to do just one more thing. Most of the time it handles the increased burden without complaint, but sometimes the demands we place upon the liver exceed its ability to cope. Too much alcohol, for example, can cause cirrhosis; excessive acetaminophen (for example, a suicide attempt using Tylenol) can cause severe liver damage.

If the liver could talk, there are probably many occasions when it would say, "What the heck do you think you are *doing?* Can't you see I'm busy already? Did you have to drink that wine *now?* I'm already working on that antibiotic you took an hour ago. I'm not sure I can handle all this."

Since the liver can't talk, it can get our attention only by means of signs and symptoms. Different underlying problems—for example, Gulf War syndrome, lead poisoning, ruptured silicone breast implants, or medication-induced liver strain—can all cause problems with detoxification that lead to similar symptoms. These include:

- Fatigue, malaise
- Headache
- Muscle aches
- Digestive disturbances, constipation
- Allergies and chemical sensitivities
- Neurological dysfunction

All of us have different detoxifying capabilities, based on the factors I mentioned earlier—age, nutritional status, hormone levels, genetic predispositions, immunological competence, lifestyle and habits, gastrointestinal health, and the presence of liver disease. People who are sluggish detoxifiers, or who are placing large demands on the liver, may feel generally unwell. Sometimes a vicious cycle sets in: they have a headache because of the bioaccumulation of toxins, so they take acetaminophen, which contributes to the body's toxic load, so they get another headache (or a persistent one) or other toxicity-related symptoms.

Diagnosing Liver Detoxification Problems

As I mentioned in Chapter 4, the liver processes toxins in two phases. Phase I is an oxidation/reduction step that involves a family of enzymes called the cytochrome P-450 enzymes. Phase I biotransforms toxins into reactive intermediates, which in some cases are harder on the body than the original substance from which they were derived. Phase II takes these intermediates and puts them through a conjugation step—using glutathione and glycine, among other amino acids—creating final end products that can be excreted. It is not necessary for all substances to go through both of these phases.

I can get a rough idea of a patient's detoxification status by taking a medical history (this will help me identify the risk factors listed above) and by reviewing signs and symptoms. In addition, there are tests we can give that not only evaluate a patient's detoxification abilities, but also tell us if Phase I and Phase II are out of sync. These tests involve relatively harmless substances that are processed specifically by Phase I or Phase II.

- The oral caffeine challenge test evaluates Phase I. Caffeine is used to test Phase I because it is metabolized almost exclusively in the liver by the cytochrome P-450 enzymes. After avoiding caffeine for at least twelve hours, the patient then takes in a measured dose of caffeine. The rate of the disappearance of the caffeine from the blood and saliva correlates with the activity of the cytochrome P-450 enzymes. If this rate is too slow, the patient is a sluggish Phase I detoxifier. If the rate is too fast, it suggests that Phase I has been upregulated by the presence of other toxins.
- The sodium benzoate challenge test was used until recently to evaluate Phase II. Sodium benzoate is converted to hippuric acid in the liver, using only the Phase II step. The patient takes a measured amount of sodium benzoate, his or her urine is collected after four hours, and the amount of hippuric acid is measured. A low percentage of hippuric acid indicates that Phase II is impaired. A high percentage suggests that Phase II is overactive, possibly because it has been upregulated by the presence of other toxins. Testing recently has become more sophisticated and is now capable of assessing different Phase II detoxification pathways.
- The urinary sulfate-to-creatinine ratio indicates the status of the liver's supply of glutathione. A low ratio suggests that the liver has a reduced reserve of sulfur-conjugating nutrients at its disposal, which suggests in turn that the liver is being subjected to oxidative stress.

LIVER DETOXIFICATION

Liver detoxification is closely related to gastrointestinal detoxification, but includes more emphasis specifically on liver support. As with gastrointestinal detoxification, the first step is to remove any sources of allergens, chemicals, and toxins (including toxic fats) from the diet, and to adopt the Immune Empowering Diet, including plenty of fiber to help escort toxins out of the gut. Again, some patients benefit from going on an elimination diet or, in more extreme cases, a nutrient-rich liquid diet. Certain commercially prepared food products (usually in the form of powders) are designed to backfill the nutrients necessary for liver detoxification. Some formulations are made specifically to even further boost the nutrients necessary for successful Phase II detoxification.

Treating any gastrointestinal problems, such as a parasitic infection or yeast overgrowth, also eases the burden on the liver. Repopulating the GI tract with beneficial microorganisms is important, so probiotics and prebiotics are a part of any liver detoxification program.

Because the liver is exposed to such an amount of oxidative stress, I give my liver detox patients plenty of antioxidants (including vitamin C, vitamin E, and beta-carotene) and mineral cofactors (zinc and selenium). Glutathione and the glutathione precursors cysteine, N-acetylcysteine, and glycine support Phase II detoxification. In fact, N-acetylcysteine is the antidote for acetaminophen overdose. This has been known for years, and is used by emergency room physicians all over the country, but most physicians have no idea of the relationship between this treatment protocol and liver detoxification.

Lipoic acid is helpful for liver detoxification because it is an enzyme cofactor in the Krebs cycle, our main energy production pathway (see Chapter 11). Other substances that boost this pathway include thiamine and alpha-ketoglutarate.

Lipotrophic factors (such as carnitine and choline) enhance the removal of fatty deposits in the liver. As I mentioned earlier, many toxins are excreted with bile, so stimulating the flow of bile from the liver is helpful. Substances called *choleretics* stimulate the liver's secretion of bile, and *cholagogues* stimulate the flow of bile from the gallbladder.

Certain botanicals helpful specifically for liver support include:

- Dandelion root, which acts as both a choleretic and a cholagogue.
- Turmeric, an antioxidant that helps to prevent lipid peroxidation in the liver.
- Artichoke leaves, which are liver protective and stimulate liver regeneration. They stimulate the liver's secretion of bile and decrease the synthesis of cholesterol.
- Catechin, a bioflavonoid antioxidant in tea.
- Barberry, which assists with liver function.
- Yarrow flower, which regulates liver function.
- Milk thistle, which contains three potent liver-protecting flavonoids—silybin, silydianin, and silychristin, known collectively as silymarin. Silymarin prevents liver destruction (it is known to protect the liver from the damaging effects of death cap mushrooms and carbon tetrachloride) and enhances liver function. Silymarin stimulates liver repair, quenches free radicals and protects cell membranes (it is a more potent antioxidant than vitamin E), inhibits the secretion of certain inflammatory leukotrienes and prostaglandins, and stimulates the secretion of bile. Silymarin not only helps offset the depletion of glutathione, but actually boosts glutathione levels in the liver. If I had to choose just one herb for liver support, it would be milk thistle. When indicated, I give my patients a product called Hepagen, which is a combination of liver protective herbs and nutrients.

RECOVERY

After liver detoxification, the body is relatively toxin-free. With the detoxification pathways cleared, the body can keep up with its toxic burden, and balance is restored. Systems that were stressed by the bioaccumulation of toxins can begin to work properly again. Functions that were depressed—for example, growth hormone secretion decreases when the body is in a stressed state—can normalize. Energy metabolism becomes more efficient. The immune system, no longer dysregulated by the presence of excessive toxins, "resets" itself. This results in immune rehabilitation, with greater immune balance and tolerance, and can be accompanied by a decrease in intolerances, such as food allergies and chemical sensitivities.

Gordon, a hardworking young man of twenty-five, had recently been diagnosed with attention deficit disorder (ADD). He had had difficulty concentrating all his life and was easily distracted, but—probably because of his great intelligence and perseverance—he had gone all the way through school without any teacher picking up on his disorder. When Gordon took a psychology course in college, he read a description of someone who sounded like him—someone who had ADD. Testing confirmed Gordon's suspicion, and his doctor recommended Ritalin (a medication that can help certain patients with ADD). However, Gordon did not want to go on Ritalin, so he ended up in my office, looking for alternatives.

Gordon's lab results indicated elevated antibodies against candida, and he also tested positive for several allergies. His liver detoxification profile indicated sluggish Phase II activity.

The first leg of Gordon's treatment regimen consisted of a three-week liver detoxification program. He found this extremely helpful. Gordon also adopted a yeast-free, allergen-free diet, started on nystatin, and received enzyme-potentiated desensitization immunotherapy as well as other immune system boosters. His head became clearer, he developed a better tolerance for stress, and he noticed that his memory no longer gave out on him when he was under stress. His overall improvement has been quite remarkable, and although Gordon technically still has ADD, he is managing much, much better than when I'd first seen him.

THE MODIFIED ELIMINATION DIET

The elimination diet is designed to eliminate foods that may provoke an immune response from the body. Sometimes the elimination diet is used as a diagnostic tool: after certain foods are scrupulously avoided for a period of one to two weeks, they are reintroduced one at a time to see if symptoms develop. The diagnostic elimination diet is extremely restrictive and needs to be followed precisely. The addition of even small amounts of restricted foods can throw off the results.

Following is a modified elimination diet that can be used to support gastrointestinal and liver detoxification. This is not intended as a diagnostic elimination diet.

1. Eliminate any foods to which you know you are sensitive.

2. Eliminate dairy products. (Possible exception: organic, unsweetened, live-culture yogurt.) Milk substitutes include rice milk and nut milks. Avoid soy milk, as soy is a common allergen.

3. Eliminate meat (beef, pork, veal) and eggs. Chicken, turkey, lamb, and cold-water

fish (salmon, mackerel, halibut) are acceptable. Legumes are another acceptable protein source.

4. Eliminate gluten. This is the most difficult part of the diet, because you must avoid anything made with wheat, spelt, kamut, oats, rye, barley, amaranth, or quinoa. Also eliminate malts, which are derived from gluten-containing sources. Rice, corn, and buckwheat are acceptable starches. Gluten-free flours include rice flour, potato flour, and tapioca flour.

5. Eliminate alcohol and caffeine.

6. Eliminate sugar, and watch your intake of fruit and fruit juice. Avoid "fruit drinks," citrus fruits, dried fruits, and canned fruits in sugary syrup.

7. Eliminate toxic fats (margarine, shortening, refined vegetable oils). Use olive oil instead.

8. Drink at least two quarts of water (preferably filtered) per day. Caffeine-free, noncitrus herbal teas are acceptable, as are vegetable juices.

You'll probably want to make homemade vegetarian soups, which are very healthful. All vegetables are acceptable on the modified elimination diet.

Read labels carefully. Over-the-counter medications can include alcohol and caffeine; processed foods can include practically anything. Fresh, organic whole foods are definitely the way to go.

This is not an easy diet, particularly for people who have been eating at the other end of the spectrum, but stick with it and you'll feel better. If you were formerly a junk food junkie, I suspect you'll feel so much better that you will not want to return to your old eating habits.

∽ ELLIE'S STORY

My patient Ellie had a candida problem for years that went undiagnosed before she came to see me. It's just incredible to me that someone with so many symptoms could have been told by her previous doctors that there was nothing wrong with her.

During our first conversation, Ellie told me that she'd started to suffer bouts of terrible nausea and dry heaves ("like I am pregnant") along with diarrhea. She also was experiencing intense headaches, hot flashes, episodic fatigue, and some light-headedness. She had consulted three gynecologists and had tried various synthetic estrogens, but her headaches had grown worse and she had discontinued estrogen replacement therapy. Her local doctor had prescribed Xanax (an anxiety-relieving medication), which made Ellie feel light-headed. She knew, and I knew, that something was indeed wrong with her. Ellie felt terrible, looked terrible, and was polite but rather grim. She had the eyes of someone who has been in chronic pain for a long time—in her case, from daily migraine headaches. The fact that she was still functional was due to her incredible strength of will.

Ellie's medical history included chronic sinusitis that had been treated with antibiotics and steroidal nasal spray. She'd also had recurrent vaginal candidiasis and repeated urinary tract infections. At one point she had been diagnosed with allergies, including a sensitivity to molds, but her allergist had discontinued her allergy shots after six months.

In the previous six months, Ellie had lost 45 pounds due to her nausea and inability to eat. A previous doctor had told her two months before that she had thrush (oral candidiasis), which is—to me—invariably a tip-off that there is a yeast imbalance in the body.

My initial diagnoses, pending lab results, were chronic allergic sinusitis, migraine headaches, and chronic candidiasis (even Ellie's toenails were affected by fungal growth). Ellie's blood work was essentially unremarkable, but a vitamin profile did reveal low levels of folic acid and biotin and high levels of vitamin A.

To combat Ellie's candidiasis, we instituted a regimen that included a yeast-free Immune Empowering Diet, environmental controls to minimize her exposure to mold, Diflucan, and intravenous vitamin C. To improve Ellie's nutritional status and gastrointestinal function, I placed her on a high-potency multivitamin/mineral supplement, probiotics (such as acidophilus and bifidus), prebiotics to support the probiotics, buffered vitamin C powder, borage oil, and folic acid and biotin supplements. For her menopausal symptoms, I prescribed a natural progesterone, supplements for glandular support, and two different combination homeopathic remedies called Klimaktheel and Feminine. To help Ellie sleep I recommended melatonin and another homeopathic remedy called Calming.

Ellie showed a marked improvement on this regimen, and I mean *marked*. When she started to feel better, I could see she was really an attractive, bright, funny, vivacious person, but I never would have known this from her first visit. Her improving health allowed her real spirit to come out, and she was ecstatic not to be suffering from daily headaches anymore.

Ellie had a serious and tenacious yeast problem, and it took a long course of Diflucan to help her. Eventually I started her on candida immunotherapy, which was very helpful, and recommended that she obtain acupuncture treatment, which was an additional help. Ellie's chronic sinusitis and fungus-infected toenails both cleared up. Her hot flashes disappeared, and she was successfully tapered off the Xanax.

Ellie's yeast problem was tough to beat. Whenever I tried to taper her off the Diflucan, her candida symptoms returned. We had trouble finding precisely the correct doses for Ellie's candida immunotherapy, so ultimately I stopped this approach and started her on intravenous hydrogen peroxide. Ellie's husband noted that she looked even better after the oxidative treatments than she had during the first part of her recovery. Once the oxidative therapy took effect, we were finally able to eliminate Ellie's prescription antifungal medication.

Ellie eventually moved south to a sunny new home that had no basement and no mold. The only trouble with her new location was that she could no longer get oxidative therapy, and as a consequence she had occasional flare-ups of candida symptoms, particularly the nausea. Ellie discovered that the hot and humid summer made her symptoms worse, but during these months she takes Diflucan and pays stricter attention to her yeast-free diet.

I cannot emphasize enough the dramatic change we saw in Ellie with treatment for her candidiasis. This success story is played out again and again, with different variations, every time I diagnose and treat chronic candidiasis. My holistic colleagues and I know that yeast overgrowth and sensitivity is a genuine health issue, and that it is one of the most underrecognized problems of today. To me it's just a shame that so many patients are living with the symptoms of chronic candidiasis when it is a problem that, when appropriately recognized, can be treated so successfully.

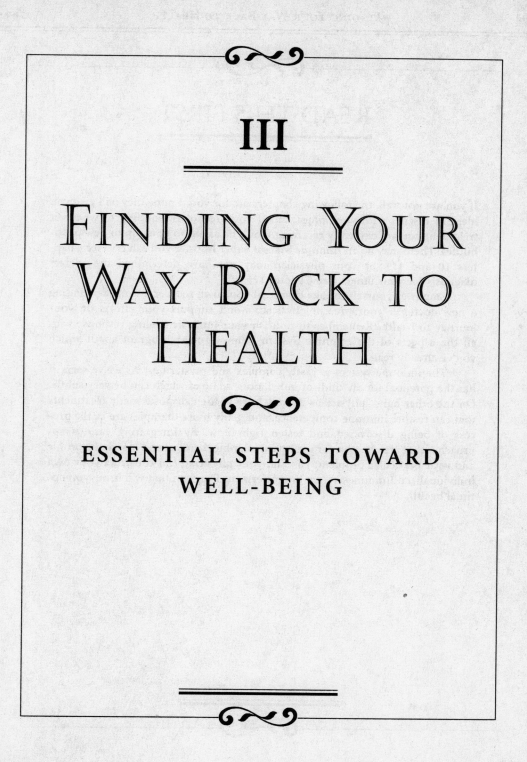

III

FINDING YOUR WAY BACK TO HEALTH

ESSENTIAL STEPS TOWARD
WELL-BEING

READ THIS FIRST

If you are not well, the following chapters are for you. I hope they will give you ideas to discuss with your physician. If you are not responding to whatever treatment you are currently receiving, don't be afraid to open up to new possibilities. There may be an Immune System Super Booster you can try (see Chapters 10 and 11), or your physician may not have determined the correct diagnosis for your illness (see Chapter 12).

Empower yourself to take charge of your own recovery. Consider finding a new doctor if your present physician won't support your efforts on your journey to health. Remember to nourish your intrinsic healing response with all the aspects of the Immune System Empowerment Program about which you've already read.

The immune system is vastly complex and mysterious. As we've seen, it has the potential for all kinds of imbalances, some of which can be very subtle. On the other hand, physicians already have at their disposal many treatments that can restore immune competence, and many more therapies are in the process of being discovered and tested right now. By integrating various approaches that are effective for your particular biochemical and metabolic profile and your particular problem, you and your physician can construct your own individualized Immune System Empowerment Program that will bring you optimal health.

Chapter 10

❧❧❧

IMMUNE SYSTEM SUPER BOOSTERS

All that we do is touched with ocean, yet we remain on the
shore of what we know.

—RICHARD WILBUR

In our increasingly toxic world, our bodies are subjected to unprecedented stresses. You are already familiar with the list—toxins (both from within and without), allergens, radiation, pollution, stress, and so on. It's remarkable how effectively our bodies cope with all these burdens, and for how long. Eventually, however, damage builds up, homeostasis is lost, and the scales tip toward ill health.

Today physicians are seeing unprecedented rates of certain kinds of illnesses—including allergies, asthma, autoimmune disorders, cancer, and degenerative diseases. These are all signs of immune system malfunction. An overburdened and underenergized immune system is far more likely to allow these disorders to develop than an immune system that is operating at peak efficiency.

In addition to seeing more chronic illnesses, physicians today are seeing more antibiotic-resistant bacteria. According to a 1996 article in *The New England Journal of Medicine*, "so far resistance has developed to all microbial drugs."[1] Discovery of new drugs that might enable us to deal with these resistant organisms is slowing down even as resistance to existing drugs is increasing. Bacteria are extremely adaptable, and a single genetic mutation can make them resistant to an antibiotic without lessening the virulence of the strain. Bacteria are also capable of taking up foreign DNA from resistant organisms and incorporating it into their own chromosomes, another way of acquiring resistance to antibiotics.

Not long ago doctors could count on vancomycin, an extremely potent antibiotic, to wipe out bacteria that other antibiotics could not touch. Today, however, bacteria that are resistant even to vancomycin are increasingly being seen in hospitals. It's time for us to reconsider treatments that encourage the body's healing response—or, to borrow Pasteur's analogy, to tend to the soil. This concept has evolved to the point where we now can evaluate the status of a patient's biological terrain. We need to "grow" good health with the Immune

System Empowerment Program and with immune-boosting therapies that enhance host resistance. We need to head off chronic diseases and infectious organisms before they have a chance to take hold in the body, and we can do this by supporting the body's own defenses.

This chapter will cover a variety of Immune System Super Boosters that can help rehabilitate and rebalance your immune system. These therapies are used in different ways for different illnesses. Some of them are uncommon, but I have found all of them to be safe and effective. They may open doors for you that you never even knew existed.

TREATING HORMONE DEFICIENCIES AND IMBALANCES

Mary Kate came to see me because she had made a definite connection between her menstrual cycle and her recurring feelings of anxiety and depression. Her intense fears would begin several days before her period and then last until ovulation, so she was spending half of every month very upset. During her periods she would be overcome by body shakes, crying, and fears. She had worsening sleep problems and was experiencing occasional hot flashes as well.

At thirty-nine, Mary Kate not only had premenstrual syndrome but also was entering early menopause, just as her mother had. I placed her on natural progesterone, natural estrogen, oral adrenal extract and nutrients to support her adrenal glands, and a high-potency, well-balanced multivitamin/mineral supplement I use for hormonal imbalances.

Within one month, Mary Kate experienced a marked improvement. Her fears became fewer and less intense, her spirits were much brighter, and she looked terrific. A couple of months later she began to show signs of excess estrogen, including breast tenderness, bloating, and cramping, so I cut back on her dose of estrogen. She did wonderfully on her new regimen.

Hormones: Small but Mighty

Mary Kate's long-suffering husband thought I was a miracle worker, but the real miracle is that today doctors can correct hormonal deficiencies and imbalances and give both men and women their lives back. Hormones are small molecules with powerful effects. They are vital for normal body functions. By means of hormones, the glands of the endocrine system can send messages to one another and to every cell of the body. Disorders of the endocrine system can cause significantly altered physiology and a wide range of signs and symptoms, from the annoying to the debilitating.

For years I listened to patients' complaints about problems that I knew intuitively were hormonal in nature, but I didn't know how to correct them. Synthetic hormonal preparations were not the answer. Referring the patients to an endocrinologist, or hormone specialist, often didn't help. Eventually, by attending conferences, taking courses, and reading the literature, I figured out which tools I needed and how to use them. Today hormone balancing is a critically important part of what I do.

Hormone imbalances can be quite problematic, as they can be subtle and difficult to measure. In addition, some modern medications used to treat hormone deficiencies create problems of their own. Fortunately, there have been recent advances in the manufacturing of natural hormone preparations that are safe, effective, and well tolerated.

I often find subtle hormone imbalances complicating other illnesses, from rheumatoid arthritis to chronic fatigue immune dysfunction syndrome (CFIDS) to Lyme disease. Correcting the underlying hormone imbalances can improve the patient's overall clinical picture.

Certain glands have overlapping duties, so if necessary they can compensate for each other—for a while. For instance, the thyroid and adrenal glands cover for each other, so if the thyroid is functioning at a low level, the adrenals may start working overtime. Eventually, however, the adrenals may become exhausted. Treating the thyroid deficiency may suddenly highlight the adrenal insufficiency. Sometimes patients have to go through a period of seesawing hormone levels before balance is restored.

Which Gland Secretes What?

Hormones are a little like the lighting at a Broadway show. Theatrical lighting changes subtly for each scene just as hormones constantly shift in response to internal and external cues. Just as lights of different colors blend to create one effect, many different hormones work together to keep the body functioning well as a whole. If one hormone flashes too brightly or dims too low, the overall synergy can be ruined.

The pituitary, located near the base of the brain, is sometimes called the "master gland" (even though it is strongly influenced by its neighbor, the hypothalamus). The pituitary secretes many different hormones, including, but not limited to:

- **Growth hormone (GH)**, which stimulates cell division and protein synthesis in soft tissue as well as bone
- **Thyroid-stimulating hormone (TSH)**, which stimulates the thyroid to release its own hormones
- **Adrenocorticotropic hormone (ACTH)**, which stimulates the adrenal cortex to produce certain hormones
- **Luteinizing hormone (LH)** and **follicle-stimulating hormone (FSH)**, also called **gonadotropins**, which stimulate the gonads
- **Melanocyte-stimulating hormone (MSH)**, which stimulates pigment cells in the skin

Of course, that's not all. The thymus secretes thymic hormone. The pancreas, as I discussed in Chapter 5, secretes both insulin and glucagon. The ovaries produce estrogen and progesterone, and the testes turn out testosterone. The adrenal glands produce several important hormones (see below), as does the thyroid.

Any one of these glands can overproduce or underproduce a given hormone. Sometimes this is due to an autoimmune problem or localized tumor that affects the gland directly. Sometimes there is a problem with the orders that are being transmitted from the hypothalamus or pituitary. In my experience, it is common for patients to have more than one endocrine insufficiency at the same time.

Glandular Support

Before individual hormones were isolated and produced synthetically, whole glandular concentrates (preparations of glandular material taken from animals) were used to help correct hormone deficiencies. Before insulin was available, diabetes was treated with pancreatic extracts. Before growth hormone was manufactured, undersized children were sometimes given pituitary gland extract. Before thyroid hormone was commercially available, desiccated thyroid was used to help control body temperature and heart rate.

Thymus glandular is used specifically to boost the immune system. You'll recall that all T cells are "educated" by the thymus, so energizing the thymus can be very helpful in strengthening T cell immunity, which in turn can help the body combat chronic infections that are T cell mediated (such as fungal and viral infections). Thymus glandulars are used to boost cellular immunity by stimulating the production, maturation, and activation of T cells.

The interesting thing about glandulars is that they contain only minute amounts of the actual beneficial hormones, but, most important, all the cellular building blocks of the organ from which they were derived. This means they provide a stressed gland with the reparative and restorative substances it needs in order to heal itself. In my experience, glandular support has been particularly useful in treating subtle adrenal problems.

One disadvantage of glandulars is that it is difficult to quantify their effects. When I give a patient a prescription thyroid medication, I know exactly what dose he or she will be receiving, and if necessary I can make adjustments (up or down) accordingly. Glandulars vary in effectiveness, due to variations in their active constituents and differences in the way in which they are metabolized and utilized. However, there are dosing guidelines for each product, so consumers do have an idea of each product's effectiveness. In general, I have not been impressed with the various thyroid glandular preparations that I have tried in the past, so therefore I give my patients a prescription preparation of desiccated thyroid instead. However, my experience with specific thymus and adrenal glandular preparations has been much more positive.

Glandulars are available over the counter, but I hope you'll consult a nutritionally oriented physician or health care practitioner before you self-medicate. When I recommend a glandular to a patient, I choose a brand I trust that has clinically proven efficacy and incorporate it into a complete treatment regimen.

Hormone Treatment

Research has come a long way since glandulars were first introduced. Today many different specific hormones have been isolated. We know what they do, how to extract them naturally, and even how to manufacture them artificially.

Most doctors prefer hormone treatment to glandular treatment. If the body is running short of a particular hormone, it's easy to make up the deficit with a prescription. Sometimes administering the correct hormone allows an overtaxed gland to take a rest for a while. And when a gland becomes diseased and has to be removed altogether, it's possible to keep the body running smoothly with hormone replacement.

Between natural hormones, synthetic hormones, hormone precursors (substances converted by the body into hormones), and hormone fractions (hormonal subsets), physicians have many options at their disposal. Protocols for some conditions are relatively standard (for example, using thyroid hormone to correct low thyroid function), while protocols for other conditions are less clear-cut (for example, hormone replacement therapy for menopausal women). To complicate the picture further, hormone treatment is very individual. While one patient may respond beautifully to a certain prescription, another may try it briefly, experience no beneficial effects or even adverse effects, and then categorically refuse to keep taking it.

Extremely complicated hormonal problems are usually handled by an endocrinologist (a doctor who specializes in hormonal disorders). However, some endocrinologists are so rigid in their outlook that they miss borderline cases of hormone insufficiency that don't present themselves "by the book." Holistic physicians who maintain an open mind about subtle hormonal imbalances may actually be more helpful to patients who present with vague or puzzling symptoms that are a result of subtle hormonal imbalances. Many times patients I have placed on hormone therapy will be told by another physician that they don't need to keep taking their medication(s). Sometimes patients I have placed on natural preparations will be told to switch to synthetic preparations. Often if these patients change their regimen—doctor's orders, after all—they feel much worse.

I have treated innumerable patients for hormone deficiencies and imbalances. My intent here is not to present you with a compendium of hormone disorders, but to alert you to a handful of treatment options that could make a significant difference to your well-being and to the functioning of your immune system.

Low Thymus Function

The thymus, located behind the breastbone, is essential to the proper functioning of the immune system. The thymus can be adversely affected by prescription steroids (more about these in a moment) as well as by steroids produced naturally by the body when it is stressed. As we saw in Chapter 8, significant stress—acute or prolonged—impairs cellular immunity, which indicates that the thymus is affected.

The thymus shrinks with age, but it still remains important. Low thymus function translates into suppressed defense mechanisms, which in turn can cause lowered resistance and increased susceptibility to viral infections. The hormone thymosin can be used to correct some of the immunologic deficiencies that result from low thymus function. In my practice, I use a specific thymus glandular preparation that contains thymosin in its natural form, which has proven to be very effective.

Low Thyroid Function (Hypothyroidism)

The thyroid gland, a butterfly-shaped gland located at the base of the neck, controls our metabolism (the rate at which our cells burn oxygen and fuel). An overactive thyroid (hyperthyroid) can rev up bodily systems, while an underactive thyroid (hypothyroid) can slow us down. I am particularly interested in borderline or functional hypothyroidism, which is serious enough to make my patients feel lousy, but which is not pronounced enough to be easily diagnosed by most physicians. According to Broda Barnes, M.D., Ph.D., who is noted for his groundbreaking work on hypothyroidism, as much as 40 percent of the population may suffer from chronic hypothyroidism, and many of these cases go unrecognized.[2] This represents a lot of people, but seems more likely when you consider that the thyroid is quite sensitive to xenobiotics, nutritional deficiencies (especially selenium), dietary influences, and immunological factors.

Because thyroid hormones affect the entire body, the signs and symptoms of low thyroid function are varied. Some of the real giveaway symptoms are:

- Fatigue, sluggishness, lack of motivation
- Low body temperature
- Sensitivity to cold, cold hands and feet
- Unexplained or easy weight gain
- Difficulty losing weight, even on a low-calorie diet
- Chronic constipation
- Dry skin and other skin problems

Other symptoms that can contribute to the clinical picture of hypothyroidism include:

- Low blood sugar, cravings for sweets or carbohydrates
- Low blood pressure
- Coarsening of hair
- Hair thinning or hair loss (including eyebrows)
- Heavy or irregular periods
- Depression

- Fuzzy thinking, memory loss
- Edema (swelling) of the eyelids, face, ankles, feet
- Muscle aches, muscle weakness
- Numbness or tingling of the extremities
- Recurrent infections

One of the reasons the signs and symptoms of hypothyroidism are so varied is that the proper functioning of the human body depends heavily upon enzymes, which are designed to do their jobs at a certain body temperature. A drop in body temperature can translate into altered enzyme function, which can show up in myriad ways, including decreased immune function.

Diagnosing Thyroid Insufficiency

Dr. Barnes believed that no health problem is more common than thyroid gland deficiency. Despite the fact that it is readily and inexpensively corrected, it often goes undiagnosed and untreated. He found a simple and affordable way to test for low thyroid function: the patient measures his or her axillary (armpit) basal (resting) temperature for ten minutes first thing in the morning before getting up for five to seven days. (Menstruating women should start on the third day of their period to avoid the temperature variations associated with ovulation.) The temperature of the mouth can be affected by variables such as a sore throat or a sinus infection, so the axillary temperature is more reliable. A normal axillary temperature is between 97.8 and 98.2 degrees F. A trend of readings above 98.2 degrees F suggests hyperthyroidism. A trend of readings below 97.8 degrees F is suggestive of hypothyroidism. This old-fashioned, low-tech test has fallen out of favor with many physicians, but it is inexpensive and noninvasive, and I find it to be quite reliable. When a patient has normal thyroid blood work (see below) but consistently has an axillary temperature between 96 and 97 degrees F, coupled with a history that is suggestive of hypothyroidism, then I am likely to place him or her on a course of desiccated thyroid.

An early blood test for hypothyroidism was the protein-bound iodine test, which measured iodine levels (iodine is needed for the synthesis of thyroid hormones). Low protein-bound iodine was found to be suggestive of hypothyroidism. However, it is possible to have normal iodine levels and abnormal thyroid function at the same time.

There are now more accurate blood tests that can be used to evaluate thyroid function. It is possible to measure the amount of the thyroid hormone T_4 (thyroxine) circulating in the blood. A low level of free-floating T_4 can be associated with hypothyroidism. It's also possible to measure the amount of thyroid-stimulating hormone (TSH) put out by the pituitary. If the pituitary is producing a lot of TSH, this could indicate that it is working overtime to get a response out of an exhausted thyroid.

An even more elaborate blood test is the TRH stimulation test, in which the patient is injected with thyrotropin-releasing hormone (TRH), the hormone secreted by the hypothalamus to stimulate the pituitary gland to produce TSH. Before and after the TRH is given, TSH levels are checked at certain intervals. This test is useful for getting to the bottom of complex endocrine problems, but it is not commonly used.

COMMONLY ASKED QUESTION NO. 19:

If my thyroid blood work results are okay, how can I be hypothyroid?

I never rely solely on blood work for a diagnosis of hypothyroidism because blood work can be misleading. For starters, thyroid hormone levels can fluctuate over a twenty-four-hour period, so test results are variable. In addition, the blood levels of thyroid hormones may not fully indicate the active amount of the hormones at the cellular level (which is most important for cellular function). At this level, thyroid hormone T_4 (thyroxin) is converted to T_3 (triiodothyronine) by enzymes that require copper and zinc as cofactors as well as selenium. While circulating levels of T_4 may look adequate, this conversion may not be taking place, perhaps due to an insufficiency of copper, zinc, or selenium.

A patient with mild to moderate hypothyroidism may have T_4 levels in the "low-normal" range and perhaps a "high-normal" TSH level. On paper, this patient is not hypothyroid. In reality, however, he or she may have a low body temperature and multiple signs and symptoms of low thyroid function. Putting this patient on a small amount of thyroid medication can make a dramatic difference in his or her well-being.

Increasingly sensitive tests are enabling physicians to pick up on subtler cases of hypothyroidism. Does this mean these cases did not exist before these tests? Of course not.

Treating Hypothyroidism

It's possible to treat thyroid problems with synthetic thyroid hormones—both T_4 (thyroxine) and T_3 (triiodothyronine) are available. I usually prescribe a pharmaceutical medication called Armour thyroid that is prepared from natural desiccated thyroid. I also add nutrients for thyroid support (including minerals such as zinc, copper, and selenium, which are important for the function of thyroid hormones at the cellular level) and make sure the patient is taking a well-balanced high-potency multivitamin/mineral supplement.

Thyroid medication should be started up slowly. It is a stimulant, so it increases the rate of metabolism and the need for oxygen. Too much too soon can be hard on the heart (especially in older people or in patients with preexisting heart problems). Once the correct dose is determined, it can take several weeks for change to become apparent. The effects of months or years of metabolic dysfunction don't just vanish overnight.

Sometimes patients who don't respond to thyroid medication actually have a problem with their adrenal glands as well. It's not unusual for people to have both low thyroid function and low adrenal function (see below). Only when both are treated together can the patient return to optimal health.

Autoimmune Thyroid Disorders

Some thyroid disorders actually originate with the instructions the thyroid is receiving from the pituitary gland (which in turn gets its orders from the hypothalamus). Two disorders of the thyroid itself are Graves' disease and Hashimoto's thyroiditis. These autoimmune disorders can be diagnosed with a specific blood test that checks for the presence of antithyroid antibodies—a blood test that is *not* part of the routine thyroid profile. Again, you need to know where to look.

Graves' disease is an autoimmune disorder that affects the thyroid. In this disorder the thyroid overproduces thyroid hormones, causing hyperthyroidism.

Hashimoto's thyroiditis is an autoimmune disorder in which the immune system develops antibodies against the thyroid. It is one of the most common autoimmune disorders I see, and is far more common than Graves' disease. Signs of Hashimoto's thyroiditis include symptoms of hypothyroidism (or, infrequently, hyperthyroidism) plus inflammation and enlargement of the thyroid. When thyroid hormone is administered, it enters into a feedback loop that causes the level of thyroid-stimulating hormone in the blood to decrease, thereby giving the thyroid gland a rest. This helps both the symptoms and the inflammation.

Many of my patients with chronic Lyme disease also have evidence of Hashimoto's thyroiditis. My suspicion is that this is due to the upregulation of the immune system that we see in chronic Lyme. A possible explanation is that antibodies created to combat the Lyme spirochete cross-react with the thyroid tissue. Another possibility is that the Lyme bacteria somehow cause the thyroid cells to be exposed to immune surveillance, thereby precipitating a response to what was previously an immunologically privileged site. Either way, the immune system perceives the cells of the thyroid as foreign antigens and reacts to them, causing autoimmune illness.

Low Adrenal Function (Adrenal Insufficiency)

The adrenal glands are almond-sized glands located above the kidneys. Each adrenal gland can be divided (functionally and anatomically) into a central region called the *adrenal medulla* and a thin outer layer called the *adrenal cortex.*

The adrenal medulla produces epinephrine and norepinephrine in response to acute stress (remember the upregulated stress response?). The adrenal cortex secretes several different hormones, including an extremely influential hormone called dehydroepiandrosterone, or DHEA (see page 308). The adrenal cortex also produces a family of hormones called glucocorticoids. The chief glucocorticoid normally produced by the human adrenal cortex is cortisol (also called hydrocortisone).

Most endocrinologists believe that if you don't have adrenal failure, then your adrenal function is fine. This kind of black-or-white thinking (what I call 100/100 thinking—see page 247) is very arbitrary and does not reflect all we know about the functional subtleties of the human body. Adrenals actually can function well some of the time, or function just adequately a large part of the time, without being healthy. The functioning of different organs of the body can almost always be placed on a continuum between "fully functional" and "nonfunctional," with multiple variables contributing to different levels of functioning.

Cortisol Insufficiency

The adrenal glands produce glucocorticoids in response to physical or emotional stress, including:

- Trauma, injury, burns, surgery
- Infection, chronic disease
- Chronic allergies
- Intense heat or cold
- Chemical exposure, toxic overload
- Overwork
- Lack of sleep
- Overtraining, too much exercise
- Fasting, plummeting blood sugar levels
- Too much caffeine
- Chronic rage
- Depression, anxiety

Cortisol helps the body maintain its homeostasis when it is subjected to stress. It also counteracts allergic and inflammatory reactions and controls the body's metabolism of protein and carbohydrates.

Most people aren't aware that cortisol is vital for immune function. Early experiments showed that rats whose adrenal glands were removed would die if they were exposed to infection, indicating that the adrenals have a beneficial effect on immunity. Eventually researchers were able to determine that the body increases its secretion of corticosteroid hormones early in the course of an acute infectious illness, and that cortisol in low concentrations enhances the synthesis of antibodies.

During a flu epidemic in Sweden in 1957, it was noted that patients with untreated adrenocortical insufficiency fared poorly. Some American doctors took this information to heart and, during a 1976 flu epidemic in the United States, administered moderate doses of cortisol to acutely ill patients with low plasma cortisol levels. The subsequent improvement of these patients was impressive.[3]

Cortisol is a misunderstood hormone. Again, balance is the key. Although cortisol is immune stimulating in the correct (naturally low) dosage, it can be immune suppressing in elevated doses. Synthetic derivatives of cortisone (such as prednisone) are undeniably useful for treating autoimmune diseases, asthma, allergies, and athletic injuries, but they need to be used with caution, as they are far more powerful than natural cortisol. Long-term use of high-dose cortisone therapy can actually suppress the ability of the adrenals to produce natural corticosteroids, which creates complications when the cortisone is discontinued. Its long-term use can also cause many other adverse side effects, including cataracts, diabetes, osteoporosis, muscle weakness, and gastritis.

When the adrenal glands do not produce enough cortisol, a wide variety of signs and symptoms can develop. Symptoms that are suggestive of cortisol insufficiency include:

- Low blood sugar, hypoglycemia, cravings for sweets or carbohydrates
- Dizziness, a drop in blood pressure upon standing (it should rise)
- Low energy, chronic fatigue, weakness
- Brain fog, depression
- Nervousness, irritability
- Low body weight, weight loss, anorexia
- Gastrointestinal cramps, nausea, vomiting, diarrhea
- Headaches

These symptoms usually develop insidiously and are not in themselves especially worrisome. Many patients with cortisol insufficiency may have a number of these symptoms, but when they are told by their doctor that they have no diagnosable illness, they accept these symptoms as their lot in life. Taken together, however, such symptoms can present a picture of cortisol insufficiency.

Medical conditions that can be associated with cortisol insufficiency include allergies, asthma, arthritis, and dermatitis. When the body does not have enough cortisol at its disposal, inflammatory conditions can proceed unchecked.

Cortisol and Blood Sugar

Cortisol plays an integral role in regulating blood sugar levels. As you'll remember from Chapter 5, when blood sugar levels go up after eating, the pancreas secretes insulin to help the body either use or store the excess sugar. As blood sugar levels go down, the adrenals secrete cortisol to modulate the activity of the pancreas, thereby preventing glucose levels from dropping too far or too fast. This helps explain why hyperinsulinism—an overenthusiastic insulin response (see page 143)—can overwork not only the pancreas, but also the adrenal glands.

Cortisol insufficiency is often associated with hypoglycemia. As the adrenals tire, they can't produce enough cortisol to prevent blood sugar levels from dropping too low. When our blood sugar level plummets, we reach for a quick fix—sweets, sugar, refined carbohydrates—to bring our circulating glucose back up rapidly. Unfortunately, this sets the hypoglycemic pendulum back into motion all over again.

The brain has a very high requirement for glucose. Nervous tissue and the retina of the eye do not store glucose. This makes these tissues especially vulnerable to low blood sugar, which helps explain why hypoglycemia is associated with headache, cognitive difficulty ("brain fog"), nervousness, shakiness, and blurred vision.

Diagnosing Cortisol Insufficiency

If the adrenals are damaged, cortisol insufficiency is likely. The permanent destruction of the adrenals—called Addison's disease—can occur for many reasons, including cancer, infection, or damage due to autoantibodies (antibodies against the self). According to a 1996 article in *The New England Journal of Medicine,* the most common cause of chronic primary adrenal insufficiency used to be tuberculous adrenalitis (inflammation of the adrenal glands due to tuberculosis). Today the most common cause is autoimmune adrenalitis (slow destruction of the adrenal cortex by the immune system's own cells).[4] The current upsurge in this autoimmune disorder (and others) is clearly consistent with my clinical experience with my patients, and has been one of the things that has required me to become a medical detective.

Sometimes imbalances in adrenal hormones are not due to adrenal dysfunction, but to dysfunctions at the level of the hypothalamus or pituitary gland. After all, the adrenal glands are just following orders. However, endocrine problems at this level and of this magnitude usually produce irregularities in multiple hormone systems.

A frank deficiency of cortisol causes distinctive symptoms such as hyperpigmentation (bronze skin), vitiligo (white patches of skin), and/or autoimmune thyroid disease. In this chapter I am not as concerned about obvious cortisol deficiency as about borderline cortisol deficiency, or cortisol insufficiency, which is subtler and therefore, I believe, underdiagnosed.

It's not difficult to test for blood levels of cortisol. The problem is that the test results aren't that meaningful. As always, there is the matter of those arbitrary cutoff points between "normal" and "abnormal." If you have an increased need for cortisol, a "low-normal" level of serum cortisol may not actually be a healthy level for you. On the other hand, your neighbor, who either does not have an increased need for cortisol or is simply more responsive to it, could be perfectly healthy with a "low-normal" result.

In addition to issues of interpretation, serum cortisol test results can be skewed by anxiety (cortisol levels increase in response to stress, and having blood work done can be stressful), pregnancy, contraceptives, hyperthyroidism, and certain medications. Also, the test measures both unbound and protein-bound cortisol, when in fact only the free cortisol is biologically active.

If I administer a cortisol blood test at midday, I might get a high reading even in a patient whose adrenals are nearing exhaustion. This paradox is mediated by low blood sugar levels. When glucose levels drop, the tired adrenals respond by pumping out cortisol. In effect, adrenal insufficiency can still be present in spite of high levels of cortisol, although if left untreated, this condition would probably progress to more severe adrenal fatigue and finally to frank deficiency.

A slightly better test is the ACTH challenge test. Adrenocorticotropic hormone (ACTH) is produced by the pituitary gland to stimulate the adrenal cortex to release cortisol (and other hormones). We can test a patient's baseline cortisol level, then inject him or her with ACTH and check the blood again to see if the adrenals were able to churn out an appropriate amount of cortisol. If cortisol levels don't rise appropriately, this suggests adrenal exhaustion.

A drawback of both the cortisol blood test and the ACTH challenge test is that the patient's adrenals may be able to rally enough to fall within a normal range, but still be unable to respond to real-life situations. This is one reason I prefer a test called the Temporal Adrenal Profile, which assesses the amount of a patient's unbound, active cortisol by monitoring his or her saliva over a twenty-four-hour period. Patients like this test because it doesn't involve blood work or urine specimens, it's economical, and it can be done at home.

Treating Cortisol Insufficiency

To support the adrenal glands, I prescribe an oral adrenal glandular extract, vitamin B_6, pantothenic acid, and vitamin C, and I make sure the patient is taking a high-potency, well-balanced multivitamin/mineral supplement. Patients with adrenal exhaustion also need to work on stress management. To avoid fluctuations in blood sugar that can stress their adrenals, they must adopt a hypoglycemic version of the Immune Empowering Diet (see page 161).

I often prescribe low doses of cortisol to my patients with cortisol insufficiency. (Moderately higher doses won't cause hypercorticism, but they do run the risk of shutting down normal adrenal production of corticosteroids. This is in contrast to synthetic cortisone preparations such as prednisone, which can cause side effects and immune suppression.) Three or four doses of 5 milligrams each, spread over the course of the day, help these patients maintain an appropriate level of cortisol in their body. This is called a *physiologic* rather than a *pharmacologic* dose. When these patients are stressed by an infection or surgery, I have them increase their dose to 10 milligrams because of the immune-stimulating effects of cortisol. Studies have indicated that raising the physiologic dose of cortisol this way can lessen the severity of an infection and sometimes can even head off an infection altogether.[5]

Paige, one of my cortisol-insufficient patients, was delighted to find out that she was pregnant. Pregnancy complicates the picture for cortisol administration, but we handled it well. We increased her dose of cortisol during her pregnancy (which places increased demands on the mother), raised her cortisol levels further during labor and delivery (which is very stressful), and then decreased her cortisol doses after birth. All went well. Mom had no problem and the baby was healthy.

For years I administered Adrenal Cortical Extract (ACE), a natural extract of beef adrenal glands, with excellent results and no problems whatsoever. One of the wonderful things about ACE is that it did not cause adrenal suppression. This was the earliest product that was used to help the adrenals, but its usage diminished greatly upon the introduction of more potent synthetic steroids. Unfortunately, the FDA recently banned the use of this product. The rationale for this decision was that some patients had experienced adverse reactions, but my understanding is that this had more to do with the administration of the ACE than with the product itself. Many holistic physicians believe that the FDA's decision has more to do with the economics of the pharmaceutical industry than with a true concern for consumer health. It's difficult for me to believe that after a half century of safe use, ACE would suddenly become a threat to public safety. While there is certainly a place in medicine for synthetic cortisone derivatives, these products are not a substitute for ACE.

DHEA

Another hormone produced by the adrenal glands is dehydroepiandrosterone, or DHEA. The most abundant steroid in the bloodstream, DHEA converts to (or stimulates the production of) many other hormones, including estrogens, testosterone, progesterone, and cortisone. Serum levels of DHEA peak at age twenty-five and decline with age. At age eighty, our DHEA production is 5 percent of what it was at age twenty.

DHEA has been getting a lot of attention lately, both from medical researchers and from consumers who are looking for an elixir of youth. I am somewhat concerned about the ready availability of DHEA in every health food store in America. I'm afraid that people will assume that "if a little is good, a lot must be better!" With DHEA, this is not necessarily the case.

DHEA has immune-stimulating effects. It strengthens the body's resistance to disease and helps to reverse the immune deficiency associated with aging. DHEA may boost the body's response to viral and bacterial infections. It has been shown to prevent infection by the Epstein-Barr virus (which causes mononucleosis), and it has been associated with a reduction in viral load in AIDS patients. A 1995 article in the *Lancet* noted that in one DHEA study, there was pronounced stimulation of natural killer cell activity.[6]

DHEA is beginning to look like a wonder drug. Therapeutic applications for DHEA include:

- **Heart disease.** DHEA blocks the development of atherosclerosis. In one study, plasma levels of DHEA were inversely related to death from cardiovascular disease in men over fifty (but not in women). Low DHEA levels corresponded to fatal heart attacks. High DHEA levels were associated not only with fewer fatal heart attacks, but with a reduction in the death rate from all other diseases as well.[7]
- **Stroke.** Because higher DHEA levels can reduce hardening of the arteries, DHEA is protective against cardiovascular disease.
- **Diabetes.** DHEA helps offset insulin resistance by increasing the sensitivity of the cells to insulin.
- **Cancer.** DHEA may help prevent cancer. Low DHEA levels are associated with the development of cancer, and one long-term study found that women with lower than normal DHEA-derived hormones developed breast cancer several years later.[8]
- **Obesity and weight loss.** It looks as if the decline in DHEA that occurs as we age may play a role in the weight gain that is associated with growing older. DHEA decreases body fat and increases muscle mass, and has also allowed some lucky people on DHEA replacement therapy to lose weight without cutting back on calories. One explanation is that DHEA causes calories to be burned more efficiently so that less fat is deposited.
- **Osteoporosis.** DHEA converts into both estrogen (which inhibits bone resorption) and progesterone (which stimulates bone formation), so it combats osteoporosis from two directions at once. Women with higher levels of DHEA tend to have greater bone mass.
- **Arthritis and autoimmune problems.** Studies show that DHEA restrains autoantibodies, which play a pivotal role in arthritis and other autoimmune diseases. This could help explain why DHEA has been useful in the treatment of lupus. In one study of lupus patients, high doses of DHEA (200 milligrams a day—not a level for routine use) resulted in fewer symptoms and lowered doses of other potent medications.[9]

DHEA seems to improve people's overall well-being. Some of my patients report increased energy and enhanced memory (perhaps because DHEA helps maintain the normal function of neuronal cells). DHEA also seems to act as a buffer against stress (it offsets stress hormones like adrenaline) and to reverse some of the deterioration of aging. Some older patients report that they have more "get up and go," and some comment that they didn't realize they could feel so good at their age.

Diagnosing and Treating DHEA Insufficiency

DHEA production in the body is affected by many factors, including stress, disease, alcohol, birth control pills, and smoking. My goal in supplementing DHEA is not to restore a patient's DHEA level to that of a twenty-year-old, but to make sure he or she has a serum DHEA level that is mid- to high-normal for his or her age. In general, I'm not convinced that those of us with older bodies should necessarily be trying to resurrect the hormone levels we had in our college years. There may be reasons, as yet undetermined, why nature chooses not to keep our hormones surging at full strength while our cells and other systems age.

I always test a patient's blood levels of DHEA sulfate (a metabolite of DHEA that is more stable in the blood than DHEA) before recommending supplementation. When I do give a patient DHEA supplements, I start him or her on a low dose (such as 5 to 10 milligrams a day for women and 10 to 25 milligrams a day for men) and work up (usually to 20 to 50 milligrams a day, occasionally higher). I also continue to monitor a patient's DHEA levels with periodic blood tests, initially two or three months after starting DHEA replacement, and then, after blood levels appear stable, annually.

DHEA isn't appropriate for everyone. Because it's a hormone precursor, it should not be given to young people (who are not sexually mature), to women with estrogen-dependent problems (such as breast or uterine cancer, endometriosis, or uterine fibroids), or to men with prostate cancer.

Hormone Replacement Therapy

While "hormone replacement therapy" usually refers to the supplementation of sex hormones, it isn't just for women. Most of this section will be devoted to hormone replacement therapy for menopause, but male readers might want to skip to page 315 to read up on testosterone replacement therapy.

Women can experience hormone deficiencies and imbalances while they're of menstruating age, while they're entering menopause, or even after they've "paused." Don't assume that painful menstrual cramps or extreme premenstrual symptoms are just a part of life, or that irregular periods are simply due to growing older. Hormone therapy might be beneficial for you if you have these kinds of symptoms.

Many doctors will address a woman's hormonal imbalances by issuing a prescription for birth control pills. After all, birth control pills are supposed to deliver the correct hormones in the right doses. This just doesn't make sense to me. It's a little like putting in a new bathroom because the handle fell off your shower door. Sure, you fixed the handle . . . but what new problems did you create?

Menopause

Menopause is very individual. Some women sail through the "change of life" without much thought, while others experience symptoms that are as wide-ranging as they are intense. Some women are forced to go into instant menopause because of the surgical removal of their uterus and ovaries (which can occur at any age). For others, the climacteric (as doctors call it) can last up to ten years. When menopause occurs naturally, it is a process, not a single event.

The mind/body connection is very important in menopause, because how a woman feels about leaving her childbearing years behind can influence her health. Seeing this process as losing reproductive capabilities, and therefore being diminished, is markedly different than viewing this transition as an opportunity to move into maturity and wisdom, with all the power and beauty inherent in this.

Women making the transition into menopause may experience:

- Hot flashes
- Insomnia, restless sleep
- Irritability, mood swings
- Depression, anxiety attacks
- Migraine headaches
- Chronic fatigue
- Decreased short-term memory
- Loss of libido
- Bone loss (osteoporosis)
- Irregular menstrual cycles
- Premenstrual-like syndrome

Menopause is brought about by declining hormone levels. Estrogen levels start to slip at around age forty and keep falling until age seventy and beyond. As the ovaries age, the amount of hormones they produce declines by up to 80 percent. The adrenal glands try to compensate by secreting androgens, which can be converted by the body into estrogens, but this is basically a stopgap measure. By age fifty or so, a woman no longer has a sufficient amount of estrogen to produce a menstrual cycle. At this point, ovulation and menstruation cease, and menopause begins.

After menopause, the adrenals continue to secrete estrogen precursors, so there is still estrogen in a woman's body. Over time, however, smaller and smaller amounts of estrogen precursors are produced, and estrogen levels fall further. Estrogen-dependent tissues (such as the breasts, urethra, vagina, and vulva) begin to atrophy, and secondary problems like inflammation of the urethra and vaginal itching can develop.

Low estrogen levels are also associated with increased cardiac risk and osteoporosis. At present 400,000 women die from cardiovascular disease each year (compared to 46,000 from breast cancer), and 300,000 women fracture their hips,[10] so clearly these are very significant health concerns.

Estrogen

Because low levels of estrogen can have an adverse effect on women's health, giving women estrogen replacement therapy (ERT) seemed like a logical thing to do in the 1960s. And in fact, ERT turned out to have many benefits. ERT may prevent hardening of the arteries (atherosclerosis), prevent the oxidation of cholesterol (remember, oxidized choles-terol is a bad thing), and have a beneficial effect on HDL (good) cholesterol. In addition, ERT decreases the risk of osteoporosis by as much as 50 percent by preventing the bone loss that accelerates at menopause. (ERT can't reverse bone loss once it has occurred.) Estrogen also can eliminate many of the symptoms of menopause, including hot flashes and tissue atrophy.

There's a connection between estrogen and the immune system that is worth noting. Estrogen seems to enhance immunity. It has been known for some time that the female of the species is immunologically stronger than the male, but the flip side of this advantage is an increased tendency toward autoimmune disorders. The fact that estrogen can activate B cells may partially explain why women are more likely to have autoimmune problems than men.[11]

Knowing, as we now do, that the neurological, endocrine, and immune systems all keep up a steady conversation among themselves, perhaps it is isn't so surprising that lymphoid cells have hormone receptors on them. Studies have shown that prior to ovulation, a wom-an's sex hormones upregulate her immune system. One theory holds that estrogen acts to increase secretions of both prolactin (a hormone primarily responsible for stimulating fe-male breast development and milk production) and growth hormones, which in turn in-crease the production of T cells and B cells.[12] After she stops menstruating, a woman's level of circulating antibodies and her general immune response become much more like a man's: steady, and not upregulated.

So is ERT the answer to menopause? Not necessarily. It turns out that estrogen supple-mentation used alone (unopposed) definitely increases the risk of uterine cancer (it causes hyperplasia, or overgrowth of the uterine lining, which is potentially cancerous), and it possibly increases the risk of breast cancer.

Another reason to be cautious is the connection between estrogen and endometriosis (a disease characterized by the growth of endometrial cells outside the uterus). Medical therapy for endometriosis traditionally consists of regimens that limit the effects of estrogen. One study found that patients with endometriosis show an inverse relationship between blood levels of estradiol (one of the estrogenic hormones) and the cytotoxicity of NK cells. Advanced endometriosis is associated with elevated estradiol and impaired NK cytotoxicity.[13]

As you know by now, balance is the key, and estrogen is naturally balanced in the body with other hormones. Since ERT was first introduced, researchers have determined that one way to minimize the risks of unopposed estrogen therapy is to administer progesterone as well (see page 313).

If you proceed with estrogen replacement therapy for menopause or for another condi-tion (for example, infertility, a menstrual disorder, or—for men—prostate cancer), you and your doctor should discuss the different forms of estrogen available. All estrogen medications are not created equal.

The ovaries produce three different types (or fractions) of estrogen: estrone (E1), estradiol (E2), and estriol (E3). Estradiol is by far the most predominant and the most powerful. The most commonly prescribed medication is Premarin, which is a mixture of conjugated estrogens extracted from the urine of pregnant mares.

Taking estrogen in pills presents some uncertainties (much of the active estrogen is not absorbed, and much of that which is absorbed is destroyed by the liver), so the continuous-supply estrogen patch was invented. Estrogen cream is also available. (Although it is applied locally, it is absorbed through the skin and can have systemic effects.)

I rarely prescribe synthetic estrogens. I am concerned about the way they are utilized by the body, and I don't like the fact that they can be associated with side effects ranging from stroke and blood clots to liver disorders. Instead, I usually prescribe a natural "triple" estrogen from plant sources that contains E1, E2, and E3. This preparation provides the benefits of ERT with fewer risks. (You'll recall from the discussion of soy on pages 139–40 that some plants contain phytoestrogens, compounds with estrogenlike activity.)

Estriol, one of the weaker estrogens, is turning out to hold great promise for ERT. Estriol used alone does not seem to cause uterine cancer, and it may even help prevent breast cancer.[14]

Patients on any kind of ERT should have regular checkups. ERT can cause a variety of side effects, including breast pain, vaginal bleeding, nausea and vomiting, high blood pressure, headaches, fluid retention (bloating), jaundice (when the liver is overburdened), and impaired glucose tolerance. An unsatisfactory experience with one type of ERT should not lead you to rule out ERT altogether.

Estrogen replacement is not for everyone. Estrogen should not be taken during pregnancy. Women with reproductive cancer, a family history of breast cancer, or any indications of precancerous conditions should not take estradiol. Women with severe fibrocystic breast disease, hypertension, or clotting disorders should be aware that added estrogen can worsen these conditions. Oral estrogen can elevate triglyceride levels and enhance gallstone formation (although the patch does not).

As you can see, there is a lot to discuss with your doctor. The subject of ERT is complicated, but you may be able to find a way of incorporating natural estrogen into your life in a way that allows you to reap its beneficial effects while minimizing its risks.

Progesterone

During a normal menstrual cycle, estrogen levels rise for about two weeks, at which point ovulation occurs. After ovulation, the ovaries produce progesterone (as in "promote estrogen") for the next two weeks or so. Both estrogen and progesterone levels drop off just before menstruation.

Progesterone, like estrogen, has immune-regulating effects, although progesterone tends to be immune suppressing (as does testosterone). This helps explain why men in their reproductive years are significantly less affected by autoimmune disorders than women. The way men's and women's macrophages are affected by sex hormones seems to influence the development of rheumatoid arthritis.[15]

During the second half of a woman's monthly cycle, when progesterone levels rise, the immune system is suppressed in anticipation of pregnancy. If this process works correctly and if conception does occur, the immune system does not reject the fetus. During pregnancy, progesterone's suppressive effects on lymphocyte proliferation and activity continue to be protective of the baby, even though the mother is more vulnerable to viral infections.

Progesterone helps offset the effects of estrogen on the body, so these two important hormones are in a perpetual dance. Sometimes the ratio between estrogen and progesterone goes out of balance. Women with an excess of estrogen may develop estrogen-related disorders such as uterine fibroids or fibrocystic breast disease. Adding a small amount of progesterone can rebalance the ratio between estrogen and progesterone and relieve symptoms. This approach also can minimize the symptoms of premenstrual syndrome, as well as the exacerbation of chronic Lyme symptoms that some women experience in the second half of their menstrual cycle.

Progesterone can help restore libido, and it plays a role in preventing osteoporosis. After menopause, progesterone levels fall even more than estrogen levels, so when I treat women who are entering menopause, I usually start them off with nutrients and herbs and some progesterone. If necessary, I'll add estrogen next. Occasionally a patient will show signs of taking too much progesterone (such as dizziness, sleepiness, and fatigue), but this is easily remedied by cutting back on the dose.

Again, I prefer natural progesterone (micronized, or finely ground) from plant sources (wild yams) over synthetic progesterone (such as Provera), which lacks the full effects of natural progesterone. Artificial progesterone has a different chemical structure than natural progesterone, so while it displaces natural progesterone, it also functions slightly differently in the body. For example, synthetic progesterone moves sodium and water into cells, which can cause water retention and hypertension. With natural progesterone, the sodium stays outside cells where it belongs.[16] Typical doses of natural progesterone are from $\frac{1}{4}$ to $\frac{1}{2}$ teaspoon twice a day of progesterone cream, or from 50 to 100 milligrams of natural progesterone orally two to four times a day. (Unlike synthetic progesterones, natural progesterone preparations need to be taken more than once a day.)

Like some of the other natural hormone preparations, it is possible to obtain progesterone cream without a prescription. However, without proper monitoring, patients may take excessive and possibly unsafe doses. Evidence has recently come to light that progesterone cream, even in typical doses, may accumulate in the subcutaneous tissue, causing an overdose of the active fraction of the hormone. It is best to have your hormone status evaluated and monitored by a knowledgeable physician.

Combination Estrogen/Progesterone Therapy

Estrogen and progesterone are, as we've seen, linked together during the normal menstrual cycle. Combination therapy does not seem to interfere with estrogenic benefits, but it modulates estrogen's risks.

There are many different approaches to combination therapy. Which one is best for you can be determined only by a physician who has a thorough understanding of your hormone profile. Cyclic hormone therapy (modeled after the changing hormone levels of a natural menstrual cycle) can cause a return of menstrual bleeding, but need not do so (especially if relatively low doses are used). Another approach for menopausal women is a continuous combined regimen (the same doses every day), which also is not associated with bleeding.

Testosterone

Both men and women have testosterone. Testosterone levels in men start to decline gradually at about age forty; in women, at about age fifty. By age eighty, healthy men have one-third to one-half the amount of free testosterone they had at age twenty.[17]

Testosterone affects metabolism. One of its functions is to ensure that the body's major source of energy is aerobic (not anaerobic) metabolism. Metabolism that uses oxygen more efficiently can combat fatigue as well as the diseases associated with aging (see Chapter 11, Redox Medicine).

Testosterone also can have anti-autoimmune effects. In one study, men with active rheumatoid arthritis were treated daily with oral testosterone. At the end of six months, they had an increase in T suppressor cells, fewer joints were affected, and their daily intake of nonsteroidal anti-inflammatory drugs was reduced.[18] Treating an autoimmune disorder with testosterone is an option not only for men but also for women.

In men, testosterone deficiency can cause a decrease in libido, erection problems, and "male menopause" (andropause). In women, testosterone deficiency can cause loss of libido and breast tenderness. Both men and women with testosterone deficiency complain of just feeling lousy.

Testosterone replacement therapy can increase sex drive in older men and women. In women, it may help menopausal symptoms when estrogen replacement therapy does not, and it may help prevent osteoporosis as well. On the other hand, giving testosterone to a woman who does not need it can cause hair growth and acne. Both men and women should have their testosterone levels checked before initiating testosterone replacement therapy, and their testosterone levels should be monitored periodically and adjusted as necessary.

There is controversy about whether or not testosterone replacement therapy increases a man's risk of prostate cancer. In Europe, according to some medical reports, low testosterone levels are associated with prostate cancer. Here in the United States, the general consensus is that excess testosterone, via its conversion to dihydrotestosterone, is associated with BPH (benign prostatic hypertrophy) and prostate cancer. Clearly we don't yet have all the answers.

Once again, I favor natural testosterone preparations over their synthetic analogues. Doses generally range from 5 to 20 milligrams a day for women, and from 80 to 160 milligrams a day for men.

Growth Hormone Deficiency

In the body, growth hormone is secreted by the pituitary gland. Growth hormone levels peak at adolescence and then gradually decline (faster in men than in women). Today interest in growth hormone is picking up because of its antiaging properties. Growth hormone holds promise for stopping or even reversing some of the degenerative changes that occur with age, and in fact there have been reports of improvement in many age-related conditions with growth hormone replacement.

Growth hormone levels can decline for reasons other than advancing age. Growth hormone is secreted predominantly during deep sleep—the kind of sleep that can be cut short by illness, medications, or age. Also, physical activity sets off the release of growth hormone, while a sedentary life may contribute to low growth hormone levels. Excess tobacco, coffee, and alcohol all decrease growth hormone levels.

Growth hormone affects the metabolism of glucose and fat. In fact, it redistributes body fat (it tends to displace belly fat, which is associated with heart disease). Higher levels of growth hormone are associated with decreased fat mass and increased lean body tissue.

Congenital growth hormone deficiency can impair cardiac growth and function. Growth hormone deficiency in a young person causes short stature. In a full-grown individual, growth hormone deficiency can cause:

- Impaired psychological well-being
- Increased fat mass, particularly in the abdomen
- Reduced muscle strength, reduced capacity for exercise
- Intolerance to cold
- Skin changes (wrinkles, thin skin)

Growth hormone replacement therapy causes a shift in metabolism, resulting in more muscle and less fat. It accelerates healing in both the skeletal and soft tissue of surgical patients, and it is used to treat heart conditions. A 1996 article in *The New England Journal of Medicine* noted that growth hormone administered for three months to patients with idiopathic dilated cardiomyopathy (a condition in which a ventricle of the heart progressively dilates and no longer pumps blood normally) increased myocardial mass and improved clinical symptoms and exercise capacity.[19] After growth hormone was discontinued, these beneficial effects were partially reversed.

In addition to these physical effects, growth hormone can affect psychological well-being. European researchers, following up on patients who had lost their pituitary gland and who were already receiving what was considered adequate hormone replacement therapy, discovered that when growth hormone was added to their regimen, there was a great improvement in psychological well-being.[20] A study of hypopituitary patients with growth hormone deficiency (almost all hypopituitary patients have this condition) found that growth hormone replacement improved their quality of life, including their energy level, emotional reactions, social interaction, and vitality.[21]

Diagnosing and Treating Growth Hormone Deficiency

Blood tests for growth hormone deficiency are unreliable because even healthy individuals can have levels below the lower detection limit of most tests. Also, there is a thirtyfold or larger range in growth hormone secretion among ostensibly healthy adults.[22] Age, body composition, physical fitness, gender, nutritional status, and sleep patterns all help determine growth hormone levels.

Stimulation tests (in which the secretion of growth hormone is artificially stimulated) can be helpful, as can tests that assess markers of growth hormone action (such as *insulinlike growth factor 1* and *somatomedin C* levels). However, there is still controversy over how reliable these tests are and what factors can skew the results. A clinical diagnosis of growth hormone deficiency can be made based on the constellation of signs and symptoms listed above. Additional factors often associated with growth hormone deficiency are pituitary disease and evidence of other hormone deficiencies.

Growth hormone is expensive, slow to take effect, and available only in injection form. It is generally well tolerated. Sometimes it can cause fluid retention (i.e., swelling of the hands or fingers), and because it antagonizes insulin, it can bring on diabetes-like symptoms. There is some question as to whether supplemental growth hormone is associated with a stimulatory effect on tumors. Researchers are working on developing ways to stimulate the body's production of natural growth hormone by administering growth hormone releasing hormone (GHRH). This may turn out to be the optimal way of raising growth hormone levels in the body.

Growth hormone used to be in very short supply because it could be obtained only from the pituitary glands of cadavers. Interest in growth hormone picked up significantly after researchers figured out how to produce it artificially.

People vary in their sensitivity to growth hormone, so dosing is individual. A common dosage regimen is one vial (4 units) per week, as an injection two times a day, in the morning and at bedtime. Injections are usually given 4–6 days per week. Patients receiving growth hormone replacement therapy should have their levels of somatomedin C periodically measured and also should be monitored for possible side effects. Usually these can be corrected with an adjustment in dosage rather than cessation of treatment.

INTRAVENOUS VITAMIN C

In Chapter 6, I discussed the many reasons why everyone should take in abundant amounts of vitamin C. In addition to recommending a daily dose of vitamin C to help prevent health problems, I also administer pharmacologic doses of vitamin C (sometimes with other nutrients included) to help patients who are ill.

When taken orally, high doses of vitamin C can cause gastrointestinal upset (gas, cramps, diarrhea). However, when high doses of vitamin C are administered intravenously, there is usually no digestive upset. The intravenous method is a more efficient way of rapidly getting an optimal amount of vitamin C into the body, for none of the vitamin is destroyed in the gut or lost due to malabsorption problems.

Even though it is extremely, sometimes dramatically, effective, high-dose intravenous vitamin C is somewhat controversial. Adding a gram of vitamin C to an intravenous solution does not upset traditional doctors as much as administering many grams at once. (I'm happy to say that some of the surgeons at my local hospital add vitamin C to the intravenous solution of their postoperative surgical patients.) A minority of doctors vehemently oppose high-dose intravenous vitamin C therapy, while the great majority just aren't persuaded that it does any good. They never learned about this protocol in medical school, they aren't hearing about it from the pharmaceutical salespeople, and they haven't read any articles about it in *The Journal of the American Medical Association* or *The New England Journal of Medicine,* so it is not one of their treatment options. Some doctors are afraid of possible side effects, but in my view as well as in my clinical experience, these have been terribly overstated, especially when you read the full description of any drug in the *Physicians' Desk Reference.*

I know that intravenous vitamin C will withstand the test of time, and that eventually the wonderful benefits of this therapy will be more broadly recognized. In the meantime, there are economic reasons why few experts are willing to champion vitamin C. The pharmaceutical companies couldn't make large amounts of money off vitamin C because it's not a patentable substance. When the cost of developing a new drug can run into the hundreds of millions of dollars, why would a drug manufacturer invest in a substance that is already cheap and readily available?

Researchers can't pursue vitamin C studies because there is no money to fund them. Physicians are slow to pick up on intravenous vitamin C because most insurance companies don't cover the cost. Also, intravenous vitamin C has become one of those symbols of alternative medicine, like chronic candidiasis. The attitude seems to be that if you give your patients intravenous vitamin C, you aren't a "real" doctor.

I think you know by now that I'm a very scientific physician who also uses effective alternative treatments. There is no doubt in my mind that intravenous vitamin C works. I've been giving it to my patients for fourteen years, and I could fill another entire book with case histories involving the benefits of high-dose vitamin C.

Why Intravenous Vitamin C?

The body's need for vitamin C increases when we are exposed to toxins or threatened by infection. A cold increases the body's need for vitamin C. Hepatitis increases the body's need for vitamin C even further. In fact, Robert Cathcart, M.D., an expert on the clinical use of high dosages of vitamin C, has correlated what doses are most beneficial for which disorders. By saturating the tissues, we can ensure that the white blood cells have enough vitamin C to function with maximal effectiveness.

Intravenous vitamin C has many benefits, including:

- **It is an excellent antiviral agent.** Intravenous vitamin C is appropriate for both acute and chronic viral infections, and it helps control reactivated viral infections, which tend to flare up when the immune system is challenged by additional stressors. I find that it is useful in treating viral hepatitis, shingles, mononucleosis (Epstein-Barr virus), and cytomegalovirus infection. Many people are now interested in the effects of intravenous vitamin C on the virus that causes AIDS, and studies are currently being done. One study conducted by Linus Pauling and his colleagues showed that continuous exposure of HIV-infected cells to noncytotoxic concentrations of vitamin C resulted in significant inhibition of virus replication.[23]

- **It is helpful in treating bacterial infections.** I commonly use intravenous vitamin C as an adjunctive treatment in my patients with severe Lyme disease. Not only does vitamin C support the immune system directly, but it also appears to broaden the spectrum of antibiotics, making them more effective against a greater number of organisms.[24]

- **It is a detoxifying agent.** Intravenous vitamin C helps the body defend itself against heavy metals, chemical pollutants, and bacterial toxins (for example, those involved in botulism, tetanus, and diphtheria). Fred Klenner, M.D., an early champion of intravenous vitamin C, used it to counteract snake and spider venom.[25] Vitamin C infusions also help protect the body against damage from high-dose antibiotics, radiation, and chemotherapy.

- **It is an effective immune modulator.** I find intravenous vitamin C very helpful for patients with recurrent infections, chronic fatigue immune dysfunction syndrome, autoimmune disorders, and allergies. The wonder of this treatment is that it helps bring the immune system back into balance whether it is upregulated (hypersensitive) or downregulated (not responsive enough). In this way, vitamin C functions like an adaptogen.

- **It helps maintain a healthy state of homeostasis.** Intravenous vitamin C helps the body "keep its balance" when it is stressed by physical trauma, surgery, burns, intense cold, or debilitating medical treatments. In general, it helps patients feel more energetic and less lethargic.

Intravenous vitamin C is generally very safe, but it may be contraindicated for people with kidney problems, iron overload, or a tendency to form oxalate stones. I usually start patients on intravenous vitamin C treatments once or twice a week and work up to a dose of 50 grams per session for four to eight treatments. Then I reevaluate the patient's condition and readjust his or her dosage and the frequency with which it is administered.

At forty-four, my patient Naomi felt as if all her life's bills were suddenly coming due. In her youth, she had used intravenous drugs, but within a few years she'd kicked the habit. Now, twenty years later, she had a busy career in academia. She also had chronic hepatitis, low-grade fever, persistent fatigue, and bouts of depression, plus many allergies and signs of decreased immune competence (tests revealed both low secretory IgA and low NK cell function).

Naomi's previous doctor had placed her on interferon, which can be helpful for hepatitis, but which was making Naomi feel lousy. She was taking Tylenol to counteract the effects of the interferon, and Zoloft to offset her depression—and she still had "zero energy."

Naomi lived in another state eight hours by car from our health center, so she made arrangements to come and stay nearby while she received intensive intravenous treatments for a three-week period. During this time she received intravenous vitamin C infusions that included several other nutrients, and in between these she received intravenous hydrogen peroxide treatments twice a week (see Chapter 11). During this period she also went through a three-week liver detoxification program.

This concentrated regimen had marked effects that were both immediate and long-lasting. After Naomi returned home, she kept up her allergen-free diet and continued to take a number of hormonal and nutritional supplements I prescribed for her, including buffered vitamin C powder and a special formula for liver support. Her temperature returned to normal, she was able to discontinue both the interferon and the Zoloft, her spirits were better, her energy was markedly improved, and she had a "whole new lease on life."

Vitamin C and Cancer

There is a tremendous amount of anecdotal evidence—innumerable case histories from doctors who use intravenous vitamin C—indicating that vitamin C therapy can be an important part of a cancer treatment regimen. There are also many studies about vitamin C and cancer, but I am not aware of any watertight double-blind placebo-controlled study published in a major medical journal. Still, clinical evidence abounds.

An article in *Oncology*[26] tells of a forty-two-year-old man with malignant tumors of the reticuloendothelial system who was placed on intravenous vitamin C until conventional medical treatment could be initiated. After two weeks he was astonishingly improved, so conventional therapy was postponed. After twenty-two days he was "cured." When he cut back on his dose of vitamin C, his cancer returned. Again, intravenous vitamin C reversed his symptoms, although the second time it took a little longer. That intravenous vitamin C played a role in inducing both of these remissions seems indisputable.

Just how helpful vitamin C will be depends upon many factors, including the dose used, the duration of each infusion, the type of cancer that is being treated, what other treatments have been tried (or are being tried), what stage the cancer is in, the patient's ability to utilize vitamin C, and how long treatments are continued. In a best-case scenario, enough of these variables will favor recovery so that the patient will improve.

When using vitamin C to treat cancer, it is vital to use high doses and to keep the tissues saturated. A study with mice showed that while lower doses of vitamin C caused no changes in cancer cells, higher concentrations were lethal (to the cancer cells, not the mice).[27] To be maximally effective against tumors, the blood concentration of vitamin C should be kept at tumor toxicity range for as long as possible. In between intravenous treatments, I have my patients take very high doses of oral vitamin C. I also have found that it is important to keep up this regimen indefinitely.

In my experience, intravenous vitamin C can be an extremely important part of a larger regimen. It usually is not The Answer, although certainly there are stories of vitamin C melting tumors away all by itself. In fact, clinicians learned the hard way that vitamin C can be *too* effective. In a few rare cases, when too much vitamin C was given too quickly, extensive tumor necrosis and hemorrhage resulted, which not only destroyed the cancer but killed the patient.

One study showed convincingly that vitamin C has preferential toxicity for malignant melanoma cells in cell culture.[28] Human studies, too, indicate that vitamin C is preferentially toxic to tumor cells.[29] When it is given in high enough doses (attainable only intravenously), vitamin C levels in the blood are cytotoxic to abnormal cells but not to healthy cells. As an added bonus, intravenous vitamin C has few side effects (if any), it appears to make it more difficult for cancer to spread, and it does not suppress the immune system the way conventional cancer therapies do.

CHELATION THERAPY

Chelation is derived from the Greek word *chel,* which means "latch on to." Intravenous chelation therapy removes heavy metals from the body by means of a chelating agent that binds with the metals (lead, mercury, cadmium, etc.) and carries them into the blood. The kidneys then filter the bound-together complexes out of the bloodstream, and they are then excreted in the urine.

With age or illness, cells have a more difficult time eliminating heavy metals, which can lead to immune-compromising accumulations of toxins. Taking steps to remove heavy metals from the body can bring immediate relief to the immune system. Some doctors routinely recommend chelation therapy for patients over forty for this reason.

EDTA

Most often when people refer to "chelation therapy," they mean EDTA (ethylenediaminetetraacetic acid) therapy. EDTA is a synthetic amino acid that is not broken down by the body, so it's a good vehicle for chelating heavy metals and escorting them out of the body.

In the 1950s, when workers were treated with chelation therapy for lead poisoning, it was unexpectedly discovered that their heart disease improved. Since then, chelation therapy has been shown to improve blood flow throughout the body, which in turn restores the body's ability to oxygenate tissues and cells. This beneficial effect on circulation helps explain why chelation therapy can help everything from cognitive function to chronic fatigue to eye problems.

Heavy metals bind with enzymes in the body and inactivate them, so removing the heavy metals normalizes the distribution of metallic elements in the body and allows enzymes to function again. This helps counteract cardiovascular disease by making arterial walls more elastic and inhibiting platelet aggregation and the formation of arterial plaques.

Even when heavy metals are not a problem, chelation has beneficial effects on the way the body uses calcium. On one hand, EDTA therapy reverses the effects of calcification, or calcium buildup inside the arteries ("hardening of the arteries") and inside the joints. On the other hand, calcium in the bones is either undisturbed or increased.

EDTA also inhibits the production of free radicals, thereby reducing the lipid peroxidation of cellular and mitochondrial membranes. As you know from reading the previous chapters, cell membranes are of the utmost importance in cell function and in cell-to-cell communication. Healthy cell membranes enable the immune system to do its job efficiently.

In addition, EDTA stimulates the enlargement of small vessels, which in turn enhances what is known as "collateral circulation" (vessels that act as a detour around a blockage). This, too, is beneficial for cardiovascular health.

Because the effect of EDTA is nonspecific—it will bind with beneficial minerals such as zinc, chromium, and selenium, to name a few—I make sure my patients on EDTA therapy are well supplemented with important nutrients. Cardiac patients can keep taking any necessary medications (such as blood thinners, blood pressure medications, and antianginal agents) while having chelation therapy. Sometimes the improvement in their health allows their medications to become more effective. The happiest situation is when improved health makes it possible for patients to decrease or even to stop taking medications altogether.

DMPS

Another chelating agent, DMPS (dimercaptoproprionsulfonic acid), binds preferentially with mercury. As I mentioned in Chapter 4, mercury is a serious health issue today not only because of mercury-contaminated fish but also because of mercury-containing dental amalgams. Some people are not particularly sensitive to mercury, but a toxic overload has accumulated in their bodies. Other people are sensitive even to small amounts.

DMPS can be used as a challenge test. After a patient is given a dose of DMPS (intravenously or intramuscularly), he or she collects urine samples for twenty-four hours. These are then checked for heavy metals at labs (such as the Mayo Clinic laboratory) that are experienced in the evaluation of heavy metals.

A positive test result indicates the presence of excess mercury in the body. It seems that more and more people are having abnormal, even toxic, results from this test. Even though this is a "provocative" test—that is, it is designed to pull mercury out of the tissues—these high test results are far from normal.

Mercury poisoning isn't usually the first thing a doctor will think of when presented with a complex clinical picture, but again, you need to know where to look for answers. It is not uncommon for patients with immune disorders, chronic skin problems, chronic neurological problems, and chronic autoimmune problems to have a major body load of mercury. Once these toxic levels of mercury are removed from their system, they can start to make significant progress.

DMPS therapy can be used when a patient has mercury toxicity, but only after he or she has had any mercury-containing fillings removed. Because the process of replacing dental amalgams can actually add to the patient's toxic burden (more mercury is inhaled and absorbed while the old fillings are removed), the patient frequently is given an injection of DMPS before visiting the dentist.

One of my patients not only had a lot of fillings, but also was a dental assistant, so she worked with mercury-containing amalgam all day. She had eczema *everywhere,* persistent fatigue, numbness in her fingers, and recurrent candida infections, and toxic levels of mercury were showing up in her urine. After she was treated for mercury toxicity, including "protected" amalgam removal, her urine levels of mercury returned to normal, her skin cleared, and her multiple other symptoms abated.

Desferrioxamine

Desferrioxamine chelation therapy is used for iron overload. It's not uncommon for people to have evidence of excessive iron in their blood, but usually not to the point where chelation is necessary. Patients with thalassemia, a hereditary blood disorder that results in abnormally low levels of hemoglobin, often receive many blood transfusions, which can cause an accumulation of excess iron. Iron overload also is not unusual in diabetic patients.

COMMONLY ASKED QUESTION NO. 20:

Why isn't chelation therapy more common?

The FDA has approved chelation therapy for heavy metal poisoning, digitalis toxicity, and hypercalcemia (increased blood calcium levels). However, once a drug is approved for one purpose, physicians may use it for another as long as there is evidence that this may be helpful. There is clinical evidence linking chelation therapy with improved immune function and improved cardiovascular health. An increasing number of holistic physicians are using chelation therapy for a variety of chronic degenerative problems with notable success. Although the major medical associations maintain that the effectiveness of chelation therapy for the treatment of cardiovascular disease and other degenerative diseases is unproven, I have seen enough evidence in my own practice to be fully convinced that chelation therapy can be invaluable to patients with these types of problems.

In fact, the effectiveness of chelation therapy may be one reason why the medical establishment doesn't approve of it. A relatively inexpensive, noninvasive therapy that improves circulation throughout the body with few side effects calls into question many of the more invasive procedures such as cardiac catheterization, balloon angioplasty, and coronary bypass surgery. Some of my patients have even been able to avoid bypass surgery with chelation therapy and lifestyle modifications.

IMMUNOTHERAPY

Back in Chapter 4, I discussed allergy shots. Although immunotherapy is very common, I handle it a little differently in my office. When we test a patient for allergies, we use various dilutions of allergy extract until we find the correct dose that will produce the desired immune response without making the patient uncomfortable. As you will recall, this dose becomes the starting point of the patient's individualized immunotherapy. Because we don't necessarily start at square one, we're able to start the patient's allergy shots at a well-tolerated, higher, and more beneficial dose.

Allergy work makes up a large part of my practice. Many of my patients have complicated clinical situations that include allergies to foods, inhalants, and chemicals. I have found that it is often possible to give a patient a neutralizing dose of an antigen or allergen that will "cancel out" symptoms. We have used this technique for foods as well as for fungal and bacterial illnesses. In the last few years, we have also become involved with a very exciting new method of immunotherapy called enzyme-potentiated desensitization (EPD) that allows us to quiet down a hyperactive immune system.

Candida and Lyme Immunotherapy

Some of my patients have nearly intractable cases of candidiasis or Lyme disease that are difficult to beat. These persistent, chronic illnesses can lead to immune-mediated problems. The immune system becomes hyperreactive to the candida yeast or to the Lyme antigen (or piece of antigen), and symptoms persist even after all the usual, and maybe even unusual, antifungal and antibacterial therapies have been tried.

Remember the sea serpent from Chapter 4—the sine curve illustrating the harmonic quality of immune reactions? Once you find the precise neutralizing dose for allergic or infectious problems, you can restore balance to the immune system and quiet an immune reaction immediately. I've had patients tell me that their headache just stopped dead, or their vaginal burning suddenly ceased, in the middle of the treatment. This kind of immunotherapy is extremely dose-dependent. It's important to find exactly the right dose, or symptoms can worsen instead of improve.

This kind of immunotherapy can be difficult to explain to patients. Rather than directly fighting the infection, here we are trying to normalize the immune system's hypersensitive response to the infectious antigen. Lingering antigens—which include dead or fragmented organisms—can continue to provoke an immune response even after an infection has been treated. When a bacterial infection is involved (as with Lyme), I do not use immunotherapy as a substitute for antibiotic treatment. However, after a course of antibiotics, immunotherapy can enhance recovery by modulating the body's overreactivity to the Lyme spirochete or to its residual components.

Lyme or candida immunotherapy is not the first treatment I'll try, but this approach can make a world of difference for patients who still have symptoms after other treatments have been utilized. My patient Roy, for example, already had many, many health issues—including fungal hypersensitivity, chronic pharyngitis and rhinitis, chronic Epstein-Barr viral syndrome, and underlying allergies—when he contracted Lyme disease. To add to his discomfort, he now had neck pain, knee pain, numbness and tingling, fuzzy thinking, and fever.

Several months of treatment with antibiotics reduced the severity of Roy's symptoms, but they did not completely go away. When I added Lyme immunotherapy to his regimen, Roy responded beautifully—so well, in fact, that he considers Lyme immunotherapy to be one of the major events in his recovering his health.

Enzyme-Potentiated Desensitization (EPD)

I have used EPD successfully for all kinds of patients, young and old, vigorous and weak, ready for anything or cautious about new treatments. What these patients all had in common was a large number of troublesome allergies and sensitivities, both overt and covert.

When I first saw Callie, she was six years old. She was a pretty little girl with a pale, thin face, dark circles under her eyes (often a giveaway for allergies), and a deep, frequent cough. Callie's medical history was already fairly involved. She'd had traditional allergy testing and had been diagnosed with asthma, for which she had been given inhalers. She'd had chronic nasal congestion, recurrent bronchitis, repeated episodes of croup, multiple ear infections, and many courses of antibiotics.

Callie turned out to be allergic to many foods and inhalants. Traditional skin testing had failed to diagnose her delayed-reaction allergies, and her local allergist—unaware of EPD—offered no treatment for her food allergies other than avoidance.

I started Callie on a yeast-free and allergen-free diet and antifungal medication, and subsequently initiated EPD treatment. The incidence of her infections diminished greatly, she stopped sneezing every morning, her nasal congestion went away, the dark circles under her eyes disappeared, and she started to gain weight. People were commenting on how much better she looked. Callie didn't mind the compliments, but what she really enjoyed was feeling so much better.

EPD is unusual because it is effective for such a broad range of allergies, including not only inhalant allergies but also food and chemical sensitivities. Many people believe that there is nothing they can do but avoid the substances to which they are allergic. This just isn't so. I have seen EPD bring relief to some of my most severely ill allergic patients, including those with multiple chemical sensitivities, and this has been a gratifying experience.

EPD was developed by Dr. Len McEwen in England over the course of many years of research. It is an ingenious technique that combines very small (that is, very safe) doses of allergens with the enzyme beta-glucuronidase, which is ubiquitous in the human body. The antigen mixture (there are different mixtures to choose from) covers a wide range of problematic substances. The enzyme part of the injection increases the effect of the small doses of antigen extracts. The combination is very powerful. For example, a single dose of grass pollen given with beta-glucuronidase can be as effective as a long course of conventional allergy shots.

Because lymphocytes take time to mature, and because EPD shots cannot be given more frequently than every eight weeks, EPD is a long-term proposition. However, its effects can be permanent. The literature on EPD associates it with an overall 70 to 80 percent success rate.

EPD shots work by stimulating the body to produce suppressor T cells that switch off allergic reactions. The enzyme beta-glucuronidase (which is released by macrophages and other types of white blood cells during an immune response) acts as a lymphokine and initiates a process that "reprograms" a new population of suppressor T cells. EPD may have other mechanisms as well (for example, enhancing cytokine production, such as the production of IL-10, which tends to downregulate inflammation and allergy). The effects of EPD do not appear to be confined to specific immunity. EPD seems to deliver a powerful autoregulatory stimulus that goes beyond the antigens in the treatment. EPD is actually proactive, as it can head off latent or hidden allergies before they become apparent.

However, EPD can also cause heightened sensitivities if it is administered on top of a large exposure to a particular antigen. For this reason, there is a careful protocol that must be followed in conjunction with EPD treatment. In order to avoid precipitating previously hidden allergies, patients need to avoid large doses of any common allergen (dust, molds, pet dander, pollens) as well as exposure to chemical fumes, smoke, aerosols, and newsprint for twenty-four hours before and after a treatment. Patients also are required to follow a hypoallergenic "EPD Diet" for a few days. There are other rules as well, all designed to enhance the effectiveness of EPD. This is quite unlike standard allergy shots, which are given without any regard for exposures to allergens either before or after.

EPD has some interesting applications. It can help rebalance an immune system that has been dysregulated by a viral or bacterial infection. Patients with allergic disorders such as asthma, eczema, rhinitis, and chronic hives benefit from EPD treatment. It can also help with hyperactivity, migraines and chronic headaches, irritable bowel syndrome, inflammatory bowel diseases, and mood swings, all of which can have an allergic component. A 1992 article in the *Lancet*[30] noted that EPD successfully treated underlying food allergies in hyperactive children. Of twenty hyperkinetic children who received EPD, sixteen became tolerant toward provoking foods. Of twenty in the control (placebo) group, four became tolerant. (Later evidence suggested that in fact only two in the control group became tolerant.)

Presently an international study of EPD is being conducted under the auspices of the Institutional Review Board of the Great Lakes Association of Clinical Medicine. I am one of the investigators participating in this study, and I look forward to the publication of its results. There are currently over six thousand patients in the study in the United States.

Remember Mikey, the autistic boy who had so many allergies? After his first EPD shot, Mikey's parents noted an increase in his awareness, attention, and the vocalizations he made. By the third treatment, his chronic ear infections had lessened. By the fourth, his ear infections stopped altogether. EPD was not the solution to all of Mikey's problems, but it certainly was an important step.

BIOLOGICAL RESPONSE MODIFIERS

As you'll recall from Chapter 3, the immune system produces cytokines for the purposes of cell-to-cell communication. Being immune system messengers, cytokines are enormously influential in an immune response. By isolating and synthesizing cytokines in the lab, researchers have been able to produce substances called *biological response modifiers* that can directly affect immune function.

Some biological response modifiers don't appear naturally in the body. For example, plants that have antimicrobial or immune-stimulating effects could be considered biological response modifiers. My purpose here, however, is to mention a few pharmaceutical biological response modifiers I use that can affect the progress of disease.

Kutapressin

Developed in the late 1940s, Kutapressin is a mixture of polypeptides derived from porcine liver. A broad-spectrum antiviral agent, Kutapressin is safe and generally well tolerated. Its beneficial effects can take several weeks to be apparent, and patients sometimes need to continue Kutapressin therapy for at least six weeks before seeing any improvement. Kutapressin is useful in controlling inflammation and is used for its immune-modulating effects in certain viral infections and psoriasis. I generally use it for patients with chronic fatigue immune dysfunction syndrome (CFIDS), particularly those with concomitant psoriasis. I frequently administer Kutapressin as an injection that includes vitamin B_{12} and folic acid, and have found this to be helpful in a subset of CFIDS patients.

Gamma Globulin

Gamma globulin provides passive immunity. It is a processed form of concentrated antibodies derived from human blood. The blood itself is pooled from many donors to provide the broadest possible immune protection.

Gamma globulin has been available as an intramuscular injection for more than forty years. It has a history of being used to protect against hepatitis and a wide variety of common infections, and is often used to protect travelers who may be exposed to these kinds of illnesses.

The shortcomings of gamma globulin injections include the fact that they can be painful, they can cause local irritation, and only a small amount can be given. In the 1980s, a form of gamma globulin was developed for intravenous use, which opened up new therapeutic possibilities. However, intravenous gamma globulin can be extremely expensive, especially in higher doses, and it is not necessarily covered by medical insurance. A theoretical drawback to gamma globulin use is the possibility of the transmission of the hepatitis C virus.[31]

Although its early use was problematic, modern gamma globulin preparations are generally well tolerated. Some patients experience dizziness, headache, nausea, and/or flu-like symptoms for up to several days after receiving intravenous treatment.

Gamma globulin is useful for immunodeficiency disorders of all types. It is especially helpful for people with antibody-deficient disorders, including IgG subclass deficiency, as it provides them with antibodies that otherwise would be unavailable to them. Gamma globulin is also used in connection with burns, HIV, CFIDS, myasthenia gravis, chronic inflammatory myopathy, ITP (immune thrombocytopenia), Kawasaki disease, cancer, and some autoimmune disorders. I use gamma globulin for patients with late-stage Lyme disease, although I reserve it for patients with severe and/or persistent symptoms and evidence of immune deficiency.

Gamma globulin has some interesting applications. Research on the connection between gamma globulin and autism is ongoing, and gamma globulin has been shown to be helpful in treating B19 parvovirus infection in the bone marrow, which destroys precursor red blood cells and causes anemia. Some people do not produce antibodies against this parvovirus, so they show few signs of infection even as their red blood cell counts fall.

The timing of the administration of gamma globulin may be important. Doctors don't rush to use this treatment, but there is evidence that giving it earlier in the progress of a disease may be more effective than waiting until later.

ON THE HORIZON

Some very promising new therapies are being researched and tested even as this book is being written. I am most interested in those treatments that augment the actions of the immune system, and I believe that many of the invasive and destructive approaches we use today will in the not-too-distant future be viewed the same way we now regard the historical use of bloodletting and leeches.

I look forward to the time when we know how to stimulate an appropriate response that maintains the correct balance within the immune system. As I mentioned earlier, biological response modifiers are so powerful that they can disrupt critical immune system balance by excessively weighting an immune response in a particular direction.

New Vaccines

Today chemotherapy and radiation are commonly used to combat cancer. Someday we may have vaccines tailor-made against specific cancers that will stimulate the body's immune system to react appropriately to cancer cells and to clear them out of the body. These cancer vaccines are currently in development, as are vaccines for specific viruses, bacteria, fungi, and parasites. A 1996 article in *The New England Journal of Medicine* called attention to these vaccines and noted that this kind of adoptive immunotherapy already has had some preliminary success for advanced cancer and for CMV (cytomegalovirus) infection in immunocompromised patients.[32]

Oral Tolerance

Researchers are pursuing treatments for autoimmune disorders based on the principle of oral tolerance. When we take in food, we ingest proteins that are not-self. The immune cells in the gut (or GALT, for gut-associated lymphoid tissue) not only tolerate these foreign proteins, but also communicate this tolerance to immune cells elsewhere in the body. By extension, this principle is being used as the basis of oral immunotherapy. When patients are given tiny doses of particular proteins, this stimulates the body's own regulatory systems and teaches the immune system to be more tolerant of them.

Oral tolerance is already being tested on human patients. For example, arthritis patients have been given chick cartilage, and multiple sclerosis patients have been given oral myelin pills (you'll recall that in multiple sclerosis, immune system cells attack the myelin sheaths around nerve cells). Early test results show that these treatments have enabled some patients to cut back on their doses of immunosuppressive drugs, or even to stop taking them altogether. Oral tolerance has been shown to affect the immune system in a way that helps suppress autoimmune disorders without suppressing normal immune function. As an added bonus, there appear to be few, if any, side effects. An interesting phenomenon with oral tolerance is that lower doses appear to be more effective than higher doses, suggesting a homeopathic type of dose response curve.

Telomere Research

Telomeres are like tiny timers on the ends of chromosomes. Each time certain cells divide, their telomeres become a little shorter. Eventually a critical point is reached and the cell cannot divide any further.

Short telomeres are a sign that a cell has led a long and active life, dividing and redividing. Researchers have found that one of the ways HIV (the virus that causes AIDS) overwhelms the immune system is by forcing CD8 cells to divide and redivide until they run through their cellular supply of telomeres, which were supposed to last a lifetime. In fact, some AIDS patients have been found to have telomeres as short as those of people one hundred years old.[33] The theoretical solution for this problem would be to find a way to lengthen a cell's telomeres.

Telomeres also figure into cancer research because of an enzyme called *telomerase* that is present in cancer cells, but not in normal cells. Telomerase automatically replaces every piece of telomere lost during the process of cell division, which enables cancer cells to become immortal. In this case, a theoretical cure for cancer would be to find a telomerase blocker.

Telomere research is ongoing, but don't look for medical applications anytime soon.

For now, telomeres only offer tantalizing possibilities as they expand our understanding of cellular processes.

Protease Inhibitors

I'd like to mention protease inhibitors here because there have been many reports about them in the media and they may turn AIDS into a manageable disease. When HIV is getting ready to replicate, it grows strands of protein that include all the components needed for a new virus. The virus also creates an enzyme called *protease,* which is designed to cut these strands into sections. *Protease inhibitors* block the action of this enzyme and therefore interfere with the replication of HIV. After taking protease inhibitors along with other medications, some patients who formerly had full-blown AIDS now have no detectable HIV in their blood.

Hyperthermia

It has long been recognized that fever can play an important role in healing. This has led to research into the stimulation of feverlike conditions to treat a wide variety of problems.

The process of heating up the body is called *hyperthermia.* Heating up one small part of the body—for example, a tumor—is called *local hyperthermia.* Heating up a larger area, such as a limb, is called *regional hyperthermia.* Many different heating techniques are being studied, from simple saunas to removing a patient's blood, heating it, and pumping it back again.

Hyperthermia may be effective against cancer cells and against organisms that literally "can't take the heat," such as the spirochetes that cause syphilis and Lyme disease and perhaps even HIV. Hyperthermia may not be able to kill every one of these invaders, but it may reduce their numbers to a level that the immune system finds manageable.

Hyperthermia also may stimulate the immune system to produce certain cytokines, increase the body's production of antibodies, and release the toxins stored in fat cells.[34] Currently being studied both alone and in conjunction with other treatments, hyperthermia may become an important tool in supporting immune system function.

Energetic Medicine

Energy is intimately related to matter. We are energetic beings. Every cell has membranes that are electrically charged. Nerve cells transmit information by means of electrical charges that create ionic currents. Each heartbeat depends upon electrical impulses firing at the right moment. We are both producers and conductors of electrical current.

Many types of sophisticated techniques in use today depend upon the principles of energetic medicine, including EEG (electroencephalogram) and MRI (magnetic resonance imaging). Newer and less common techniques are also being used to detect imbalances in the body's energy fields so that early intervention can head off disease.

Whenever I think about the future of energetic medicine, I am reminded of Bones, the ship's physician on the old *Star Trek* shows, who would place a kind of diagnostic computer on the patient's neck, immediately learn what was necessary to return the charges and energy of the patient's cells to normal, and supply the appropriate treatment on the spot. I believe the time is near when developments in the field of energetic medicine will allow us to reliably and consistently determine subtle disturbances in each individual's energy field, even before noticeable symptoms develop. Picking up subtle imbalances at the earliest levels will allow us to make the necessary corrections before problems progress to symptomatic clinical illness.

Although other fields of medicine, such as acupuncture, have long paid attention to these early movements in the disease process, traditional medical doctors show little interest in correcting problems that are not yet at the level of organ system dysfunction. Probably because the earliest cellular imbalances aren't visible, it's difficult to persuade most doctors that this kind of energetic intervention is useful, let alone effective. Even if the patient is noticeably better after energetic treatment, his improvement may be viewed as "all in his head."

Sometimes our own limitations prevent us from being able to see, touch, or accept what is nonetheless real. For example, for years no one knew the planet Pluto existed because no one had seen it. Some observant astronomers, however, noticed the effect of Pluto's gravitational pull on the *other* planets, and they started looking harder. By keeping an open mind and continually pushing the envelope, we may find similarly indirect evidence of cellular mechanisms that may ultimately lead us to universally accepted, quantifiable, and reproducible applications of energetic medicine.

Electroacupuncture

One of the most common forms of energetic medicine is electroacupuncture, which combines the ancient art of acupuncture with modern diagnostic machinery. Using a special device (there are several different kinds, mostly manufactured in Germany), practitioners of energetic medicine measure the electrical resistance of a patient's skin at certain acupuncture points. Each point has a standard measurement for anyone who is in good health. Changes in these readings can indicate energy imbalances and the need for appropriate treatment.

If a patient already has developed symptoms, certain practitioners use electroacupuncture to determine which bacteria, virus, toxin, or nutrient deficiency is the culprit. They feel they can also diagnose food allergies with electroacupuncture, as well as determine the precisely correct dose of a homeopathic remedy. A patient who is unwell registers an abnormal reading on the feedback equipment, but when he or she holds the correct treatment in his or her hands, this reading will return to normal.

I am very interested in these applications of energetic medicine, but it concerns me that many of the bioelectrical devices are not completely consistent, and that many depend upon the interpretative skills of the practitioner. This would differentiate electroacupuncture from an EEG, which generally gives the same result regardless of the technician or physician performing the test. I look forward to a time when these devices are more refined and universally consistent as well as integrated into everyday medicine.

Energetic Healing

Human beings have a long tradition of healing one another through the "laying on of hands" or "healing hands." (Related forms of energetic healing include "psychic healing" and "spiritual healing.") Somehow the healer exerts a bioenergetic force on the patient and reverses the course of his or her illness.

Dolores Krieger, Ph.D., R.N., became interested in this kind of healing and eventually developed a technique she calls Therapeutic Touch. Using Therapeutic Touch, a trained healer can use his or her own vitality to "jump-start" or redirect the energy of someone who is ill. There do appear to be true energy effects that occur between patients and healers, including measurable and statistically significant increases in hemoglobin.[35] There are innumerable anecdotes of remarkable recoveries that support the importance of energetic healing.

Trained energetic healers are still in relatively short supply. Barbara Brennan, an internationally acclaimed teacher and healer, has started a school that teaches healers how to do another type of deep energetic healing. Practitioners not only learn how to access and treat energy imbalances, but also are required to do deep personal growth work to facilitate the effectiveness of their healing. Also, because of the nature of some of these healing treatments, there is a limit to how many patients one healer can see. I look forward to a time when this type of healing becomes more widespread.

Magnetic Field Therapy

Magnetic field therapy certainly is another type of energetic medicine because it is based upon making corrections in human energy fields. However, magnetic therapy is different from electroacupuncture and Therapeutic Touch because it uses therapeutic magnets.

Magnetic fields are generated by gravity, by changes in the weather, by power lines, by everyday electrical appliances, and by the human body. We produce subtle magnetic fields in various ways, including by means of the electrical charges of our cells and the ionic currents used by the nervous system to transmit information.

Magnets and electrical devices can be used to generate controlled magnetic fields that penetrate the human body and affect cellular processes. Magnetic therapy is used to treat everything from broken bones to stress to infections. If every illness represents a bioenergetic breakdown, then it stands to reason that magnets could in fact be beneficial on a wide scale.

I am most interested in the application of magnetic field therapy to disorders of the central nervous system. When there is too much electrical activity in the brain, for example, the correct magnetic field can be used to subtly reestablish order in the energy system and normalize nerve function. This discovery has profound implications for pain management as well as for the treatment of diseases such as multiple sclerosis and Parkinson's.

A 1996 editorial in the *International Journal of Neuroscience* noted a novel treatment for multiple sclerosis in which patients were exposed to extracerebral applications of low-frequency electromagnetic fields. The "pulsed" nature of the treatment seemed to improve and even, in some cases, normalize the functioning of neuronal pathways.[36]

There is a window of efficacy with magnetic field therapy, just as there is with other therapies. Only the correct electromagnetic amplitudes will correspond to the currents within the body. Magnetic field therapy often uses amplitudes that are extremely low, but the key to its effectiveness may lie in a sympathetic electrical resonance that is created between the magnet and the body's cells.

Harmonic Resonance

Remember the sine curve back on page 98? I use this curve to explain why there are multiple points in immune therapy that can reverse hyperreactive immune responses. As we've already seen, lower treatment doses of certain preparations—for example, a homeopathic remedy, an oral tolerance immunotherapy dose, a dilution used for provocation/neutralization testing, or a dose of antigen used for Lyme immunotherapy—can have more powerful effects than higher doses. Another fascinating and related phenomenon is the way in which the body is able to communicate certain kinds of information instantaneously to every cell. This is not an immune-mediated type of communication. It can be described as immediate, simultaneous perception, and it encompasses every cell of the body at once.

It has been proposed by William Rea, M.D., and others that the cells of the body are able to communicate by means of a common harmonic resonance through the fluid that bathes them, like a fluid-filled ground system. When a substance is introduced into this ground system, it instantaneously affects the homeostasis of the entire ground system. I have seen, for example, that drops placed under a patient's tongue can immediately turn off a systemic allergic reaction and alleviate a whole complex of symptoms. This cannot be explained by the current dogma about immune system function. In fact, this even challenges our current ideas about the nature of time.

This concept of harmonic resonance holds vast promise for healing—not only in terms of being healed by others, but also in terms of learning to heal ourselves (see Chapter 13, Healing Begins with Acceptance). By gaining a better understanding of energetic medicine, we may learn to influence the energy systems of the body in a way that promotes health and well-being.

᎒᷍᷍᷍᷍᷍᷍ DOROTHY'S STORY

Dorothy—nicknamed Dot—is an example of a patient who needed several different Super Boosters to rehabilitate her immune system. By the time she came to see me, she had been on many courses of powerful antibiotics, and she needed a new approach to reestablishing her health.

Dot had started feeling fatigued in the spring of 1991. Accompanying her fatigue was back and leg pain, but a neurological workup revealed nothing out of the ordinary.

In the fall of 1991, Dot developed a circular rash behind her left knee and swelling of her left foot and toes. Doctors at her local emergency room diagnosed ringworm. The rash subsided, but my clinical suspicion is that it was caused by Lyme disease, not ringworm. Left untreated, rashes caused by Lyme disease can disappear—but the spirochete that causes the illness remains in the body.

By the spring of 1992, Dot still had back and leg pain, and she also had developed nausea and dizziness. After visiting several different physicians, she eventually consulted an infectious-diseases doctor who ordered a Lyme titer. When the results came back positive, he treated Dot with four weeks of intravenous Rocephin (a strong antibiotic), followed by two weeks of oral antibiotics. The antibiotics helped Dot's symptoms, but when she stopped taking them, her symptoms returned. The infectious-diseases doctor told her there was nothing else to do.

Thoroughly worried, Dot then consulted a Lyme specialist, who first treated her with high doses of Biaxin and then added a second antibiotic, Ceftin, on top of that. Dot was unable to tolerate this combination therapy. Unfortunately, she still had symptoms.

By the time Dot came to my office in 1994, simply moving was painful for her. She'd had to stop working, as her symptoms had steadily worsened. She still had back and leg pain, plus the dizziness and nausea, and now she felt numbness "everywhere" (including her legs, arms, and face). Her joint pains would move around from place to place or side to side. She was perpetually exhausted, had difficulty sleeping, and sometimes had trouble thinking straight.

I felt that Dot's problems could not all be attributed to Lyme disease. Although Lyme does cause both psychological and musculoskeletal symptoms, Dot had been on potent antibiotics for years. I felt that we needed to look for other explanations and treatments.

Testing revealed that Dot had reactive hypoglycemia, food allergies, candida hypersensitivity, and suboptimal levels of several nutrients. Dot also tested positive for Lyme, but I did not want to start her on antibiotics again without first rehabilitating her immune system.

I started Dot on Diflucan (an antiyeast medication) and a yeast-free diet for her candida problem, plus intravenous vitamin C with added nutrients for nutrient repletion and immunomodulation. I also started her on oral supplements. After several months, Dot was feeling much better, but then she caught a viral infection that knocked her flat. She just couldn't seem to recover fully.

Further tests showed that Dot had a deficiency of one of the subclasses of IgG antibodies, plus a decrease in the number and function of her NK cells. At that point, I started Dot on intravenous gamma globulin. She felt it was extremely helpful. In fact, when she ran out of her usual anti-inflammatory medication, she didn't need to replace it. For the first time in quite a while, she was off anti-inflammatory medications altogether.

Dot reported that the combination of intravenous vitamin C and intravenous gamma globulin treatments gave her more energy than she'd had in years. She was able to do much more walking and shopping, and without pain.

To see if she could clear the last hurdle without having to resort to antibiotics again, I started Dot on Lyme immunotherapy. I also started her on candida immunotherapy. These treatments helped her reach a new level of well-being and alleviated her remaining nausea, fatigue, and nerve pain.

One year after her first visit, Dot stated she was "just feeling wonderful!" She is still receiving Lyme immunotherapy and needs to be careful about her diet, but her general health is so much better that she is back to work full-time. Traditional doctors had been able to offer Dot little hope, but progressive medicine provided new avenues that led her back to good health.

Chapter 11

REDOX MEDICINE

Excessive peroxidation and free radical activity may need
inhibiting. Inadequate peroxidation and free radical activity
may need boosting. Normal peroxidation and free radical
activity should be left alone.

—DR. T. L. DORMANCY

You'll remember from Chapter 4 that human life is based on the processes of oxidation and reduction. Two sides of the same coin, these processes together are called *redox.*

Until this point, I've been talking a lot about the body's need for antioxidants to protect our cells from oxidant stress. Now I'm going to switch gears and talk about the body's need for oxygen and the therapeutic benefits of controlled bursts of oxidative activation. A contradiction? Not really. As always, maintaining homeostasis in the body is a process of balancing opposing reactions without letting one or the other inappropriately predominate.

All cellular functions can be classified as building up or breaking down, biosynthesis or biodegradation. If one of these processes constitutes a melody, then together both of them create the harmony of life. The 50/50 rule still applies: neither process is all good, nor all bad. Each can be used constructively or destructively. The process of building up is not always beneficial (for example, the growth of a tumor is not healthy), and the process of tearing apart is not always harmful (for example, destroying dead cells is a part of good health).

The more we explore how the body works, the more we learn about the exquisitely sensitive feedback mechanisms it uses to continuously monitor opposing forces. Day in and day out, through stress and strain or relaxation and rejuvenation, the body maintains innumerable internal balances by making continuous fine adjustments to our cellular machinery. Occasionally, balances are lost and need to be restored. When our oxidative processes go out of balance, our energy production can be adversely affected. Redox medicine plays a role in rebalancing the body's metabolic processes and restoring efficient energy production.

WHAT IS REDOX MEDICINE?

First, we need to review some terms. You'll remember that *oxidation* is the loss of electrons. When oxygen combines with another substance, electrons are transferred, and the other substance is changed, or oxidized. Corrosion, decay, combustion, rust, and respiration are all examples of oxidation.

Reduction is the addition of electrons. When one molecule is oxidized (loses an electron), another is reduced (gains an electron). Sometimes the oxidation/reduction process goes around in cycles, as when synergistic antioxidants regenerate each other.

Oxygenation is not the same as oxidation. Oxygenation is simply the process of providing oxygen where it is needed. It is now clear that a broad spectrum of diseases, both chronic and acute, are in some way related to oxygen deficiency (more about this in a moment).

Oxygen is the foundation of human existence. It makes up 21 percent of the air we breathe, it constitutes 65 percent of all the elements of our body, and it is involved in all body functions.[1] Again, balance is the key. Too much oxygen can be harmful—for example, it can cause a fire to rage out of control and burn down a house. However, too little oxygen also can be harmful, and can cause the fire to go out and the house to go cold.

I use the term *redox medicine* to cover those therapies that specifically affect the body's use of oxygen. Redox medicine includes both oxygen therapies and oxidative (sometimes called bio-oxidative) therapies. Oxygen therapies focus on delivering higher amounts of oxygen to cells, and range from deep breathing to the use of oxygen chambers (hyperbaric oxygen). Oxidative therapies are treatments that deliver a carefully measured burst of strong oxidants. They are effective because of the highly reactive nature of the oxidants they employ.

While most people are aware that free radicals can be harmful, few people know that not all oxidants are free radicals, and that oxidants can also be healthful when used under properly controlled circumstances. The whole concept of oxidative treatments is often met with alarm because of the misconception that all oxidants are free radicals that cause free radical damage. In this chapter, I hope to clarify—for physicians and for patients—how oxidative therapies can promote health. Once you understand how they work, they make perfect sense.

One of my patients, Shelly, was a prime candidate for oxidative therapies, but she was very resistant to the idea. She was a little afraid of the procedure itself, but more important, she was just very skeptical. Shelly was not convinced that oxidative therapies could help her. Shelly had many allergies, with accompanying allergic rhinosinusitis. She also had chronic candidiasis that was associated with many symptoms, most notably irregular menstrual periods with cramps and heavy bleeding. In fact, her menstrual problems were so severe that her gynecologist had recommended a hysterectomy—which is what brought Shelly to my office.

Shelly responded well to traditional immunotherapy plus a program of allergen avoidance and EPD therapy. However, treating her candida was more complicated. She could not tolerate antifungal medications, but when she stopped taking them, all her symptoms would return.

Shelly eventually read the literature I'd given her on oxidative therapies, and she also spoke with other patients who had been greatly helped by these treatments for difficult candida problems. After hearing these testimonials, Shelly consented to try a course of four treatments. (I encouraged her to commit to four because the effects of oxidative therapy are not always immediately apparent.)

Since Shelly started on oxidative therapies, her menstrual periods have been almost normal. She has more energy, she is concentrating better, and she is generally more resilient. As time went on, she gained more confidence and trust in this unfamiliar treatment, which actually had the effect of making her more receptive to other therapies as well. She has continued to improve.

METABOLISM: THE BIG PICTURE

Metabolism is that long journey from food to energy. We need a constant supply of energy to fuel our cells, to support the body's processes of defense and repair, and to enable us to move and to think. How *does* that plate of rice and beans end up as energy? And how is energy stored in the body so that it is available when we need it?

After we eat, digestive processes break down large particles of food into smaller ones. Proteins are broken down into amino acids, fats are metabolized into glycerol and fatty acids, and complex sugars are turned into simple sugars. At this stage of the game, no energy is generated.

As metabolism continues, foodstuffs are further broken down or chemically rearranged so that the body can release the energy within each molecule. Through a process I'll discuss shortly, ATP (adenosine triphosphate) is formed inside cells to store energy. When ATP is broken down, energy is released.

All metabolic processes depend upon the proper functioning of myriad enzymes, the presence of many necessary cofactors, and appropriate feedback mechanisms to ensure that the right steps are taking place at the right time. Of course, things can go wrong. Enzymes can function too slowly, nutrient cofactors may be in short supply, and feedback mechanisms can go haywire. When metabolic processes are disrupted, the body may not be able to generate enough energy to keep functioning optimally. This is why metabolic disorders are at the heart of many chronic and degenerative diseases.

Metabolic problems can be likened to a plane that runs out of gas in midair. As the plane goes into a dive, the ground gets closer and closer. Unless the engine can be restarted, the plane will crash. Redox therapies can jump-start metabolic processes and put the plane back on the right flight path again.

THE METABOLIC STEPS

Now that you've got the big picture, let's narrow the focus a little further. In aerobic organisms (organisms that use oxygen for metabolism), metabolism *usually* goes like this:

Step 1. During *glycolysis,* small molecules of glucose (a six-carbon sugar derived from food) are broken down into single units of pyruvate, which is a three-carbon sugar. Glycolysis begins and ends with sugars. (Although fats and amino acids can be metabolized, they do not go through glycolysis.)

Step 2. Next the units of pyruvate are converted into units of acetyl CoA (acetyl coenzyme A). Each acetyl CoA is a two-carbon molecule with a CoA attached. These two-carbon molecules are needed for the next step. (Fats also can be oxidized into acetyl CoA if necessary, but not through glycolysis.)

Step 3. During the *citric acid cycle* (also called the *Krebs cycle*), acetyl CoA is oxidized. This process spins off carbon dioxide (CO_2), NADH (the reduced form of NAD—technically NAD^+—or nicotinamide-adenine dinucleotide), and $FADH_2$ (the reduced form of FAD, or flavine-adenine dinucleotide). NADH and $FADH_2$ are needed for the next step to take place.

Step 4. During *oxidative phosphorylation,* two processes take place at the same time. The electron transport chain transfers electrons to oxygen (yielding water, or H_2O), and ATP is generated (energy is stored in high-energy phosphate bonds).

METABOLISM REEXAMINED

Let's take an even closer look at the different metabolic steps. You need to know what occurs at each step in order to understand redox therapies. This discussion won't even come close to my biochemistry textbook from medical school, I promise.

Close-Up: Glycolysis

Glycolysis is a ten-step sequence of reactions that results in the conversion of glucose into pyruvate. Some energy is freed up during this process, for one molecule of glucose yields two ATP and two pyruvate molecules. During later steps of aerobic metabolism, pyruvate enters the mitochondria (little energy factories) inside the cells so that ATP can be generated. Ultimately pyruvate is completely oxidized to carbon dioxide and water.

All of the intermediate substances in glycolysis between glucose and pyruvate are phosphorylated (converted into phosphate-containing compounds). This is important because energy is held in the phosphate bonds. Each intermediate step in glycolysis requires enzyme activity, so the steps can't proceed without the appropriate enzymes and cofactors (most of which happen to be vitamins and minerals) in the necessary amounts. Now you see why I keep talking about the importance of good nutrition!

During glycolysis, NAD is converted to NADH. With all this NADH production going on, where is the body going to find a constant supply of NAD? The answer lies in the last step of aerobic metabolism, during which NADH gives up its electrons to oxygen via the electron transport chain. NAD is regenerated from NADH, and is then free to reenter glycolysis. Nature thought of everything.

Anaerobic Metabolism

Glycolysis is not actually aerobic. However, it requires substances generated by aerobic processes further down the metabolic line to keep it going. If a cell's supply of oxygen is inadequate—for example, during intense exercise, when available oxygen is used up quickly—the body will shift gears and move into *anaerobic metabolism.*

During anaerobic metabolism, glucose is converted into ATP and lactate in the cytoplasm of the cell. (For this reason, anaerobic metabolism is also called *lactic fermentation.*) Anaerobic metabolism is faster but less efficient than aerobic metabolism, for a molecule of glucose yields two ATP and two lactate molecules. Unlike pyruvate, lactate is a waste product—a by-product of incomplete combustion. When lactate builds up during strenuous exercise, it makes muscles stiff and sore. A buildup of lactate in cells can be a sign that aerobic metabolism is not proceeding well, and that the body has been forced to use anaerobic metabolism to meet its energy needs.

Close-Up: The Conversion of Pyruvate

This step doesn't have a handy name, but it is the link between glycolysis (which generated pyruvate) and the next step in aerobic metabolism. The body has to change pyruvate into acetyl CoA in order to fuel the citric acid cycle. Amino acids that were rearranged into pyruvate also need to run through this conversion process.

You might think that two-carbon sugars could enter the citric acid cycle all by themselves, but the enzyme cofactor A (the CoA part) makes it easier for each two-carbon sugar to be processed. Cofactors are facilitators that help get the job done.

This juncture in aerobic metabolism is a regulatory step. If there is a lot of acetyl CoA already on hand in a cell, the creation of new acetyl CoA will slow down. Similarly, if there's a lot of ATP on hand (the energy charge of a cell is high), the cell's demand for acetyl CoA falls and less is produced.

Close-Up: The Citric Acid Cycle

During the citric acid cycle, acetyl CoA is completely oxidized to carbon dioxide. In the process, energy is "trapped" in NADH and in $FADH_2$. The rate at which the citric acid cycle operates is adjusted to meet a cell's needs for ATP. It's a very tidy process: two carbons enter the citric acid cycle in the form of acetyl CoA, and two carbons exit in the form of CO_2.

During the citric acid cycle, six electrons are transferred to NAD, yielding three NADH, and one pair of hydrogen atoms (two electrons) is transferred to FAD, yielding $FADH_2$. Both NADH and $FADH_2$ are essential for the last step of aerobic metabolism.

Each spin of the citric acid cycle produces a total of twelve high-energy bonds. These high-energy bonds yield molecules of ATP when they are oxidized in the next step. The grand total of high-energy phosphate bonds looks like this:

$$\begin{array}{lr}
\text{Each NADH has 3 (3} \times \text{3 NADH)} & = 9 \\
\text{The FADH has 2} & = 2 \\
\text{GTP (guanosine triphosphate) has 1} & = \underline{1} \\
& 12
\end{array}$$

The Citric Acid Cycle

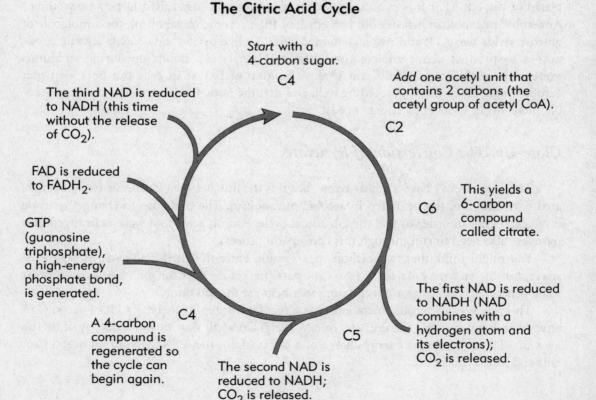

Start with a 4-carbon sugar.

C4

Add one acetyl unit that contains 2 carbons (the acetyl group of acetyl CoA).

C2

The third NAD is reduced to NADH (this time without the release of CO_2).

FAD is reduced to $FADH_2$.

GTP (guanosine triphosphate), a high-energy phosphate bond, is generated.

This yields a 6-carbon compound called citrate.

C6

A 4-carbon compound is regenerated so the cycle can begin again.

C4

C5

The first NAD is reduced to NADH (NAD combines with a hydrogen atom and its electrons); CO_2 is released.

The second NAD is reduced to NADH; CO_2 is released.

The citric acid cycle takes place inside each cell's mitochondria. Like glycolysis, this cycle doesn't use molecular oxygen. However, it can operate only under aerobic conditions because the substances upon which it depends (NAD and FAD) are regenerated by the next step in aerobic metabolism.

Close-Up: Oxidative Phosphorylation

Oxidative phosphorylation consists of two closely linked processes that are the major source of energy (ATP) in aerobic organisms. Basically it goes like this: When the electrons on NADH and $FADH_2$ are transferred to molecular oxygen via the electron transport chain, a large amount of energy is liberated. The oxygen accepts the "spent" electrons, which creates water (H_2O). The energy that is released while the electrons are being transported is used to generate ATP.

The electrons are escorted from NADH and $FADH_2$ to the waiting molecular oxygen by a series of electron carriers (including CoQ10). After they give up their electrons, NADH and $FADH_2$ are regenerated to NAD and FAD. The NAD can then return to the citric acid cycle to participate in these metabolic processes all over again.

As the electrons are moving down the electron transport chain, ADP (adenosine diphosphate) is phosphorylated into ATP (adenosine triphosphate) at three sites. Each NADH yields three ATP, while an $FADH_2$, which enters at a later stage, yields two ATP.

ADP and ATP regulate each other. ADP enters the mitochondrial matrix only if ATP exits. The presence of a lot of ADP is a signal to cells to make more ATP. On the other hand, the presence of a lot of ATP is a signal to downregulate ATP production. These feedback mechanisms ensure that cells are generating the correct amount of energy.

ENERGY FAILURE

It takes a lot of energy to get through each day. Of course, some days are harder than others, but many of us juggle several demanding roles all at the same time. We're trying to get ahead (or just keep up) at work, we're raising our kids, we're taking care of our parents, we're stressed by financial and societal problems . . . no wonder we're tired!

Not everyone bounces out of bed in the morning bright-eyed and raring to go. Many people have chronic metabolic problems that, combined with their draining lifestyle, leave them in a constant low-energy state. When energy production is less than ideal and energy demands are great, our health suffers. Imbalances and interruptions in ATP production aren't associated just with fatigue; they're also associated with disease, immune dysregulation, cancer, and other disorders.

Energy production can be compromised if a step is blocked, if enzymes or cofactors are not present in sufficient quantities, or if feedback loops stop functioning correctly. Any of these problems can cause "mitochondrial brownout." In addition, there are two other metabolic disruptions worth noting.

Uncoupling Oxidative Phosphorylation

Oxidative phosphorylation is said to be "uncoupled" when NADH and $FADH_2$ are oxidized, but ADP is not simultaneously phosphorylated into ATP. Usually these processes occur together, but it's possible to release energy via the electron transport chain without binding it up into ATP. This generates heat, but no stored energy. Occasionally the uncoupling of oxidative phosphorylation can be beneficial (for example, it keeps hibernating animals warm), but usually it is a sign that proper metabolic regulation has been lost.

If oxidative phosphorylation is uncoupled and the body needs ATP, it will keep shuttling electrons into the electron transport chain in a futile attempt to generate energy. This will increase the body's consumption of oxygen and the oxidation of NADH and $FADH_2$, but it won't produce energy. Obviously, this counterproductive state is not beneficial for health.

Known uncouplers of oxidative phosphorylation include mercury (absorbed from dental amalgam, for example), mycotoxins (toxins from fungi and molds—this is one reason why correctly diagnosing and treating candidiasis is so important), xenobiotics (foreign substances, including environmental toxins and drugs), and malonate (a competing enzyme that poisons respiration). Nonsteroidal anti-inflammatory drugs have also been associated with the uncoupling of mitochondrial oxidative phosphorylation.[2]

Oxidant Stress Within the Mitochondria

Because it is single-stranded, mitochondrial DNA is more sensitive than nuclear DNA. Also, the repair enzymes for mitochondrial DNA are less effective than those for nuclear DNA. This means that free radicals generated during metabolism—especially those free radicals that act very fast—can do damage within the mitochondria and even can cause mutations in mitochondrial DNA. It's as if the mitochondrial DNA is burned by the fire.

We tend to have energy levels resembling that of our mothers because the mother's genes largely determine mitochondrial DNA. Whether the mitochondrial DNA we received is superefficient or slow and sleepy, we can end up worse off than we started if we acquire DNA defects created by oxidant stress.

Paradoxically, oxidant stress is *more severe in a low-oxygen environment.* People usually think the opposite—that abundant oxygen would be associated with abundant amounts of free radicals. Actually, when energy production is inefficient and oxygen levels are low, *more* free radicals are produced. So mitochondrial problems can build on themselves.

Greg Lemond, a world-renowned competitive long-distance bicycle racer, is believed to have blown out his mitochondria with years of training and vigorous competition. He now has a rare form of mitochondrial myopathy, perhaps caused by accumulated oxidative damage to his mitochondrial DNA.[3]

Low Cellular Energy

A cell with a low energy charge is in trouble. If it does not have enough ATP to maintain its cellular processes correctly, a cascade of damaging events can be initiated. When cellular work doesn't get done:

- Cellular repairs aren't made.
- Toxins build up (poisoning, among other things, the immune system).
- Calcium gets inside the cell (setting off other imbalances).
- Free radicals cause more oxidant stress (within the mitochondria, within the cell, and elsewhere).
- Nitric oxide builds up.

Nitric oxide is an interesting substance. Depending upon the concentration, it can protect or harm us. It is the main determinant of blood pressure, it is released by macrophages in large amounts when they are stimulated, and it acts as a neurotransmitter in the brain and peripheral nervous system. On the other hand, excess nitric oxide is associated with oxidant stress, mitochondrial problems, and programmed cell death (apoptosis).[4]

Energy failure, therefore, is the culprit behind all manner of diseases and disorders. How do we combat it? With the growing number of treatments in redox medicine.

OXYGEN THERAPY

It's kind of amazing to me that although oxygen is more important to us than food or water, the only time we receive it is when we're lying in an ambulance. Unless, that is, we happen to be in an "air bar"—an establishment that, instead of alcohol, serves up oxygen. Already familiar in smoggy Asian cities, air bars are making inroads elsewhere, and the first one in North America recently opened up in Toronto.

Oxygen therapies use oxygen in various ways and at various concentrations. Following are some techniques for improving oxygen levels in the body.

• **Deep breathing.** Yes, this counts. The ancient traditions of Ayurvedic medicine and Yoga included deep breathing for good health. This oxygen therapy costs nothing!

• **Aerobic exercise and normal air.** The air we usually breathe is 21 percent oxygen. (In a crowded room or airplane cabin, there's less oxygen in the air.) Breathing hard helps oxygen exchange.

- **Aerobic exercise followed by concentrated oxygen.** First the patient exercises, then he or she breathes oxygen. Different concentrations of oxygen can be used.
- **Aerobic exercise with concentrated oxygen.** With this therapy, the patient exercises—for example, on a stationary bike—while breathing concentrated oxygen.
- **Medications and/or nutrients** can be used to increase the utilization of oxygen in tissues and cells.
- **Medications to increase blood flow** can help with oxygenation. Sometimes it is helpful to give a patient who cannot exercise a medication to increase blood flow, followed by concentrated oxygen.
- **Hyperbaric oxygen.** With this technique, patients are placed in a chamber and given 100 percent oxygen at two to three times atmospheric pressure, usually for one and a half to two hours. This counteracts low oxygen levels in tissues and reverses some disorders, such as smoke inhalation or carbon monoxide poisoning, on the spot.

Recently I have gotten very interested in the effects of hyperbaric oxygen. Oxygen chambers have been in use since the 1800s, and most people are aware that they are used for "the bends"—when deep sea divers surface too fast and get decompression sickness. However,

---

COMMONLY ASKED QUESTION NO. 21:

Why do I need oxygen therapy? Isn't breathing enough?

First of all, polluted air is obviously a problem. If you can get out in truly fresh air for some vigorous exercise every day, that would be a very good thing. For many of us, though, this is not possible.

In addition, the problem of low oxygen levels in cells builds upon itself. Low oxygen leads to even lower oxygen because cellular processes become so inefficient. When the body's ability to use oxygen declines, the situation calls for something more than normal breathing.

To reverse poor utilization of oxygen, you need to cross an oxygen threshold for a certain period of time. (How long this period should last depends upon the severity of the problem.) When the body has a lot of oxygen at its disposal, it can improve its utilization of oxygen at the cellular level. Also, the administration of oxidative therapies (see p. 347) will jump-start its metabolic processes.

Once you cross this threshold, you can look forward to long-lasting results. Like making a positive attitude adjustment, the body makes a metabolic adjustment that allows it to utilize oxygen in an improved way.

hyperbaric oxygen has many other uses as well. It can enhance phagocytosis and speed the healing of problem wounds. It is helpful in killing anaerobic organisms (which do not do well in a high-oxygen environment) and can be protective against reperfusion injury (the return of blood flow to a previously ischemic area that generates free radical damage). It helps tissue that does not receive good circulation (including skin grafts and irradiated tissue with decreased vascularity), and it helps keep blood oxygenated after exceptional blood loss when transfusions are either unavailable or refused by the patient.

Hyperbaric oxygen therapy does not cause tumors[5] (which was initially a concern), and used correctly it has few side effects. One drawback is that not many physicians are trained in hyperbaric oxygen. Another is the expense: from $150 to $400 for one ninety-minute treatment. Despite the cost, hyperbaric oxygen therapy seems to have many positive effects and may be helpful to patients with energy failure and chronic illness.

OXIDATIVE THERAPIES

Oxidative therapies don't use concentrated oxygen. Instead, they use ozone (O_3) or hydrogen peroxide (H_2O_2). These substances activate oxidative processes in the body, with a wide range of beneficial results. Oxidative therapies are counterintuitive—you wouldn't expect them to be helpful—which is probably one reason they are not better accepted.

Oxidative therapies are not endorsed by the major medical associations, they are not discussed in the big-time medical journals, they do not involve drugs manufactured by the pharmaceutical giants, and they are not administered by the majority of American physicians. On the other hand, they have a long history of use dating from the turn of the century, they are widely used in other countries, there is plenty of medical literature supporting them, and there are innumerable case histories about their effectiveness.

Oxidative therapies are probably the most controversial aspect of my practice, not because they are in any way harmful (unless administered incorrectly), but because they are unfamiliar and misunderstood. I use oxidative therapies judiciously, follow strict protocols, and have seen excellent results with my patients, including some of my sickest patients. Clearly these treatments work.

A Brief History of Oxidative Medicine

Ozone has been used clinically in Europe for over a century, and the first scientific article about hydrogen peroxide therapy, written by T. H. Oliver, appeared in the *Lancet* in 1920.[6] Despite a rather dry title ("Influenzal Pneumonia: The Intravenous Injection of Hydrogen Peroxide"), this paper was as dramatic as it was groundbreaking.

During a severe outbreak of the flu in Basrah, doctors found the usual remedies useless. As a measure of last resort, they decided to try intravenous hydrogen peroxide. They chose the sickest man in the hospital, who was near death and who had been delerious for two days (he was, in fact, tied to the bed for this reason). Within six hours of the hydrogen peroxide treatment he was sitting up in bed. He made a full recovery. (Charles Farr, M.D., Ph.D., the world's leading proponent of hydrogen peroxide therapy, calls this aspect of the treatment—watching desperately ill patients return to life—the "Lazarus phenomenon.") After the epidemic ceased, the mortality rate with hydrogen peroxide treatment (48 percent) compared very favorably to the mortality rate without it (80 percent), particularly in light of the fact that only the most severe and apparently hopeless cases were treated with the oxidative therapy.

Medical ozone (not the same as atmospheric ozone) is one of the most powerful oxidants in existence, and has long been used for its purifying effects. It is a potent detoxifier and is used to sterilize instruments and to oxidize pesticides, detergents, and chemical manufacturing waste products.

In his book *Oxygen Healing Therapies,* Nathaniel Altman reports that ozone is currently used to purify many large public water systems, and that it has been used to purify the water in public swimming pools since 1950. During the Olympic Games in Los Angeles in the summer of 1984, the European teams refused to participate as long as there was chlorine in the pool instead of ozone.[7]

Oxidative therapies are currently in general use in Germany, Cuba, Russia, Austria, Switzerland, and Italy. They are used to treat a wide range of illnesses and disorders, including viral and bacterial infections, wounds, ulcers, burns, circulatory problems, eye disorders, migraines, chronic fatigue, and diseases of old age. They are also used as an adjunctive treatment with radiation and chemotherapy. I am particularly interested in the use of oxidative therapies to combat problems with energy metabolism and for mitochondrial resuscitation.

What Oxidative Therapies Are Available?

As of this writing, I use two kinds of oxidative therapies in my office: intravenous hydrogen peroxide and ultraviolet irradiation of the blood. Ozone is used primarily in Europe, as political considerations have contained its use in this country. I suspect as we see a greater appreciation and understanding of oxidative therapies we will see an expansion in the use of ozone in the United States.

• **Intravenous hydrogen peroxide.** White blood cells use hydrogen peroxide to kill invading microorganisms. The kind of hydrogen peroxide you get in the drugstore, which is a 3 percent concentration, is used as a topical antiseptic. Intravenous hydrogen peroxide is administered as a dilute sterile solution, usually in a concentration of 0.03 percent (although sometimes higher concentrations are used). Giving hydrogen peroxide (or ozone) is the opposite of giving antioxidants. It amounts to giving a blast of an oxidant, which the body eventually breaks down to oxygen and water. The body does have antioxidant defenses, and it knows what to do with a burst of hydrogen peroxide.

- **Ultraviolet radiation of the blood (UVB).** Exposing the blood to ultraviolet light causes the formation of singlet oxygen, which in turn has all the benefits of intravenous oxidative therapies. In addition, irradiation actually puts energy into the blood. This light energy is transduced into chemical energy, and after several treatments, patients feel more energized. UVB is discussed on page 352.

The effects of the different oxidative therapies available—intravenous ozone, intravenous hydrogen peroxide, and ultraviolet blood irradiation—can be additive. Combination oxidative therapies include:

- **Tri-ox therapy,** which combines intravenous vitamin C, then EDTA chelation, then intravenous hydrogen peroxide. Tri-ox was proposed by Charles Farr, M.D., as a way to maximize the oxidative burst by combining three modalities in the same treatment session, one after the other. Tri-ox is presently being studied for its effect on chronic illnesses such as cancer.
- **Photo-ox therapy,** which combines intravenous hydrogen peroxide or ozone with ultraviolet blood irradiation (see page 352). I often combine intravenous hydrogen peroxide and UVB for their synergistic effects. This combination seems to be the most powerful and has been quite useful in many of my sickest, chronically ill patients.

Administering Oxidative Therapies

Like any effective medicine, oxidative therapy has a window of efficacy—I call it the "oxidative window"—that needs to be respected. Too little is not helpful; too much can cause adverse effects to normal cells. Oxidative therapies use controlled oxidation to promote healing.

As a rule, I prepare my patients for oxidative treatments by giving them antioxidants ahead of time. Usually I give them multiple antioxidant supplements orally as well as some high-dose intravenous vitamin C with other added antioxidants such as glutathione. If the patient has low levels of antioxidants and this is not corrected, it can cause a higher level of cellular die-off during oxidative therapy and make him or her uncomfortable. However, too many antioxidants, such as large doses of vitamin C or vitamin E, administered too close to the oxidative treatment could conceivably undermine its effectiveness.

The Benefits of Oxidative Therapies

Oxidative therapies have a broad range of benefits. In the medical literature they are grouped and described in different ways, but here are the basic effects:

Improvement of Antioxidant Defenses

The burst of the oxidant delivered by oxidative therapy gives a wake-up call to the body's antioxidant defenses and activates the antioxidant enzyme systems glutathione peroxidase, catalase, and superoxide dismutase. Over several treatments, this "rebound effect" enhances the body's capacity to deal with free radicals. Exercise follows the same principle. Each time you exercise intensely, you generate a storm of free radicals, but the more you train, the more you strengthen your antioxidant defense systems, and the less of a problem oxidant stress becomes.

Improvement of Oxygen Utilization

Oxidative therapies upregulate aerobic metabolism and counteract hypoxia (low oxygen). They improve the rate of glycolysis, activate the citric acid cycle, accelerate the interim step during which pyruvate is changed into acetyl CoA, speed up the rate at which acetyl CoA is used, and stimulate the electron transport chain. This helps oxygenate tissues and also cuts back on anaerobic metabolism. (Studies show that oxidative therapies are associated with a significant decrease in lactate production.) The energy gained from the upregulation of metabolism can then be put to use in the body for immune processes, detoxification reactions, hormone synthesis, protein metabolism, etc.

The most common cause of oxidant stress is, in fact, low oxygen (hypoxia). Inadequate oxidative metabolism in the mitochondria leads to cellular fatigue, which leads to oxidant stress. The answer to this problem is not to avoid oxygen! Nor is it a good idea to avoid treatments that can enhance oxidative metabolism.

Improvement of Oxygen Transport Mechanisms

Oxygen is transported to cells by hemoglobin, a protein found in red blood cells. This is an excellent way of conducting oxygen from the lungs to the tissues because the oxygen can't react to anything along the way—it's all bound up with hemoglobin. However, the hemoglobin has to know when to let the oxygen go.

Oxidative therapies stimulate red blood cells to produce more 2,3-DPG (diphosphoglycerate), a substance that stabilizes hemoglobin after it gives off oxygen. When metabolism is impaired, hemoglobin has an abnormally high oxygen affinity. Higher levels of 2,3-DPG mean more oxygen is given up by hemoglobin, so you get improved oxygen release and better oxygen transport to cells. The *amount* of hemoglobin isn't changed, just the way it functions.

Fighting Infections

We need oxidants to fight disease. All the antioxidants in the world won't help with an active infection.

Oxidative therapies help destroy anaerobic organisms that thrive in a low-oxygen environment. These anaerobic organisms—including bacteria, viruses, fungi, and parasites—don't have the same level of antioxidant enzymes as healthy cells. A blast of therapeutic oxidants causes fatty acid peroxidation in their cell walls and/or membranes that they are not equipped to handle. The susceptible cells die when their walls are ruptured. Viruses with lipid envelopes are more susceptible to oxidative stress.[8]

Oxidative therapies also upregulate phagocytosis. In response to infection, phagocytes consume one hundred times the amount of oxygen they require in a resting state.[9] Providing cells with intravenous hydrogen peroxide supports a natural body process, and the added hydrogen peroxide has a synergistic effect with the cellularly formed hydrogen peroxide. Even better, the body knows how to handle the by-products of its own weapon.

Traditional medicine holds that all bacteria behave in certain accepted ways. One of the things you're supposed to be able to do with bacteria is grow them in culture. In her book *Cell Wall Deficient Forms: Stealth Pathogens,*[10] Lida H. Mattman, Ph.D., indicates that certain bacteria do not divide and grow in classical ways and therefore can't be cultured—but they can be seen under a microscope. These difficult-to-detect pathogens could underlie many conditions. This helps explain why oxidative treatments are helpful for so many disorders, from inflammatory bowel diseases to CFIDS to various forms of arthritis. The oxidative therapy successfully combats the stealth pathogens.

Fighting Cancer

In 1966, Nobel prize winner Dr. Otto Warburg delivered his "Lindau lecture" to the meeting of Nobel laureates in Lindau, Germany. His lecture was entitled "The Prime Cause and Prevention of Cancer."[11] While there are countless secondary causes of cancer (carcinogens), Dr. Warburg believed that there is only one primary cause: a lack of oxygen on a cellular level. Cancer cells meet their energy needs in great part by fermentation. Dr. Warburg felt that replacing aerobic metabolism with fermentation is the prime cause of cancer. Robert Olney, an early proponent of oxidative therapies, also theorized that cancer was a result of what he called "blocked oxidation."[12]

An early experiment with mice helped to prove Dr. Warburg's point. Tetanus requires a low-oxygen environment in which to thrive, which is why it can be a problem in deep puncture wounds. When tetanus organisms were injected into healthy mice, none of them got sick—there was no low-oxygen environment in which the tetanus could take hold. On the other hand, when mice with tumors were injected with tetanus, they developed the disease. The tetanus was able to flourish in the low-oxygen environment of the tumors.

One way to fight cancer cells is with oxidative therapies. Cancer cells have minimal amounts of the antioxidant enzyme catalase, so when they are confronted with a burst of hydrogen peroxide, the oxidant stress kills them. Healthy cells are not affected. The benefits of oxidative therapy for cancer are dose related—that is, higher doses are more effective.

Detoxification

Hydrogen peroxide, ozone, and ultraviolet light are all powerful detoxifiers. Oxidative therapies have been used to combat bacterial toxins (including botulism, diphtheria, and tetanus), snake venom, petrochemicals, and even biological warfare weapons.

Immune Enhancement

Oxidative therapies cause an increase in gamma interferon (an antiviral), an increase in interleukin-2 (which initiates a cascade of immune events), and an increase in tumor necrosis factor (which has antitumor effects).[13] They also stimulate the production of white blood cells by increasing the rate at which aged white blood cells are broken down. In addition, they revive immune functions previously depressed for genetic, sexual, hormonal, or nutritional reasons or due to senescence.[14] These immune-enhancing effects help to prolong the benefits of oxidative therapies.

Improved Blood Flow

Oxidative therapies help keep cell membranes flexible, which enhances circulation. In addition, they help prevent *rouleaux,* a condition in which red blood cells develop a kind of "static cling" and pile up together like a stack of coins.

Ultraviolet Blood Irradiation (UVB)

Ultraviolet light has long been known to kill germs. For example, almost all bacteria can be killed by ultraviolet rays, and UV light has been used in water purification for some time.

UVB was first developed in the 1930s as a treatment for polio. In 1933, Emmett Knott, a pioneer of UVB, used blood irradiation on a woman who was dying of postabortion sepsis (remember, no antibiotics back then) and who was considered untreatable. She recovered.[15] There are many other spectacular case histories like this in the medical literature—stories of hopeless cases saved by UVB, including patients with conditions from peritonitis to toxemia

COMMONLY ASKED QUESTION NO. 22:

Does ultraviolet blood irradiation affect only the blood that is irradiated?

During UVB, some of the patient's blood (usually 100 to 200 cc) is drawn into a syringe or a sterile bottle, run out through IV tubing, and then through a clear glass cuvette, where it is irradiated. Then the blood is reinfused.

Why does this small amount of irradiated blood have such large effects? Because the irradiated cells provoke a whole-body response.

There are several proposed mechanisms that may explain this. First and probably foremost is the point of view that UVB supplies photon energy to the cells, and specifically to hemoglobin in red cells. Irradiated cells carry photon energy throughout the body, where it is gradually released over time, continuing to stimulate the immune system and the body's physiology.

Another proposed mechanism is through the induction of cytokines and interferons. This would also explain the amplification of UVB's biochemical and physiological effects.

When UVB is used to treat certain types of cancer cells, it's possible that the irradiated cells are altered in some way that makes them recognizable to the immune system as "foreign" after they are reinfused. This in turn may stimulate the immune system to attack the nonirradiated cancer cells as well.

---

of pregnancy. One patient with botulism who was in a coma and who could neither swallow nor see was treated with one irradiation treatment. After seventy-two hours, she could swallow, see, and was mentally clear.[16]

Robert Rowen, M.D., refers to blood irradiation as "the cure that time forgot." In a 1996 article he traces the history of ultraviolet blood irradiation from its early origins to its present state.[17] In the 1930s and 1940s, UVB was increasingly used in infectious conditions with much success, but since the age of antibiotics, interest in this has waned and today few physicians offer it.

Dr. Richard L. Edelson extensively studied blood irradiation and came up with a technique he called "photopheresis" to combat cutaneous T cell lymphoma (a rare form of malignant skin cancer). During photopheresis, a patient ingests a drug that is activated by light. Then some of his or her blood is removed and the white blood cells are concentrated.

Finally, the blood is irradiated and reinfused. This treatment has been extensively researched and studied, it is approved by the FDA, and it is offered at Yale, so it has an impressive pedigree. However, it is more expensive, more elaborate, and more time-consuming than basic UVB, which I do in my office.

During UVB, ultraviolet energy turns molecular oxygen into singlet oxygen, which leads to a burst of oxidant activation and the benefits already listed above. These effects are impressive enough, but there's more. Because energy is transferred during this procedure, UVB energizes the body's biochemical defenses. It has been suggested that ultraviolet photons are absorbed into the blood and released at a later time, perhaps deep in tissues where pathogens are lurking.

I should mention that ultraviolet blood irradiation, although abbreviated UVB, does not use UVB light. The Knott technique (pioneered by Emmett Knott) actually uses light in the UVC spectrum with a peak frequency of 253.7 nanometers.[18]

UVB holds great promise for the treatment of persistent viruses (such as Epstein-Barr, hepatitis virus, and HIV), antibiotic-resistant bacteria (which, as discussed, are becoming more of a problem), and many toxins that are unstable in the presence of ultraviolet light.

᧒ CINDY'S STORY

When I first met Cindy at her initial visit, she was very subdued. It was difficult to get a feeling for what kind of person she was or what she really thought about things. She was always very polite and compliant in the weeks ahead, but she remained somewhat enigmatic until her health started to improve markedly with intravenous hydrogen peroxide treatments. Then it became clear that when she felt well, Cindy had the energy to be cheerful and motivated. Successfully treating Cindy's symptoms was like unwrapping a present.

Cindy had plenty of reasons to be down. She had many, many symptoms and basically never felt well. After a bout of a flu-like illness nearly ten years before, she had started experiencing periods of fatigue that became longer and longer as well as more and more frequent. By the time she consulted me, she felt "achiness all over" and was plagued by lethargy, migraine headaches, frequent sore throats, a low-grade temperature, and back and leg pain.

To complicate things further, Cindy had many allergies. She could not tolerate perfumes, and the smell of a musty old book would make her throat tighten up. She had allergic rhinitis almost year round, plus recurring respiratory infections and pharyngitis, for which she had been placed on repeated courses of antibiotics.

After I heard about the antibiotics, I wasn't surprised when Cindy told me that she experienced recurrent vaginal yeast infections. She also had chronic constipation, plus episodes of nausea, gas, and bloating. All of these symptoms can be associated with yeast overgrowth due to antibiotic treatment. In addition, Cindy told me that if she didn't eat, she felt "terrible" and became light-headed and shaky.

Cindy already had been diagnosed with hypertension. After talking about her life for a while, I could see that stress undoubtedly contributed to her clinical picture. She had money worries, job worries, boyfriend worries, and now health worries as well.

Cindy had consulted a multitude of doctors. I gave her credit for her doggedness. Time after time she had tried to get help and had reached a dead end until eventually she had found her way to me. I assured her that there were many other treatments to try, and that I expected she would feel better in several months.

I suspected that Cindy had chronic fatigue immune dysfunction syndrome (CFIDS), chronic candidiasis, reactive hypoglycemia, allergies (food, chemical, and inhalant), allergic rhinitis, and perhaps hormonal imbalances as well. Testing proved these initial diagnoses to be correct, so the next step was to set up a regimen to restore Cindy's health.

I wanted Cindy to pursue stress management immediately, but she could not handle the additional expense of consulting a professional in this area. I urged her at least to meditate on her own, but she seemed noncommittal about it.

Right away we implemented a yeast-free, allergen-free, hypoglycemic diet. At the same time, I prescribed an antifungal medication and also started Cindy on intravenous vitamin C. Many of her yeast-related symptoms improved on this regimen, but her fatigue and migraines persisted.

When I started Cindy on intravenous hydrogen peroxide, she reported that she had more energy and that her headaches were less intense. She said, "It's just so wonderful to have some days where I feel almost normal!"

Next I initiated candida immunotherapy. This helped relieve Cindy's achiness and fatigue. She was definitely beginning to see a light at the end of the tunnel.

At this point I switched Cindy to a higher-dose intravenous hydrogen peroxide protocol. She had a marked response to this, saying, "This is the best I've felt in ten years!"

When Cindy eventually did pursue stress management, it dovetailed nicely with her improved health. Her increased energy, combined with certain attitude adjustments and stress management techniques, made it possible for her to contemplate making changes in her life that had seemed impossible just a few months before.

Today Cindy takes a variety of nutritional supplements (these include a high-potency, well-balanced multivitamin/mineral supplement for CFIDS support, buffered vitamin C, Eco Adrenal, Para Microcidin, and a thymus glandular) and continues to receive candida immunotherapy as well as the higher-dose hydrogen peroxide treatments. She is far happier than when I first met her, and in fact has a lot to be happy about. Her health is vastly improved, and she just got married!

Chapter 12

∼◦∽

GETTING THE RIGHT DIAGNOSIS

Discovery consists in seeing what everybody else has seen and
thinking what nobody else has thought.
—ALBERT SZENT-GYÖRGYI

By the time she came to see me, Nancy had been suffering from terrible migraine
headaches for eight years. Her aunt and her sister had migraines, too. Nancy had
medications to take when she had a migraine attack, but none of the doctors she'd consulted
had been able to determine *why* she was getting headaches—so she kept getting them.

I didn't consider "migraine headaches" to be a diagnosis. To me, headaches are a symptom. I wanted to get a real diagnosis, one that would help explain where Nancy's headaches
were coming from.

Every patient has a story, so I listened as Nancy told me hers. She had seen several
doctors about her headaches, including a prominent neurologist who had told her, "It's a
progressive disorder. You'll feel better at menopause." At thirty-six, Nancy did not find this
thought reassuring.

She also had been to a gastroenterologist for her almost constant GI upset. He had
suspected milk intolerance, but a milk-free diet had not given Nancy any relief. In addition,
she had consulted a nutritionist, who suspected Nancy had an overgrowth of candida. She
tried a yeast-free diet, but it helped her only a little.

As I talked with Nancy, I learned that her headaches were worse on rainy days. I also
learned that she had a family history of food allergies, and that she had made an attempt to
diagnose her own food allergies by going on a rice-only diet and then slowly reintroducing
foods. When she seemed to be developing new intolerances to foods she had previously been
able to eat, Nancy felt overwhelmed and made an appointment with me.

I felt certain that Nancy's gastrointestinal symptoms and her headaches were related.
The neurologist had looked at Nancy as a walking migraine, and the gastroenterologist had
viewed her as another case of irritable bowel syndrome (another "grab-bag" diagnosis).
Neither one had suggested to her that there might be a common allergic basis for her mi-

356

graines and her GI problems. The fact is that each human body is an indivisible organism made up of billions of cells that all talk to one another. Why shouldn't different symptoms be tied together by a common cause?

The next step for Nancy was to obtain certain tests to see if the results correlated with my suspicions. Allergy testing revealed that she had multiple food and inhalant allergies, and Nancy tested positive for candida hypersensitivity as well. Molds were definitely a problem, which would help explain her headaches on rainy days.

To treat Nancy, I started her on allergy shots, placed her on a low-carbohydrate, yeast-free diet (see page 161), and prescribed Diflucan (an antiyeast medication). Because of all her food sensitivities, I eventually started Nancy on EPD treatments. Gradually her migraines lessened, and with consistent EPD treatments she got to a point where she no longer needed her migraine medications at all.

Nancy's real diagnosis was fungal hypersensitivity, complicated by extensive allergies. By using this diagnosis as a starting point, we were able to put into place a truly beneficial treatment regimen for her headaches.

TAKING A FRESH LOOK

When I first started practicing medicine, I treated migraines the way everybody else did, with certain preventive medications that were seldom entirely successful, and with prescriptions to manage the headaches as they occurred. Even though I was doing everything "right," I was not bringing about lasting improvement for my migraine patients. I was helping them a little, but not a lot—which was unsatisfactory for me as well as for them.

Today I almost always can make a difference for a patient with migraines, not with the standard protocols, but by looking for underlying conditions and resolving them. This is the principle I apply to all of my patients with long-term or complex problems. When I am searching for the correct diagnosis, I am constantly reminded that:

1. If you don't ask the questions, you won't get the answers.
2. If you ask but don't listen, you won't hear the answer.
3. If you don't look, you won't find the information you need.

On the other hand, if you do ask, and listen, and look, you may see things no one has seen before. This is what excites me about clinical medicine, and what keeps me constantly pursuing new avenues and directions in my search for answers to tough clinical problems. Using these principles, I am often able to shed new light on conditions that have either evaded diagnosis or persisted in spite of conventional medical treatment. My practice is now largely made up of patients with complex conditions, many of whom travel quite a distance to seek this type of medical detective work.

If you have strep throat or need stitches, most traditional medical doctors should be able to take care of you just fine. If your problem is less acute, a traditional doctor may be able to treat your symptoms. However, please know that this is not the same as helping you get well. Doctors often treat the disease instead of the patient.

Here's a pretty typical scenario. Suppose you've had joint pain, fatigue, and muscle aches on and off for weeks. You go to your family doctor, who attempts to rule out autoimmune disorders by ordering the appropriate lab work. The lab results are inconclusive, so he (or she) prescribes symptomatic medications (medications to treat your symptoms)—for example, an anti-inflammatory drug for your aches and pains. When your symptoms persist, your family doctor refers you to a rheumatologist. He (or she) performs an extensive diagnostic evaluation, but unfortunately it does not yield any particular diagnosis. So he prescribes a stronger anti-inflammatory medication. When your symptoms still persist, he tries a different one. When eventually none of his prescriptions are effective, he suggests that the problem is in your head and refers you to a psychiatrist. At this point your immune system may have been ravaged by some of the medications you've tried, you've spent a lot of money, and you're feeling worse.

In my practice, I see people every day who already have been to see highly qualified traditional doctors, but who still aren't well.

"But he (or she) is the best!" they'll say. "He's well known, he's the chairman of his department at a respected medical school, he's published six articles, he's expensive, his waiting room is always full, and I had to wait two months for an appointment!"

"Are you feeling any better?" I'll ask.

The answer, of course, is that they are not. Despite all the tests they've had, and the hundreds or even thousands of dollars they've spent, these patients are still sick. This does not mean they are either crazy or incurable; it just means that conventional medical protocols have failed them.

You don't have to accept a diagnosis of "that's life" or "it's all in your head." Your real problem may be that your doctor is out of ideas. This does not mean that he or she is a bad or incompetent physician or an uncaring person. What it may mean is that you have come to the end of this particular leg of your journey.

So you're at a juncture. Many people arrive at this train station and sit on the platform with their luggage, unaware that there are any number of trains leaving every hour and they can make the choice to take any one of them. Recognize that you do have options—yet if you don't look, you won't find them.

FINDING THE RIGHT DOCTOR

When someone in my family gets sick, we go to a doctor just like everybody else. My father has been cared for by numerous doctors for his chronic medical conditions since his bypass operation twenty years ago, and I feel fortunate to have a good orthopedic surgeon who has helped me through a couple of skiing injuries. So I know from personal experience how important it is to have the right doctor—someone in whom you have confidence, and with whom you can speak freely.

My concern in this chapter is readers who have long-term problems, and readers who are in medical limbo. If you have a chronic condition, there may be steps you can take to feel better. You may have obtained one medical diagnosis (for example, multiple sclerosis) without realizing that you have other problems as well (say, allergies or nutritional deficiencies). If you don't have a textbook case of anything, then you're living in the Land of No Diagnosis. (This adjoins the Land of Misdiagnosis, where you are also free to wander.)

If you have a chronic, puzzling, or serious health concern, I recommend that you review your relationship with your current physician. Maybe there are questions you haven't asked, concerns you haven't expressed, or options you haven't raised. On the other hand, if your present doctor doesn't seem to be able to help you make any further progress, then consider finding another doctor who may be better for you.

Your current physician should not stand in the way of your consulting with another doctor. Patients visit other doctors all the time. As you undoubtedly know, many insurance companies *require* a second opinion before certain procedures are performed. Also, consider this: If you aren't getting better, your doctor may be feeling discouraged, too.

One of my patients had been going to the same obstetrician/gynecologist for twenty years. He placed her on synthetic hormones, and she started getting bothersome side effects. When I placed her on natural hormones instead, she felt much better. However, when she returned to her regular gynecologist for a checkup, he was angry that she had changed her regimen and put her right back on the synthetic hormones. The fact that they made her feel sick was irrelevant to him. Now, is this a physician who is truly looking after the well-being of his patient?

This patient was very confused, and we had a lengthy talk. Her gynecologist had performed some procedures that I didn't consider necessary and had not explained what he was doing or why. I suggested that it might be in this patient's best interests to find a more open-minded and communicative gynecologist. She felt loyalty to this doctor because of all the years that had gone by, but she did say, "Sometimes it's time to move on and make a change."

If it is in your best interests to find a new doctor, then do it. To get the most out of your next doctor's appointment, look for a doctor with the following qualities. A helpful physician:

- **Is willing to listen.** It is essential that your new physician take the time to review your complete medical history. Find a caring and open-minded doctor who will listen to your whole story, from the beginning, and note all of your symptoms. He (or she) should be interested in all of them, even if you've been told in the past that they are not related to your primary complaint. An open-ended medical interview can make all the difference in the world. This process alone can reintroduce you to hope and healing. During your discussion, you shouldn't have to repeat things or vie for the doctor's attention. Ideally you should have a chance to talk in an office, not while you're sitting (or lying) in an examining room. A wise doctor will listen not only to what you are saying, but also to what you are *not*.

• **Is easy to talk to.** It's important that you feel able to tell your doctor anything, because communication is everything. What if you're too embarrassed to mention a particular symptom or part of your past, but the doctor can't make an accurate diagnosis without this information? Also, communication goes both ways. A helpful physician is willing to express the most complex concepts in simple terms. If you don't understand what is wrong with you, what is required of you, or why your treatment regimen should help, you won't have much incentive to follow through on the doctor's recommendations.

• **Sees the big picture.** How you are handling your particular problem is intimately connected with your lifestyle, genes, support systems, marriage, job, attitudes, coping skills, etc. A heart attack for one patient may mean an escape from an unbearably stressful job and a much-needed restful period filled with the love and attention from a devoted family. For another patient, a heart attack may mean panic over makeshift child-care arrangements and financial ruin due to lack of insurance and loss of work. Your illness is not occurring in a vacuum, and it is essential that your doctor show an interest in this aspect of your care.

• **Is open to alternative therapies and other healing modalities.** He (or she) doesn't have to provide you with "one-stop shopping," but he should understand the value of alternative treatments, of beneficial lifestyle changes, and of other healing modalities. I routinely refer patients to other experts for stress management, nutritional consultation, and acupuncture. Sometimes I recommend psychotherapy or yoga or joining a support group. A true healing regimen extends beyond a single visit to the doctor and can include the help and support of a number of people.

• **Understands the mind/body connection.** Even if your doctor were able to examine every one of your cells under a microscope, he (or she) still would not have the complete picture of your health. We are both physical and metaphysical beings, so any diagnosis and any cure must take both levels into account. You'll want to find a physician who respects the importance of feelings as well as the value of emotional support.

• **Is willing to enter into a partnership with you, the patient.** As I said earlier, I view the doctor/patient relationship as a kind of dance. As a patient, you will be playing an active role in your recovery. Taking the medications (and other supplements) prescribed by your doctor is only the beginning. You also will be making choices, pursuing alternative treatments, finding information about your disorder, and doing whatever else it takes for you to achieve optimal health. This is true empowerment, and it is necessary for your recovery.

• **Is open-minded about others.** It is not in your best interest to consult a doctor who is judgmental about your lifestyle choices or anything else. I don't always like what my patients are doing, but I don't think it's my job to be judgmental. For example, I always strongly counsel patients to stop smoking, but I don't believe in making them feel guilty about smoking, even though I know it is terrible for their health and I greatly want them to stop. The truth is, most people are doing the best they can.

- **Is well-informed and up-to-date.** You want to find a doctor who is willing to look, and then look further. He (or she) will gather the latest information, read the medical literature, attend conferences and seminars, and incorporate new approaches into his practice. This physician's quest for knowledge will serve you well.

- **Understands biochemical individuality.** As we've already seen, every patient is unique, so "cookie-cutter" medicine just doesn't make sense. Each patient has his or her own nutrient needs, metabolic profile, sensitivities, etc. I usually give each one of my patients a different treatment regimen, even for the same illness.

- **Knows when to be flexible and when to be committed.** A helpful physician is flexible on a personal level, just the way a healthy blood cell or arterial wall or spine is flexible. On the other hand, there will be times when a doctor must be willing to stand firm, not because of personal brittleness, but because something needs to be done.

- **Is humble.** My favorite physicians are humble in their dealings with patients. They also have a grounded sense of their importance in the great scheme of life. Some of the smartest doctors I've met are also the most humble. A humble and honest physician treats patients with respect and is willing to say, "I don't know." He (or she) is also willing to learn from his patients.

- **Has a hopeful outlook.** Being sick is scary. In addition, medical information is often terrifying. Test results can be alarming, a diagnosis can be frightening, and living with uncertainty can be stressful. We've all heard stories about doctor callousness that are just unbelievable. One cancer doctor took a stick out of his desk, waved it at his patient, and told her it was a magic wand—the only thing that could help her![1] You want a doctor who will be truthful with you, but who also will support you on your healing journey. This kind of doctor focuses not just on disease, but on wellness.

Following are some warning signs that could indicate that a physician is *not* the best one for you. Be cautious if he (or she):

- Believes in the "magic bullet" (and will keep prescribing stronger medicines until it is found)
- Will not let you consult alternative healers, and/or refuses to be held accountable for your health if you consult other doctors
- Asks leading questions, or categorizes your problem too quickly
- Refuses to continue treating you if you buy any remedy from the health food store
- Insists that you follow only one rigid protocol
- Will not take your preferences into account
- Overvalues lab tests and undervalues intuition
- Refuses to explain a diagnosis, medication, or procedure in an understandable way
- Is unfeeling, uncommunicative, or difficult to speak freely with
- Gives doomsday prognoses

It should be noted that not all holistic physicians are wonderful. I know some alternative doctors who are fanatical on certain subjects (for example, candidiasis, hypothyroidism, and oxidative treatments) and have lost their objectivity. They make excessive claims for certain protocols and see every patient in terms of their favorite issue. Remember the expression, "If you're a hammer, everything else is a nail"? Too often doctors see what they believe, rather than believe what they see. Beware of zealots, and try to find a doctor who will "wipe the slate clean" of any preconceived ideas before taking care of you.

Nobody is perfect, so in your search for the best physician, be prepared to compromise on some fronts. I know one warm and brilliant diagnostician who *always* keeps his patients waiting. This is very tiresome for his patients, but they all know that when their turn comes, they will have this doctor's complete attention for as long as they need it.

Some of history's greatest physicians took their patients' symptoms so seriously that we now use diagnoses that use these doctors' names. For example, because of doctors Robert Graves, Thomas Addison, James Parkinson, and Thomas Hodgkin, we now are aware of disorders called Graves', Addison's, Parkinson's, and Hodgkin's diseases. Did people suffer from Graves' disease before Dr. Graves made his observations? Absolutely. So I have to wonder what disorders we are overlooking today.

Sometimes I liken our current medical knowledge to a big "humble pie." There's a lot doctors know. There's even more we know we don't know. But the biggest part of the humble pie is that part of knowledge of which we are totally unaware. Think of the power and possibilities for healing if we only could access that incredible fund of knowledge.

THE PATIENT'S ROLE

I've already said that a physician and a patient have a partnership. What can patients do to uphold their end of the bargain? I appreciate patients who:

• **Are willing to take responsibility.** The old-fashioned mind-set was simply to turn your body over to the doctor and follow his (or, occasionally, her) orders. The doctor would prescribe a pill or surgically remove something, and all the patient had to do was be completely compliant. I greatly prefer an approach that not only respects the preferences of patients, but also holds patients partly accountable for their own health. I appreciate a motivated patient who is willing to make changes—even uncomfortable ones, like giving up chocolate milk or pizza or coffee—and who will devote the time, energy, driving, and whatever else is required to do what needs to be done.

• **Are open to both alternative and traditional treatments.** I have patients who are resistant to standard therapies, and patients who are suspicious of progressive therapies. You have more options if you're not entrenched in any one point of view.

• **Are willing to engage in some self-examination.** Illness can have meaning, or bring meaning, on a very deep level (more about this in Chapter 13). It can be extremely healthy for the patient to examine the psychosocial backdrop against which his or her illness is being played out. Patients who refuse to reflect upon their innermost thoughts, beliefs, attitudes, and emotions are not doing all they can to heal themselves.

• **Stay in the present.** A number of my patients have had bad experiences with their previous doctors, and some of them have been guarded or even angry when they first met me. It's important not to allow previous experiences to distract from the opportunity for a fresh start. One of the first things I might tell a patient like this is to let go of his (or her) past negative medical experiences and open up to the possibility that his journey for healing may be very different from this point on. This would allow for the creation of a fresh, healing partnership, not hindered or burdened by past experiences.

COMMONLY ASKED QUESTION NO. 23:

What questions should I ask the doctor?

Many of my patients also go to other doctors for specialized care. I encourage them to ask lots of questions, in an appropriate way. Some doctors don't like to answer questions, as if educating the patient might take too much time, or diminish their own importance and expertise. A good way to approach this kind of doctor is to start with, "Can you tell me about . . . ?" or "What are your thoughts about . . . ?"

To get better, or at least to improve, it's important that you understand all aspects of your illness. The sicker you are, the more questions you need to ask. Some questions include:

• What is my diagnosis?
• What is the natural course of this disorder?
• What complications might develop?
• What treatment options are available?
• What are the benefits of each option?
• What are the potential side effects of each option?
• What about risks, complications, and drug interactions?
• What literature is available on this subject?

Some of my patients write down their questions, which I happen to think is a great idea. It's certainly better than getting home and wishing you'd remembered to ask something.

The most valuable thing a patient can do is help me practice preventive medicine. It's far better to stop a disease from developing than to try to treat it after it has taken hold in the body.

People have incredibly different points of view about this. Some of my patients are extremely health conscious. They follow the Immune System Empowerment Program in every way, they come in for regular checkups, and they plan to live to be a hundred. Other patients who already have had warning signs of illness refuse to do anything about it until they have a health crisis. For example, one of my patients needed chelation therapy to enhance his circulation, but he didn't pursue the treatments. Then he had a heart attack—and a much bigger problem to deal with. Then he couldn't wait to start!

Ask yourself how far you are willing to let things go before you make whatever changes you still need to make. Where are you on the continuum between good health and poor health? How many symptoms will it take before you reverse the trend? How many infections? How tired or sore or depressed do you have to feel before you'll adopt the Immune System Empowerment Program or take yourself to the doctor?

Most parents are quick to bring their children to the doctor but slow to make appointments for themselves. This is actually ironic, because the older we are, the more vigilant we need to be. I know many baby boomers who are tremendously responsible when it comes to work and family, yet they haven't had a physical exam in decades. They put more energy into the upkeep of their cars than into their bodies—a disturbing concept no matter how you look at it.

Being Well-Informed

Once upon a time, one of my patients with a rash asked a dermatologist about a certain skin condition. The doctor said, "Where did you hear about that?" The patient answered, "I read about it." And the doctor said, "You read too much."

This patient was insulted, and I have to say I can understand why. I encourage my patients to find out more about their illness(es), as usually this knowledge is helpful in their healing. However, there are times when they read conflicting reports or hear one too many anecdote from friends or family. Usually we can clear up any confusion during an office visit. However, it's something to be aware of and to try to avoid getting entangled in.

Bernie Siegel calls patients who insist on getting information "respants," for "responsible participants."[2] These are the patients who come in to the doctor's office with a list of questions, who want to understand their options, and who insist on learning how they can participate in their recovery. These patients can be obstinate and demanding, but they also tend to get better.

THE ROLE OF DIAGNOSTIC TESTS

My purpose here is not to discuss all the different diagnostic tests that doctors use today. There are more tests available than I could even list, let alone describe. Instead, I want to talk about how I approach diagnostic tests in general.

When I first see a new patient, it's not unusual for me to order a lot of tests. This is because I need to compile the necessary information to individualize the patient's Immune System Empowerment Program. After that I usually don't need to order very many tests except to follow up on significant abnormalities. Most physicians ask for the following blood work fairly routinely:

- CBC (complete blood count)—yields the number of white blood cells, the percentage of each kind of white blood cell (this is called a *differential*), the number of red blood cells, some characteristics of the red blood cells, and the number of platelets
- SMAC (also called a chem profile)—indicates liver function, kidney function, blood sugar levels, electrolytes, serum calcium, serum magnesium, serum cholesterol, serum uric acid, and more
- Sedimentation rate—used as a nonspecific measure of inflammation

Other body fluids, such as saliva, plasma, spinal fluid, and urine, can also be used for different tests. Urinalysis checks the urine for proper pH (acidity), signs of infection, and indications of sugar or protein irregularities.

All these tests give general indications of the health of the patient. I often order additional tests that will help me either rule out or verify different diagnoses. You already know what many of these tests are because you've read about them in the previous chapters. They include:

- Allergy tests
- Immune profiles (both cellular and antibody)
- Tests that determine hormone levels
- Tests that help determine thyroid function
- Tests that help determine adrenal function
- Test for candida antibodies
- Tests for chronic hidden infections (including Lyme disease and viral infections)
- Stool analysis (including tests for parasites)
- Tests for intestinal permeability
- Liver detoxification profile
- Tests for nutritional status (checking nutrient levels in the blood, cells, and urine)
- Tests for antioxidant status

- Tests that help determine metabolic status
- Glucose tolerance tests
- A procedure that measures stomach acidity
- Tests that evaluate cardiovascular function

These tests (and others) help me pinpoint disorders that are often overlooked by other doctors, including subclinical (or functional) hypothyroidism, adrenal fatigue, reactive hypoglycemia, chronic candidiasis (fungal hypersensitivity), hidden allergies, chemical sensitivities, digestive problems, hormonal imbalances, nutritional deficiencies, metabolic imbalances, Hashimoto's thyroiditis, parasites, and Lyme disease. I order some tests that traditional doctors do not simply because they wouldn't know what to do with the test results if they were abnormal. For example, if one of my patients has elevated levels of Lipoprotein-a [Lp(a)], I know that even though there is no prescription drug for this condition, I can prescribe nutritional supplements such as vitamin C, lysine, proline, niacinate, and N-acetylcysteine that will help bring these levels back to the normal range. Traditional doctors won't ask for this test because presently there's no pharmacologic treatment for an abnormal result, even though elevated Lipoprotein-a has been proven to be a very significant risk factor for heart and blood vessel disease.

As of this writing, we've just begun using a new piece of equipment that assesses biological terrain—the "soil" of which Pasteur spoke. This equipment allows us to determine a patient's pH level (this is important because enzymes in the body function only within a certain range of acidity), redox status (this would help reveal oxidation/reduction imbalances, including clues to mitochondrial dysfunction), and resistivity (how well the patient's tissues conduct electrical current, which is influenced by the presence of proper levels of minerals in the tissues). I'm very excited about this testing, for it can be done rapidly and noninvasively, it paints a comprehensive picture of the patient's strengths, weaknesses, and predispositions to problems, and it allows us to monitor patient response to treatment. In my view it truly represents progressive medicine.

Most of my patients have complex or undiagnosed long-term problems of unknown origin. Because health problems tend to build on themselves (remember the Illness Spiral?), one untreated disorder can lead to several more related problems. Getting the right diagnosis in this case is like peeling an onion: I treat one layer at a time until I finally reach the core problem and can address it.

When a patient with a multisymptom, multisystem illness first comes to me, I do a complete history and physical exam and then begin compiling a list of potential contributing or underlying problems. Then I start administering diagnostic tests in a logical sequence. Depending on the patient's symptoms, I might check for food allergies, hormonal and/or metabolic imbalances, or infections such as chronic candidiasis or chronic viral or parasitic infections. Usually at least one, if not several, of these test results comes back positive, and then we initiate appropriate treatment. Sometimes that's all that is needed.

However, some cases just aren't that simple. Even after dealing with the imbalances and sensitivities just listed, the patient still feels unwell. Then we need to go even further and rule out other diseases and conditions one by one and even consider empirical treatment trials, which are based on clinical considerations more than lab results.

Evaluating Immune Function

When patients show signs of immune deficiency, they can undergo tests to help determine their immunocompetence. If they are immunocompromised, these tests can help identify which component of their immune system has gone awry.

As you've already read, low secretory IgA (protective immune antibody in our mucosal secretions) is very common. It's possible to evaluate secretory IgA levels with a simple saliva test; serum IgA can be measured with blood work. As I've also already discussed, some people have specific IgG subclass deficiencies. These, too, can be measured with serum testing. It's not enough just to measure overall IgG serum levels.

Because white blood cells are so important to immune function, tests have been developed to evaluate lymphocyte function. These include:

- **Measuring the number of helper T cells (CD4).** Different labs use different cutoff points, but usually a level of 600 or higher is healthy. A level lower than 400 indicates a problem.

- **Measuring the percentages of T cells and B cells.** These percentages can get skewed if either part of the immune response is underactive or overactive.

- **Calculating the ratio of helper T cells (CD4) to suppressor T cells (CD8).** A good ratio would be in the range of 1.2:1 (depending on the cutoff point used by the lab). AIDS attacks helper T cells, resulting in a lower ratio (say, 0.4:1). Autoimmune disorders work the other way and suppress the suppressor T cells, yielding an abnormal ratio in the other direction (for example, 4.2:1).

- **Measuring the levels of natural killer cells (NK cells) and their functional activity.** As mentioned before, NK cells are important in fighting cancer cells and cells infected by viruses. It's possible to have a normal number of NK cells but decreased NK cell activity. (One of the conditions with which we frequently see this is CFIDS.)

People with HIV/AIDS follow their T cell counts very closely. However, T cells are just one aspect of overall immunocompetence, so a low T cell count need not be a death sentence.

Lyme Disease

I have many patients with chronic Lyme disease, and I think it represents a good example of a diagnostic problem. This is a disease that often goes undiagnosed, in part because lab tests are unreliable and some doctors won't treat patients for Lyme unless the patient has a positive test result. Left untreated, Lyme wreaks havoc in the body, for it can affect every body system. Once it takes hold, it can be extremely difficult to eradicate.

The basic test for Lyme disease is called a *Lyme titer*. There are different kinds available, but they all measure the presence of antibodies in the blood against the Lyme spirochete (that is, evidence of the body's fight against Lyme). A patient with a negative Lyme titer may still have the disease, partly because of lab errors, partly because of false-negative results, and partly because of inconsistencies in and among labs. Some patients have seronegative Lyme—that is, Lyme that never shows up in their blood work. As you can imagine, this is a hotly debated subject in medical circles, particularly when you consider that many doctors depend almost entirely on lab tests to make their diagnoses.

Other tests for Lyme include:

• **The Lyme Western blot tests.** These tests measure the presence of antibodies to specific components of the Lyme spirochete. There are two Western blot tests to measure two different types of antibodies: IgM antibodies (which usually show up earlier in an infection) and IgG antibodies (which usually show up later in an infection, indicating that the disease has been around for a while). The antibodies are measured in bands, and a certain number of positive bands are considered indicative of Lyme disease. As we've seen in many of the case histories throughout this book, patients without the requisite number of bands can nonetheless have symptoms of Lyme and respond to appropriate treatment. Sometimes the Western blot test is used to override misleading test results from a Lyme titer that was positive (known as a *false-positive*) due to the phenomenon of cross-reacting antibodies. Other times, contrary to popular medical dictum, we can see a positive Western blot in spite of a negative Lyme titer. When this occurs, I consider the Lyme titer to be a *false-negative*.

• **The Lyme urine antigen test.** For this test, the patient takes an antibiotic for five days. The principle of the test is that if any Lyme spirochetes are killed by the antibiotic, they will be shed into the urine. The patient's urine is checked on days 3, 4, and 5 for the presence of Lyme antigens (that is, actual components of the spirochete itself, not antibodies against it). I usually reserve this test for very complex cases. It is still relatively new and mainly considered a research tool.

• **The polymerase chain reaction (PCR) test.** This is an amplification technique used to detect the DNA of Lyme spirochetes in the joints, blood, urine, or spinal fluid. This test, useful in certain situations, is considered mainly a research tool at this time.

• **A spinal tap.** This technique can be used to detect Lyme antibodies, antigens, and/or immune complexes in the spinal fluid. A spinal tap (also called a lumbar puncture) is fairly invasive, and thus it isn't a test I order lightly.

• **The T cell lymphocyte proliferation response test.** This test exposes a patient's T cells to Lyme antigens and measures the response. If the T cells recognize the Lyme antigen and actively proliferate (a positive result), this can indicate the presence of a Lyme infection even in the absence of antibodies. It's possible that the patient has been exposed to Lyme but is not making the correct antibodies, so all the Lyme titers in the world are not going to detect his or her Lyme disease. We refer to this scenario as seronegative Lyme disease.

You can see that medical testing has gotten extremely sophisticated. You also can see that there is incredible individual variation in how people respond to Lyme. Testing is important, but it isn't everything.

COMMONLY ASKED QUESTION NO. 24:

Why are test results so often unreliable?

Both false-negative and false-positive results can be caused by dietary factors and medications. In addition, human error and poor workmanship account for many incorrect lab results. Some laboratories are better than others, but the only way for a physician to find out which labs are better is by published reports, by learning from the experiences of colleagues, or even by trial and error.

A 1992 article in *The Journal of the American Medical Association* discussed a study in which researchers took blood from six people with known Lyme disease and three people without Lyme disease and sent these samples to forty-five labs over a period of six months.[3] High levels of antibodies were missed by up to 21 percent of the labs. Low levels of antibodies were missed by 55 percent of the labs. Several of the labs gave false-positive results for the people who did not have Lyme.

As part of the study, researchers sent out the same samples more than once to see if a lab would get the same results when they repeated the test at a different time. Amazingly, the reproducibility of results ranged from 27 to 94 percent, meaning that some labs got the same results only 27 percent of the time! I find this an utterly staggering statistic.

Diagnostic tests are becoming more sensitive, but many of them still can't determine what is happening inside our cells—which is where the action really is. In the future, we'll need tests with enhanced sensitivity and specificity to pick up cases overlooked by today's tests.

MAKING A CLINICAL DIAGNOSIS

Sometimes lab work simply isn't enough. As I already discussed in Chapter 10, problems like adrenal insufficiency and borderline hypothyroidism may not be detected by the standard tests. Patients with chemical sensitivities and other disorders that evade the usual tests are often regarded as nutcases because their "proof" is almost entirely anecdotal. If test results are resoundingly positive, that makes my job easier, but in my experience, it is frequently appropriate to treat a patient based on a clinical diagnosis—that is, the patient's symptoms and medical history. Sometimes I rely on my gut-level intuition. After twenty years in medicine and many years of personal growth work, I have gained more confidence in my clinical intuition and have come to rely on it, especially in difficult or confusing cases.

Obviously, we don't have tests to measure those essential components of good health, love and emotional support. Similarly, blood work can't reveal a patient's social isolation or spiritual deficit. Only listening can uncover these problems—and more. *The key to making a correct diagnosis is, and always will be, listening to the patient.*

One of my patients, nicknamed J.P., was a fourteen-year-old who had been diagnosed by a psychiatrist as depressive. His parents were despairing when they brought him to me. Six months before, they explained, J.P. had been energetic, outgoing, and motivated. Now he was withdrawn and listless. He had various aches and pains and headaches, and he couldn't summon the energy to do much of anything except listen to music.

No great changes had occurred in J.P.'s life or in his family. Because he used to be so well-adjusted, I suspected that some physical problem was behind his symptoms. I ordered a Lyme titer for J.P., but the results were negative.

The more I talked to J.P. and his parents, the more I believed Lyme was still a possibility. Before he became ill, he had taken regular walks with his dog through the countryside in an area endemic for Lyme, and he could easily have picked up a Lyme-infected tick without being aware of it. Based on J.P.'s medical history and my clinical observations, I decided to treat J.P. for Lyme in spite of his negative test results.

J.P. recovered. His energy returned, his aches and pains and headaches disappeared, and his depression lifted.

It can be extremely difficult to diagnose diseases like Lyme that can affect many body systems at the same time and can cause both physical and psychological changes. Lyme can cause both neurologic symptoms (memory loss, fatigue, numbness, tingling) and musculoskeletal symptoms (joint aches, swelling, muscle pain), which immediately complicates the clinical picture. These symptoms can resemble those caused by multiple sclerosis, chronic arthritis, fibromyalgia, and other disorders. When you throw in the fact that many lab tests are inconclusive or inaccurate, and that many patients suffer from more than one condition at the same time, it becomes clear that determining a correct diagnosis in some of these multisymptom, multisystem disorders can sometimes be a daunting task.

Dr. William Osler, who was considered the most eminent diagnostician of the late 1800s, once said, "It is better to know the patient that has the disease than the disease that has the patient." I think one of the reasons I love medicine so much is that it is both a science and an art. The scientific part is challenging, complex, and even mysterious. The intuitive part, however, is what moves the soul of both the doctor and the patient.

6〜9 *SARAH'S STORY*

At her worst—just before I met her—Sarah thought she was going to die. On the days when she was in constant pain, unable to get out of bed and unable to see, she had moments when maybe dying didn't seem like such a bad idea. She was almost seventy, after all; perhaps, she thought, this was just the end of the line.

It was not. What a difference a diagnosis can make! When Sarah received the correct diagnosis and the appropriate treatment, she got her life back.

Sarah's first sign of illness was a "bull's-eye" rash on her abdomen. She also developed flu-like symptoms, including severe headaches and neck stiffness, but she figured the whole episode would blow over like most viral illnesses.

A month later, she was even sicker. The rash had disappeared, but she was now terribly tired, particularly if she exerted herself in any way. Sometimes she couldn't even stand up.

When she developed chest pain, Sarah went to a cardiologist. He diagnosed angina and prescribed the typical medications for angina. They didn't help.

At this time, Sarah happened to see a program on television about Lyme disease that showed a bull's-eye rash exactly like hers. Sarah went to the doctor with the intention of being treated for Lyme disease. She was very hopeful that this would be the answer.

When her Lyme titer test came back negative, her doctor refused to treat her for Lyme disease. Instead, her referred her to a rheumatologist, who gave her a prescription anti-inflammatory drug. It didn't help.

Sarah became even more exhausted and developed more symptoms, including difficulty sleeping, frequent headaches, frequent crying, aching all over, and difficulty walking and climbing stairs. Her resistance to illness was low, and it seemed as if she picked up every "bug" to which she was exposed.

By now Sarah's symptoms had been worsening for three years. She consulted an orthopedist for the pain in her arms, and he performed bilateral surgery for carpal tunnel syndrome.

When Sarah's stiff neck and fatigue worsened, she sought medical help again. This time her rheumatologist diagnosed fibromyalgia. A month later, Sarah had such severe pain in her arms that she was treated not only with anti-inflammatories but also with steroid injections.

Sarah developed a long-term low-grade fever. She was unable to close her hands and would sometimes be bedridden. She was losing her hair, losing her memory, and even losing her sight.

Finally Sarah consulted a doctor who was willing to treat her for Lyme disease even in the absence of a positive Lyme titer. He prescribed oral doxycycline, which is an appropriate treatment for Lyme. However, by now Sarah's Lyme disease had been entrenched for three and a half years. The doxycycline helped her, but she was still very sick.

It was my belief, after listening carefully to Sarah's story, that she had seronegative Lyme disease. She presented a classic history of Lyme, despite the absence of any positive test results. I ordered another Lyme titer, but was not surprised when it came back negative.

I started Sarah on intravenous Rocephin (a powerful antibiotic), and she felt definite improvement. Unfortunately, she started doing so much more that one day she fell and fractured both of her wrists, which was a setback. However, the Lyme-related pains in her arms and legs had disappeared.

Sarah was not familiar with alternative medicine, and she was not interested in pursuing intravenous vitamin C, but she was happy to follow through with the nutritional supplements I recommended as adjunctive therapy to her course of antibiotics. After twelve weeks of antibiotics (four weeks on intravenous Rocephin, and eight weeks on oral Biaxin) and nutritional therapy for about a year, Sarah was walking regularly and was delighted to have her life back. She was constantly amazed at the difference that had occurred in her health over a period of just twelve months. She has become a very loyal and grateful patient, and continues to use her nutritional supplements to maintain her good health and vitality.

Chapter 13

---◆❧◆---

HEALING BEGINS WITH ACCEPTANCE

Come to the edge,
No, we will fall.
Come to the edge,
No, we will fall.
They came to the edge.
He pushed them, and they flew.

—GUILLAUME APOLLINAIRE

This chapter marks an end, but also a beginning. Although it is written specifically for those of you with chronic illnesses, it also holds many truths for everyone. For all of us, life is a process of healing and discovery.

Included in this chapter are spiritual concepts that complement the scientifically oriented information in the previous chapters. These concepts include attitudes of love, openness, acceptance, and equanimity. Because I feel strongly that the balance between the physical and the spiritual is essential for immune system health, I hope everyone will take this chapter to heart. However, I know some readers will be more comfortable with these concepts than others.

If you have difficulty with this chapter because it contains more spiritual concepts, please know that these principles are ageless. Perhaps at another time in your life they will hold more meaning for you. For many of you, I trust that this chapter will be very timely and will hold great significance.

WHAT IS HEALING?

Nobody likes being sick. Who would want to be sick for an hour, let alone for months or years? Illness means pain, and it is human to want to avoid pain.

373

On the other hand, I have learned from my patients that there can be opportunity in illness. Sickness is a signal that something needs to be changed. Usually sickness is the expression of some kind of imbalance.

Healing is the process of making the changes we need to make in order to mend ourselves physically and spiritually. Healing consists of:

- Finding out what you need, but aren't getting
- Finding out what you have or are holding on to, but need to let go

You can see that taking charge of your healing is not the same thing as just taking pills. True healing requires personal change. So, while most of us move away from the pain of illness, it is actually this pain that obliges us to seek the help we need to heal ourselves, not only physically but also on a deeper level.

On this deeper level, strange as it may seem, the experience of illness can actually be good. If you approach your sickness with fear, resentment, and anxiety, your experience of your illness will be bad. With a different attitude, your experience of your sickness may include some of these feelings, yet still have a positive and meaningful impact on your life and make you stronger and healthier in ways you never imagined.

I know many of you may have chronic problems, such as arthritis, diabetes, migraines, or colitis, or you know someone who does. Some of you will have life-threatening diseases, such as cancer or AIDS. The point of departure for this chapter is that you have found an open-minded physician with whom you are comfortable, who has diagnosed your "main" problem, and who has possibly discovered some other underlying disorders as well. Where does your healing journey go from here?

INITIAL TASKS

The following will serve you as guideposts on your journey to health:

- **Know that there is not going to be one magic cure.** No one therapy works all the time, just as nothing is 100 percent preventive. When my patients start out with an attitude of *"This is it!"* I counsel them that healing frequently is the result of hard work at many levels, and their healing regimen may involve many different treatments and approaches used simultaneously.
- **Recognize that healing is not the same as regaining physical well-being.** Most of my patients initially come to see me to be cured. They want to feel as good as they used to feel, and they want to be able to do all the things they used to do. Much of our early work together has to do with defining and refining expectations. Because healing has such a strong spiritual aspect to it, you might actually be better off with your illness, but with an increased awareness and a newfound pursuit of wellness, than you were before—when you didn't have

these symptoms, but you also weren't paying much attention to that which is most important in your life. Some of my patients become spiritually well (i.e., accept life on its terms), yet they never return to complete physical health. Some become both spiritually and physically healed. *Healing is an ongoing process of acceptance leading to self-love and spiritual well-being that might not be synchronous with physical well-being.*

• **Know that whatever happens, you can handle it.** Many of my patients are afraid, and understandably so, that a difficult surgical procedure or an emotional loss will be unbearable. Even so, with support and guidance they find the capacity to accept what they previously feared was unacceptable, and to bear what they thought would be unbearable. As you will see throughout this chapter, this acceptance is a crucial aspect of healing.

What Are the Doctor's Responsibilities?

In addition to making a diagnosis, the doctor presents the patient with treatment options. Sometimes there are statistics involved, such as rates of cure or the likelihood of side effects. The doctor will know what has been effective for other patients and will have suggestions about which treatment to try first.

The doctor's job is to make sure that the patient can make a well-informed decision. It is not the doctor's job to impose a treatment regimen on a patient. Together, patient and doctor decide upon a healing program. When establishing this regimen, I never say "always," and I never say "never."

Some patients are really more comfortable being told what to do. I try to draw them into the decision-making process so they can help take responsibility for both their healing regimen and the results they achieve.

One of my elderly patients was brought to me with severely advanced pancreatic cancer. She was very ill, and her prognosis was not good. There were certainly treatments to try and ways of improving her general condition, but this can be a very nasty form of cancer, and her case was already very far advanced. Her husband had been caring for her every need for a very long time, which was a heavy burden for an old man.

What troubled me about this couple was that the husband was certain I could cure his wife. He regarded me as a god, and was sure that the treatments I recommended would save his wife. I tried to warn him that this might not be the outcome, but he couldn't hear me. He needed to believe that she would recover, and he was not capable of the kind of 50/50 thinking that would have enabled him to see the situation in a more balanced way.

Eventually the wife died. The husband became very upset with me. Where once he thought I could do no wrong, now he thought I could do no good. This is a classic example of dualistic thinking. Talking to the husband candidly and at length about his difficult experience helped him to perceive the situation more clearly. We both had tried to do our best. This experience made me even more aware of the importance of trying to achieve a realistic and balanced understanding before initiating treatment. Preventing misunderstandings like this is far easier than trying to resolve them after they have occurred.

What Are the Patient's Responsibilities?

In the last chapter, I talked about the patient's role (see page 362). When it comes to handling chronic illness, I would add that it is especially important for you, the patient, to take an interest in developing your healing regimen and to commit to doing whatever needs to be done. Don't "yes" the doctor if you know you don't intend to do something.

It's a good idea to develop a timetable for meeting certain goals. For example, "This week I will throw out all the junk food in the house. Next week I will start walking to the end of the road and back." And so on. This is *not* the same thing as a timetable for recovery! Avoid saying to yourself, "I *must* be well in time for my daughter's wedding." This sets you up for real disappointment. Instead, tell yourself, "I am doing everything I can to be well in time for my daughter's wedding. If I am not well by then, it will still be a wonderful event and I will take part in it as best I can."

I've found that it is essential for patients to stop obsessing over how healthy they used to be. This kind of brooding guarantees a long period, maybe even a lifetime, of frustration and anger. Even though your health has changed, it is important to remember that you are still a valuable human being—an important thread, a golden thread, in the fabric of humanity.

Healing begins with acceptance—not resignation, but simple acceptance of where you are at this moment. Acceptance allows you to live in the present, not in the past, not dwelling on who you were or what you could do. With acceptance, we peel off our defenses, uncover our misconceptions, and move to experience our true selves. Only after we come to accept what is here now can we ask the questions, "Where do we go from here?" and "What do we need to get there?"

ENERGY

The universe is made of energy. It is full of vibrations at all different levels. This isn't something most of us dwell on, but we are familiar with the idea that there are different frequencies of light and sound waves. There are also other types of vibrations—of spirit, of thought, of matter.

We are more than our physical bodies. Our body is condensed energy. Einstein tied physical matter and energy together in his equation $E = mc^2$. Each of us has an energetic field that provides a matrix upon which our cells are laid. The terminology for this concept varies: some people say "life field," others say "life force" or "human energy field."

The human energy field also extends around our body. Many people are capable of seeing the auras around living things, and healers are able to derive information from what they see in a patient's aura. The aura is thought to mediate between our physical self and higher energy levels in the universe. Our auras take in energy from the greater universe, and this energy is metabolized through successively denser vibratory fields, ending with physical matter. Our belief system exists at a higher energy level and comprises our personal answers to questions such as, "Do I feel safe?" "Is the universe friendly?" "Will my needs be met?" and "Am I in abundance?" Successively denser levels include our thought patterns and our feelings, which surround and can nurture our physical selves.

What is most important about this concept of energy is that *consciousness and energy create matter*. Our physical self is an expression of our beliefs, thoughts, feelings, and attitudes, all of which exist on these higher vibrational levels. Our attitudes can play a role in our becoming sick, and addressing them can affect our healing. Because counterproductive thought patterns based upon distorted belief systems interfere with health, physical problems may keep reemerging until these deep distortions and misconceptions are cleared. When we finally align with our deepest truth, healing on all levels becomes possible.

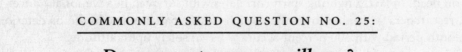

COMMONLY ASKED QUESTION NO. 25:

Do we create our own illness?

There's a lot of debate about this. Some people say we bring everything in life upon ourselves. Others say life events, including illnesses, are totally random. In my opinion, it doesn't really matter. What does matter is what you do with your illness now that you have it, and whether or not you find opportunity within it. Regardless of its cause, illness provides an opportunity for deeper healing.

I believe that we all come into this world with a life task. Illness may play a role in leading us to more awareness and acceptance of ourselves, more awareness and acceptance of others, and greater acceptance of life on its terms. This in turn moves us forward on our life task.

Wherever your illness came from, it is now a problem that you need to deal with. You aren't responsible *for* your illness, but you are responsible *to* your illness. The first step in dealing with it is to accept it.

In the process of accepting illness, we uncover core wounds that have led to emotional upsets and misconceptions that have followed us throughout our adult life. The attitudes and efforts that we bring to healing these wounds, which are layered in sadness, pain, anger, and fear, are ultimately what bring us to our deeper truths.

ACCEPTANCE

I've already said that healing begins with acceptance. The attitude of acceptance creates a state of equanimity—of being at peace with yourself, with others, with your illness, with the world.

We usually think of our self and our life as being two distinct things. This is me, this is my life. All these things that are happening to me aren't really me, right?

Not exactly! It took some deep spiritual work for me to realize that life is not something we are "put into." The life we are leading *is us.* We cannot be separated from it. We need to accept it on its own terms, because otherwise we are in some way rejecting ourselves.

Accepting and Fighting

Acceptance does not mean capitulation. It is possible to accept an illness and still work to change it. Strange as it may seem, accepting your illness can make you stronger and healthier. However, it is very important that you take control of your situation and get the help you need. In fact, a fighting spirit correlates with survival. In a National Cancer Institute study, researchers were able to predict which cancer patients would die or deteriorate in a two-month period with 100 percent accuracy based solely upon attitude.[1]

This concept of fighting and accepting at the same time is puzzling for patients at first, but I've found that it becomes clearer when I describe their task as a fight *for* life, not a fight *against* illness. Fighting for life generates energy, while fighting against illness depletes energy. Fighting for life is seeking health, not fleeing disease. Fighting out of resentment, anger, and fear is unhealthy struggle. Fighting for life is healthy struggle.

When you are faced with a difficult illness, you need to save your energy for the real fight. Don't waste your energy by frantically trying to outwit your illness. You will only churn out stress hormones and fear. Avoid fighting against the condition of your body, which sends a "die" message. Instead, sit quietly and make room for love, warmth, and compassion. Try to attain peace of mind, which sends a "live" message. When you arrive at this place, where you are totally accepting of your self and your illness, and simultaneously in each moment fighting for life with all your resources, you are well on your way in the healing process.

The Physical and Spiritual Fight

A healthy, balanced immune system parallels a healthy, balanced attitude. When both your immune system and your spiritual self are healthy, it's like riding the perfect wave.

As we've already seen, the responsiveness of the immune system can be placed on a continuum from underreactive to overreactive. Our attitudes, too, can be placed along the same continuum.

Immune system is undervigilant (cancer)	Immune system is appropriately assertive and flexible (capable of quick, strong response; accepts the self; able to distinguish between real and perceived threat)	Immune system is overvigilant (autoimmune disorders, allergies)
Weak ego (defenseless, resigned, sacrificial, overly tolerant)	Healthy ego (good boundaries, self-acceptance)	Overgrown ego (fear of losing autonomy; nothing is to be trusted)

The individual with a balanced immune system and a healthy sense of self does not waste physical or emotional energy on battles that don't need to be fought. This frees up more energy for both physical and emotional defense and repair. By living in this focused, efficient, and balanced state, we can avoid the great fatigue that so many people experience with age. If more of us were able to direct our energies only toward what is truly important, I'm sure that fewer of my patients would have mitochondrial problems, burnout, and chronic fatigue immune dysfunction syndrome.

At either end of this continuum, there is a basic misconception that shows up in many ways, both emotional and physical. The person with an underactive immune system and weak ego has a misconception that he or she is worthless, and therefore any effort won't make a difference. The person with the overactive immune system and overgrown ego has a misconception that all struggle, no matter how small the issue, is a matter of life and death. He (or she) can't let go and must fight all the time out of fear that if he stops, everything will fall apart. You can see that not much is going to improve for these people until their underlying misconceptions are addressed.

The immune system's acceptance of self parallels our emotional acceptance of self. Both are forms of self-love, or unconditional love for the self, which is tremendously important in healing. I like to think that this acceptance translates from the cellular level on up—to tissues, to organs, to the organism (that's us), to humanity, and to the universe. It could even go the other way as well, from the cellular to the intracellular contents to the subcellular. It's a powerful message.

Accepting Setbacks

The road to recovery has ups and downs. I tell my patients to picture a chart from the stock market. There are good days and bad days, gains and losses, but most of the time the overall movement of the stock market is upward.

Sometimes there are no particular signs of progress for a long while, and then suddenly there is improvement. It's difficult to get through these long plateaus unless you remember that the journey is what's important, not the destination.

Expect to go through some turmoil, particularly at the beginning of your healing regimen. Don't expect just to wake up one day fully prepared to accept each moment as it comes. If you've just been handed a difficult diagnosis, you may go through a period of anger, denial, or bargaining before you can reach acceptance. Go easy on yourself and give yourself time.

One of my patients, Elliot, was unbelievably persistent in his quest to reverse his severe rheumatoid arthritis. Elliot is an incredible gentleman with a jovial personality, always cheerful in spite of a difficult life and much physical pain.

When he first came to see me, Elliot was sixty-five years old. He had been placed on a powerful anticancer drug that can be helpful for rheumatoid arthritis. Elliot said his goal was to "get off this damn medication," and he wanted to try a nutritional approach. He did a lot of reading, he listened to health programs on the radio, and he had patience.

Elliot did everything. We pinpointed his allergies and started him on an allergen-free diet. I prescribed numerous supplements, including high doses of essential fatty acids (which can be anti-inflammatory and thus beneficial for his condition). I started Elliot on intravenous vitamin C, then added chelation therapy.

Everything improved—except his arthritis. Elliot had more energy and more appetite, but the chronic swelling of his joints persisted. At this point, on his own accord, Elliot had his amalgam fillings removed just to see if that would help. In his case, there was no immediately apparent change.

From here we moved on to a liver detoxification program. Elliot added fresh-squeezed vegetable juices to his regimen. By this time he was feeling "like a million bucks"—except for his arthritis.

Finally, I started Elliot on photo-oxidative therapy, and he definitely saw the most change in his arthritis after that. He no longer had any acutely inflamed joints. He was able to do much more, and to decrease his "damn" medication at the same time. Two years after he started treatment, Elliot was like a new person.

What was so inspiring about Elliot is that he never lost faith in what we were doing, and he never lost patience. He came in steadily for his treatments, hoping for the best but accepting whatever came along, even during times of little apparent progress. Elliot is certainly in far better shape than he has been for years, and he is committed to doing whatever he needs to do to maintain or even improve his current level of health.

When to Stop Fighting

At a certain point, even healthy fighting can turn into unhealthy fighting, and then it's time to let go. One of my desperately ill cancer patients went to Mexico in search of yet one more treatment that might help her. She became so ill there that she was unable to return home, and died in a hospital in a foreign country. The family was torn apart not only by her death, but by its circumstances.

Doctors can play into this kind of struggle, too. I have seen terminally ill patients in the hospital who are being physically preserved for as long as possible. They are tied up with restraints, they've been given drugs to paralyze them, they have tubes in and out of multiple orifices, they're isolated and often subjected to very invasive procedures. The medical profession has almost perfected how to keep us living at all costs and against all odds. I would argue that this isn't really living at all.

Although it sounds contradictory, dying is not incompatible with healing. We are all living and dying at the same time. Life and death are two sides of the same coin. Personally, I believe that life is a continuum, that there is a spirit world, and that dying represents both an end and a beginning.

For all of us, sick and well, immortality is not the goal. Instead of trying to avoid death, we need to concentrate on how to live life to the fullest. Then death becomes less fearsome.

I have a patient with late-stage cancer who is a great example of this acceptance of life and death. As of this writing, she is in a hospice program, where in all likelihood she will soon die. However, she is still very much in life. She has been speaking with friends, spending time with her family, and preparing openly and calmly for her death. Because of her lack of fear of her impending death, she has an incredible impact on all who come in contact with her.

50/50 Thinking

In Chapter 8, I introduced the concept of 50/50 thinking. This kind of thinking is important in healing, where nothing is black or white.

According to the Pathwork, a course based on inspired spiritual writings, 100/100 thinking—either/or thinking—sees only duality and extremes. When we are locked into this point of view, we are very threatened by life because we see every issue as a clash of the titans—good versus evil, life versus death, being totally perfect versus being totally worthless, being completely lovable versus being completely unlovable. We take very defensive positions because we believe there is so much at stake, so much to protect, so much to lose.

When we move away from 100/100 thinking, we move toward 50/50 thinking. Here we are still seeing extremes, but we are able to accept that they coexist. Things can be good *and* evil, we can be lovable *and* unlovable, and so on. By transcending either/or thinking, we can accept that illness is a part of life, that we can be healthy and sick at the same time.

When we are in 100/100 thinking—which we often are, and these thoughts need to be acknowledged—each of us is afraid of different things. What I consider totally hurtful, for example, might not trouble you at all. So while I'm doing everything in my power to avoid whatever my perceived nightmare is, you'll be doing everything in your power to avoid something else.

The defenses we erect all depend upon pride, self-will, and fear. If we work on diminishing our pride, and self-will, and fear, an interesting thing starts to happen. We begin to become less defensive or, as the Pathwork calls it, "undefended." Being undefended allows us to truly fight for life because we are not desperately trying to protect ourselves from hurt.

Being undefended is not to be confused with being defenseless. This is just a semantic problem. When we are undefended—meaning we are accepting of life on its terms—we are still very much able to defend ourselves. In fact, we are *better* able to properly defend ourselves when we aren't so busy wasting our energy on needless defenses against imagined threats of old. When we come from our true selves, we are better able to maintain healthy boundaries and we have more energy to fight for life.

COMMONLY ASKED QUESTION NO. 26:

Can I cure myself with a positive attitude?

Love, laughter, hope, and peace of mind are definitely healthful. You'll recall that Norman Cousins cured himself of a terminal collagen disease with humor and then wrote an influential book about his experience called *Anatomy of an Illness.*

While a positive attitude is important for healing, we do not experience only positive feelings. All of us have a darker side (sometimes called a "lower self," a "child self," or a "shadow self") that is aggressive, destructive, angry, and impatient. We need to accept *all* of our feelings in order to be whole and in order to avoid fighting the self. By recognizing our dark feelings, we can actually access their energy and use it constructively for healing.

While a positive attitude won't necessarily cure you, a negative attitude might kill you. Pessimism and powerlessness correlate with illness and death. Researchers have discovered a negative twist on placebo that they call *nocebo.* Nocebo is testimony to the power of negative beliefs and lethal words. For example, in one study, 30 percent of women given placebo chemotherapy lost their hair simply because they believed they would.[2] Similarly, patients who believe that they are not going to recover often don't.

A positive attitude isn't everything, but patients who use realistic hope as a foundation for growth and change can achieve wonders.

While 100/100 thinking is based on duality, 50/50 thinking is based on nonduality (that is, acceptance of duality). The next step up is 100 thinking—unity. The ultimate paradox is that we need to maintain healthy boundaries on the physical and psychological levels and simultaneously lose our boundaries on the spiritual level when we totally accept that everything is One. This state holds no fear of failure, no fear of life, no fear of death. There are no defenses, only total surrender to life. Few of us hold this concept in our everyday consciousness, but it is through continuous awareness and self-acceptance that we dissolve the blocks within ourselves and the boundaries between one another, thus arriving at unity consciousness.

THE INTERNAL HEALING FACTOR

The "internal healing factor" is a concept that I feel nicely expresses the mysterious wellspring of healing that is within each of us.

The body has a stunning ability to heal itself. For reasons we do not yet understand, it cannot always heal itself completely, but there are incredible examples of people recovering from illness against all reasonable expectations.

Earlier I mentioned the placebo response, a phenomenon in which patients respond to an inert substance as if it were curative. Herbert Benson, the originator of the relaxation response and the author of *Timeless Healing,* calls a placebo "remembered wellness." I like his idea that within each of us is a memory of perfect health. Healer Barbara Brennan, author of *Hands of Light,* refers to healing as the process of remembering who we are.

The placebo effect, considered rather trivial by the medical profession, is testimony to the power of the living spirit. One of the most remarkable examples of the placebo effect is provided by a patient named Mr. Wright, whose story is often included in the medical literature, but which bears repeating here because it is so extraordinary.

Mr. Wright had generalized and far-advanced cancer of the lymph nodes, including tumors the size of oranges all over his body. He was bedridden, he had difficulty breathing, and he had a fever. All known treatments had failed, and his condition was considered terminal and untreatable. Still, Mr. Wright held out hope that a new drug named krebiozen might be helpful for him.

Mr. Wright's doctor gave him his first injection of krebiozen on a Friday. On Monday morning, the doctor returned to the hospital expecting to see Mr. Wright moribund or dead. To his surprise, he found Mr. Wright happily walking around the hospital ward. The tumors had actually melted and were already half their original size.

The other patients who had received krebiozen did not seem to be experiencing any benefit, but the doctor kept giving Mr. Wright his injections of the medication. Within ten days, Mr. Wright was discharged from the hospital. He enjoyed two months of practically perfect health until conflicting reports about the effectiveness of krebiozen began to appear. Mr. Wright began to lose faith in his treatment, and he relapsed into his former state.

At this point, Mr. Wright's doctor knew of absolutely nothing he could do that would help his patient. However, he had an idea. He told Mr. Wright that a new, fresh, superstrong version of krebiozen was due to arrive shortly. After pretending to wait a couple of days—during which time Mr. Wright became very optimistic and eager—the doctor administered the first injection of the new preparation, which was in fact water.

Mr. Wright's second recovery was even more dramatic than his first. Again his tumors melted and he became the picture of health. His doctor continued the water injections, and Mr. Wright remained symptom-free for over two months.

Then, unfortunately for Mr. Wright, an announcement appeared in the press to the effect that krebiozen was a totally worthless treatment. Within a few days, Mr. Wright was readmitted to the hospital, and he died within two days.[3]

While this story has an unhappy ending, it is still incredible that Mr. Wright's total belief in the effectiveness of krebiozen enabled him to return from the brink of death to good health in one weekend. For some reason, certain patients like Mr. Wright are able to directly access their internal healing factor. So the question becomes: Can we access this healing response directly, without a placebo?

WAYS TO SUPPORT HEALING

It appears that Mr. Wright did not do a tremendous amount of work in order to get better. In a way, he was lucky—he had tremendous powers of rejuvenation. On the other hand, his remarkable recovery did not last. In my experience, most people have to work harder than Mr. Wright in order to experience sustained healing on any level.

Your internal healing factor needs biochemical, psychological, emotional, and spiritual support. With that in mind:

• **Take advantage of the therapies that are available.** Your options include medications, surgery, acupuncture, nutritional supplements, Chinese herbs, homeopathy, and other forms of healing. Immune System Super Boosters include hormone balancing, intravenous vitamin C, chelation therapy, immunotherapy, biological response modifiers, oxidative therapies, and other emergent therapies, such as energetic healing.

• **Make appropriate lifestyle changes.** Now, more than ever, you need the Immune System Empowerment Program. You need good nutrition, good circulation, and good oxygenation. Get what your body needs and eliminate what harms you. Take your supplements and avoid toxins, smoke, and allergens. Lower the level in your Immune System Kettle as far as you can. Add stress management techniques into your life if you haven't already, including biofeedback, breathing exercises, deep relaxation, meditation, and/or hypnosis. (See Healing Visualizations, page 386.)

• **Seek emotional support.** This is more important now than ever. Don't wait for support to come to you. Ask friends and family for their help. Seek out those who have been healed of your condition. Join a support group. In one study, a group of women with metastatic breast cancer were divided into two groups. All received standard medical care—radiation, chemotherapy, drugs—but half met once a week in a group therapy session. This group reported less depression, anxiety, and pain than the other group, which was not too surprising to researchers. What was amazing, however, is that the women who took part in the group psychotherapy lived twice as long after they entered the study than the women who received only standard medical care.[4]

- **Reexamine the relationships in your life.** You can't change other people, but you can change yourself and your responses. Sometimes it takes a serious illness for us to recognize that we have been engaging in an unhealthy relationship with another human being. Ask yourself why you have been vulnerable to this person (or people), and work on developing psychological immunity to defend yourself more healthfully and appropriately.

Spiritual Work and Attitude Adjustment

This is the time to use psychotherapy or spiritual work to get out of your own way. You may be blocking certain emotions or putting up certain defenses that are counterproductive to your healing. You need to confront yourself in order to accept yourself.

Many of my patients have a difficult time with this part of their healing regimen and would rather believe that a physical problem just needs the right physical cure. After an initial period of resistance, they often go on to get the help they need (this is not the time for do-it-yourself enlightenment) and as a consequence, they become much more at peace with themselves and their circumstances.

As a starting point, picture your mind as a vessel, and empty out the cluttered thoughts—not unlike emptying your Immune System Kettle. Now consider giving up blame, residual anger, guilt, old hurts, and outdated defenses. Find any misconceptions that are skewing the way in which you see the world and exchange them for true concepts.

In order to get these things out of your life, you will need to dredge them up first. This can be uncomfortable, particularly because most of us have been living with our cherished defenses for many, many years. Keep in mind that many healing processes, physical and mental, begin with a period of discomfort. Liver detoxification often makes patients feel worse before they feel better, as does candida or Lyme die-off as treatment begins to take hold. Here you are letting your misconceptions "die off" in order to fully live in the present. In actuality, you are replacing your misconceptions with truth.

One of my patients, Marianne, came to see me suspecting that she had chronic candidiasis. She had already been to see a number of other doctors and healers, and had tried Prozac, chiropractic, dietary changes, acupuncture, herbs, applied kinesiology, and more. I ordered a number of tests to get to the bottom of Marianne's problems and we worked out a healing regimen to deal with her candidiasis, allergies, hypoglycemia, and intestinal dysbiosis. What struck me the most about Marianne, however, was her anger. It would emanate from her during each visit, but whenever I tried to bring it up, she would change the subject.

Eventually I asked Marianne why we were never able to address her anger, and she admitted that she always avoided it. She attributed this to growing up with alcoholic parents. It was clear that she had many issues to address left over from a difficult childhood experience, and I believed that her hidden anger was interfering with her progress. I really felt that this was a big part of the puzzle.

Marianne went for counseling and developed significant insight into her emotional states, both past and present, and their effect on her health. The difference in her was dramatic. I feel sure her physical improvement would not have been as great if she hadn't put this effort into giving up her anger.

Back in Chapter 8 I reviewed some important aspects of attitude adjustment. These concepts now take on added meaning:

- Recognize that nothing is 100 percent.
- Recognize that there is no absolute reality.
- "Cook" your feelings, rather than serving them up raw.
- Dig up what you've been hiding from yourself.
- Don't get trapped in unhappiness.
- Drop outdated behavior.
- Don't borrow trouble.
- Avoid woulda/coulda/shoulda.
- Avoid the "if only" trap.
- Let your anger dissipate.
- Avoid blaming yourself or others.
- Recognize your idealized self-image.
- Look for solutions.

Forgiveness is particularly important during the healing process. It's beneficial for both the forgiver and the forgiven. Give yourself a break; you have done and continue to do the best you can. While you're at it, forgive others for being imperfect, too. None of us can really know what it is like to be another person, so we are not in a position to judge others, even if we think we are. I try determinedly, on a daily basis, not to make judgments and assumptions about my patients. Sometimes it's pretty hard. On the other hand, when you are not busy judging people, you can find humanity in the most unexpected places.

Healing Visualizations

In addition to your stress management techniques, try healing visualizations several times a day. As you already know, visualizing positive states can benefit both your health and your peace of mind. During a healing visualization, the mind thinks in pictures, like waking dreams. Some people refer to the effects of guided imagery as "dreams come true."

To practice a healing visualization, first you enter a state of light relaxation (Gerald Epstein, M.D., author of *Healing Visualizations: Creating Health Through Imagery,* calls this stage "quieting"). Then you introduce a positive thought or image into your mind. Some people with cancer or chronic infections visualize a beam of shining light searching throughout their body. Some people imagine white blood cells like Pac-Men on a search-and-destroy mission, gobbling up unhealthy cells. Others who don't like violence picture something less disturbing, like little police cars escorting the diseased cells out of the body. People with an autoimmune disorder picture the calming of their inflammation.

There are books available on guided imagery, and scripts for healing visualizations are included in many books about healing. You can record these scripts, if you wish, to help you with your visualizing. Some patients find this helps their concentration. The optimal way to approach guided imagery, however, is to get assistance from an expert who can create an individualized visualization exercise just for you.

The tricky thing about healing visualizations is that you don't want to *insist* on wellness. If you are terrified of your illness, desperate to get well quickly, and afraid of not getting what you want, you will sit there earnestly trying to make the cells of your body do what you want them to. Ironically, this will short-circuit the effect you're after.

Losing Fear

After observing thousands of patients, and after reflecting upon my own life and the lives of those near and dear to me, and after doing some personal and professional healing and spiritual work, I've learned that death is not the opposite of life. The opposite of life is fear.

Fear takes us out of the present and sends us on a wild ride through what happened before or what might happen ahead. It drives us to expend all kinds of energy on futile or unnecessary tasks. Fear causes us to put up all our defenses and hide behind our shields. It blocks the free movement of energy and the movement of love into our lives.

Giving up fear—or at least choosing not to let it control us—allows us to live in the present; it opens our hearts and helps us to accept ourselves and to receive love from others. To live life to the fullest, we need to give up the fear of dying, the fear of doing things imperfectly, the fear of being hurt, and the fear of our shadow self. The list goes on and on, and each of us has our own darkest fears.

Healing has everything to do with giving up fear. Life's real task, and the real task of healing, is to connect with the heart. Healing is a deeply fulfilling journey that is physical, emotional, and spiritual. You can take the first step of that journey right here.

ᏗᏗ *MEGHAN'S STORY*

Meghan is one of my patients who physically is not yet back to normal. However, I still see her as a real success story. By redefining her concept of what healing really is, Meghan has come to find opportunity in her illness, even though it is still somewhat limiting.

When I first saw Meghan, she had daily headaches, psoriasis, difficulty concentrating, and fatigue. She also had recurrent sinusitis and pharyngitis, and had been on multiple courses of antibiotics. Meghan was a true Type A stockbroker, so she relied on having good health to be able to turn in a good performance. She also was used to being able to exercise regularly, plus maintain a full schedule of social activities. There was no place in her life for fatigue.

Testing revealed that Meghan had reactive hypoglycemia and chronic candidiasis. We implemented a yeast-free, hypoglycemic diet, antifungal treatments, and intravenous treatments for adrenal support and her condition gradually improved. Meghan found that she definitely felt better when she stuck to the proper diet and also ate every three to four hours to keep her blood sugar levels steady.

A year after her first visit, Meghan came to the office because of extreme fatigue. She'd actually been exhausted for a couple of months, but she'd tried to ignore the problem because she had been working so hard. Meghan was under tremendous stress. She was not exercising, and she was being much less careful about eating every three to four hours. She always felt cold, she had frequent headaches, and she often felt shaky. There was burning in her stomach, she had intestinal gas, and her menstrual periods were heavy and painful.

We did more testing and found that Meghan was allergic to wheat. In addition to avoiding wheat, she started a stronger antifungal medication for her candida symptoms.

Meghan's fatigue deepened, and it began to interfere with her work. A successful, hardworking, and driven professional, Meghan actually had to take a temporary leave from her job. Her boss regarded her so highly that he kept her position open for her.

When Meghan was diagnosed with chronic fatigue immune dysfunction syndrome (CFIDS), everyone had to adjust to the idea that she would have to remain off work. If Meghan had been able to drag herself through even one more workday, she surely would have done it—but her body refused to cooperate.

At this point we added thyroid medication to Meghan's regimen, plus Kutapressin injections (with B_{12} and folic acid added) three times a week. These were definitely helpful. I encouraged Meghan to try oxidative therapies, but she was resistant to this idea. I asked her to give up high-impact exercise and switch to gentler yoga exercises to maintain her physical strength and flexibility. I also urged her to seek therapy to help her deal with her difficult transformation from fast-paced corporate professional to the disabled list.

Each of Meghan's treatments helped a little bit, but she still had the fatigue. Eventually she could not fight her exhaustion any longer. She learned how to rest, and started taking naps when she needed them. Eventually she came to realize that taking a nap is just taking a nap, not a sign of failure. This simple act of acceptance was a pivotal point for her. Meghan's attitude completely turned around. She saw her life and the world in a different way, and she became attentive to things she had never attended to before. Once Meghan accepted her disability and the fact that she could no longer work, she stopped resenting her illness and was able to find opportunity in it. She started to relate to people in a new way—including her friends, family, and fiancé (who would later become her husband)—and she no longer felt the need to be pushing and driving and running and working all the time.

In spite of her ongoing illness, Meghan is emotionally and spiritually in much better shape than she has ever been, and has a much greater appreciation of life. Today she has improved to the point where she can function, but not yet work, and she has become accustomed to her new lifestyle. Meghan has become very involved with CFIDS support groups, and counsels many people with this illness. Today her "work" is to give help and support and to touch the lives of others.

Endnotes

INTRODUCTION

1. Jane Goldberg, *Deceits of the Mind and Their Effects on the Body* (New Brunswick, New Jersey: Transaction Publishers, 1991), p. 56.

CHAPTER 1

1. Andrew Pollack, "U.S. Officials to Shift Funds Toward Basic AIDS Research," *The New York Times*, August 10, 1994.

2. Andrew Pollack, "Meetings Lays Bare the Abyss Between AIDS and Its Cure," *The New York Times*, August 12, 1994.

CHAPTER 2

1. Leonard A. Sagan, *The Health of Nations: True Causes of Sickness and Well-Being* (New York: Basic Books, 1987), pp. 11–12.

2. Patrick Quillin with Noreen Quillin, *Beating Cancer with Nutrition* (Tulsa: Nutrition Times Press, 1994), p. 96.

3. E. Reimund, "The Free Radical Flux Theory of Sleep," *Medical Hypotheses*, Vol. 43 (1994): pp. 231–233.

4. Russell Jaffe, "Immune Defense and Repair Systems in Biologic Medicine I." Personal communication; in press, 1996.

5. ———, "Jury Awards $8.9 Million to Plaintiff in Johnson and Johnson Case," *The Wall Street Journal*, October 21, 1994.

6. Philip J. Hilts, "Liver Patient Wins Suit Against Maker of Tylenol," *The New York Times*, October 21, 1994.

7. Andrew Weil, *Spontaneous Healing* (New York: Alfred A. Knopf, 1995), pp. 81–82.

8. Jeffrey Bland, *Medical Applications of Clinical Nutrition* (New Canaan, Conn.: Keats Publishing, 1983), p. 42.

9. William R. Beisel et al., "Single-Nutrient Effects on Immunologic Function," *The Journal of the American Medical Association*, Vol. 245, No. 1 (1981): pp. 53–58.

10. Patrick Quillin with Noreen Quillin, op. cit., p. 62.

11. Jon Kaiser, *Immune Power: A Comprehensive Treatment Program for HIV* (New York: St. Martin's Press, 1993), p. 29.

12. Thomas G. Wilcox and Donna M. Gray, "Summary of Adverse Reactions Attributed to Aspartame," Department of Health and Human Services memorandum, April 20, 1995.

13. ————, "Over 7,000 Aspartame Complaints Since '81, FDA Says; Controversy Remains," *Nutrition Week*, Vol. 25, No. 20 (1995): pp. 1–2.

14. Mary K. Serdula et al., "Fruit and Vegetable Intake Among Adults in 16 States: Results of a Brief Telephone Survey," *American Journal of Public Health*, Vol. 85, No. 2 (1995): pp. 236–239.

15. Jon Kaiser, op. cit., p. 37.

16. Patrick Quillin with Noreen Quillin, op. cit., p. 49.

17. P. Beitsch et al., "Natural Immunity in Breast Cancer Patients During Neoadjuvant Chemotherapy and After Surgery," *Surgical Oncology*, Vol. 3 (1994): pp. 211–219.

18. John Allen Paulos, *Innumeracy: Mathematical Illiteracy and Its Consequences* (New York: Vintage Books, 1990), p. 111.

19. Samuel S. Epstein, "Losing the War Against Cancer: Who's Responsible, and What to Do About It." Keynote address at the American College for Advancement in Medicine conference, fall 1994.

20. Tony Brown, "Sick of Your Job? It Could Be Stress," *Reporter Dispatch* (Gannett Suburban Newspapers, Westchester, NY), February 22, 1995.

CHAPTER 3

1. Patrick Quillin with Noreen Quillin, *Beating Cancer with Nutrition* (Tulsa: Nutrition Times Press, 1994), p. 80.

2. Yoram Elitsur, "Vitamin A and the Mucosal Immune System," *Nutrition Report*, Vol. 12, No. 11 (1994): pp. 81–88.

3. John Alverdy, "The Effect of Nutrition on Gastrointestinal Barrier Function," *Seminars in Respiratory Infections*, Vol. 9, No. 4 (1994): pp. 248–255.

4. Institute of Noetic Sciences with William Poole, *The Heart of Healing* (Atlanta: Turner Publishing, 1993), p. 71.

5. Sandra Blakeslee, "In Immune System Model, Fittest Antibodies Survive," *The New York Times*, October 24, 1995.

6. Valentin Popa et al., "IgG Deficiency in Adults with Recurrent Respiratory Infections," *Annals of Allergy*, Vol. 70 (1993): p. 422.

7. Tetsuya Gatanaga et al., "Identification of TNF-LT Blocking Factor(s) in the Serum and Ultrafiltrates of Human Cancer Patients," *Lymphokine Research*, Vol. 9, No. 2 (1990): pp. 225–229.

8. Henry G. Herrod, "Interleukins in Immunologic and Allergic Diseases," *Annals of Allergy*, Vol. 63 (1989): pp. 269–272.

9. M. Rigdon Lentz, "The Phylogeny of Oncology," *Molecular Biotherapy*, Vol. 2 (1990): pp. 137–144.

10. Kimberly A. Rumsey and Paula Trahan Rieger, eds., *Biological Response Modifiers: A Self-Instruction Manual for Health Professionals* (Chicago: Precept Press, 1992), p. 39.

11. Jane E. Brody, "New Leads in MS Fight," *The New York Times*, May 3, 1995.

12. Dan Hurley, "Studies Confirm Diabetes Risk from Cow's Milk in Infants," *Medical Tribune*, February 2, 1995, p. 11.

13. Gina Kolata, "Study Tracks Psoriasis Symptoms to Activation of Immune System," *The New York Times,* May 2, 1995.

CHAPTER 4

1. Frank Edward Allen, "One Man's Suffering Spurs Doctors to Probe Pesticide-Drug Link," *The Wall Street Journal,* October 14, 1991.

2. Ibid.

3. U.S. Environmental Protection Agency National Human Adipose Tissue Survey (NHATS), August 1990.

4. Ellen Silbergeld, "Evaluating the Success of Environmental Health Programs in Protecting the Public's Health." Address at the Hazardous Waste Conference, 1993.

5. Parris M. Kidd and Wolfgang Huber, *Living with the AIDS Virus: A Strategy for Long-Term Survival* (Berkeley, Calif.: HK Biomedical, 1990), p. 120.

6. Rebecca Voelker, "Ames Agrees with Mom's Advice: Eat Your Fruits and Vegetables," *The Journal of the American Medical Association,* Vol. 273, No. 14 (1995): pp. 1077–1078.

7. Gina Kolata, "Studies Suggest That Genes Define a Person's Nutrient Needs," *The New York Times,* October 20, 1995.

8. Interview with Francis Collins, conducted by Giovanna Breu, "Breaking the Code," *People,* November 11, 1995, pp. 107–111.

9. Natalie Angier, "Gene Hunters Pursue Elusive and Complex Traits of Mind," *The New York Times,* October 31, 1995.

10. Debra Lynn Dadd, *Nontoxic, Natural and Earthwise: How to Protect Yourself and Your Family from Harmful Products and Live in Harmony with the Earth* (Los Angeles: Jeremy P. Tarcher, 1990), p. 78.

11. The Burton Goldberg Group, *Alternative Medicine: The Definitive Guide* (Puyallup, Wash.: Future Medicine Publishing, 1994), p. 169.

12. C. M. Gwynn et al., "Bronchial Provocation Tests in Atopic Patients with Allergen-Specific IgG$_4$ Antibodies," *Lancet,* January 30, 1982, pp. 254–256.

13. J. C. Breneman, *Basics of Food Allergy* (Springfield, Ill.: Charles C. Thomas, 1978), p. 155.

14. Ibid., p. 8.

15. Hugh A. Sampson et al., "Food Allergy," *The Journal of the American Medical Association,* Vol. 258, No. 20 (1987): pp. 2886–2890.

16. F. Shakib et al., "Study of IgG Sub-Class Antibodies in Patients with Milk Intolerance," *Clinical Allergy,* Vol. 16 (1986): pp. 451–458.

17. Michael Rosenbaum and Murray Susser, *Solving the Puzzle of Chronic Fatigue Syndrome* (Tacoma: Life Sciences Press, 1992), pp. 52–53.

18. Donald P. Tashkin, "Is Frequent Marijuana Smoking Harmful to Health?" *Western Journal of Medicine,* Vol. 158, No. 6 (1993): pp. 635–637.

19. Carl Sherman, "Summer Clothing May Not Provide Sun Protection You Expect," *Family Practice News,* March 15, 1995.

20. Jayne Garrison and Patricia Long, "Danger in the Tanning Booth," *Health,* October 1995, pp. 22–24.

21. Parris M. Kidd and Wolfgang Huber, op. cit., p. 128.

22. ———, "Vital Statistics," *Health*, September 1995, p. 16.

23. George J. Spilich et al., "Cigarette Smoking and Cognitive Performance," *British Journal of Addiction*, Vol. 87 (1992): pp. 1313–1326.

24. ———, "Do I Need to Install a Carbon Monoxide Detector in My Home?" *Health*, September 1995, p. 132.

25. ———, *Journal of Agriculture and Environmental Ethics*, Vol. 8, No. 1 (1995): pp. 17–29.

26. ———, "Pesticide Usage," *Nutrition Week*, Vol. 25, No. 20 (1995): p. 7.

27. Patrick Quillin with Noreen Quillin, *Beating Cancer with Nutrition* (Tulsa: Nutrition Times Press, 1994), p. 107.

28. Samuel S. Epstein, "Losing the War Against Cancer: Who's Responsible, and What to Do About It." Keynote address at the American College for Advancement in Medicine conference, fall 1994.

29. ———, "Over 50 Million Drink Water Failing Health Standards," *Nutrition Week*, Vol. 25, No. 22 (1995): p. 6.

30. David Sharp, "A Clean Drink of Water," *Health*, September 1995, p. 89.

31. Jane E. Brody, "Aggressiveness and Delinquency in Boys Is Linked to Lead in Bones," *The New York Times*, February 7, 1996.

32. Michael Rosenbaum and Murray Susser, op. cit., p. 80.

33. Ralph Golan, *Optimal Wellness* (New York: Ballantine Books, 1995), p. 279.

34. Ellen Silbergeld, op. cit.

35. P. G. Marino et al., "Lead Paint Poisoning During Renovation of a Victorian Farmhouse," *American Journal of Public Health*, Vol. 80, No. 10 (1990): pp. 1183–1185.

36. Sandra Denton, "The Mercury Cover-Up," *Health Consciousness Magazine*, June 1989.

CHAPTER 5

1. Karen S. Scheider and Joyce Wagner, "Recipe for Hope," *People*, April 17, 1995, pp. 54–57.

2. Patrick Quillin with Noreen Quillin, *Beating Cancer with Nutrition* (Tulsa: Nutrition Times Press, 1994), p. 65.

3. Lourdes C. Corman, "Effects of Specific Nutrients on the Immune Response," *Medical Clinics of North America*, Vol. 69, No. 4 (1985): p. 761.

4. Patrick Quillin with Noreen Quillin, op. cit., p. 67.

5. David L. Brandon, "Interactions of Diet and Immunity," *Advances in Experimental Medical Biology*, Vol. 177 (1984): p. 70.

6. Ranjit K. Chandra and Shamim Tejpar, "Diet and Immunocompetence," *International Journal of Immunopharmacology*, Vol. 5, No. 3 (1983): p. 177.

7. David L. Brandon, op. cit., p. 69.

8. Ibid.

9. Sandra Blakeslee, "Complex and Hidden Brain in the Gut Makes Stomachaches and Butterflies," *The New York Times*, January 23, 1996.

10. S. Boyd Eaton and Melvin Konner, "Paleolithic Nutrition: A Consideration of Its Nature and Current Implications," *The New England Journal of Medicine*, Vol. 312, No. 5 (1985): pp. 283–289.

11. Peter D'Adamo, "Gut Ecosystem Dynamics III," *Townsend Letter for Doctors*, August/September 1990, pp. 528–534.

12. Patrick Quillin with Noreen Quillin, op. cit., p. 61.

13. Samuel S. Epstein, "Losing the War Against Cancer: Who's Responsible, and What to Do About It." Keynote address at the American College for Advancement in Medicine conference, fall 1994.

14. Patrick Quillin with Noreen Quillin, op. cit., p. 62.

15. Gladys Block, "Vitamin C and Cancer," lecture at the May 1994 conference of the American College for Advancement in Medicine.

16. Patrick Quillin with Noreen Quillin, op. cit., p. 64.

17. John M. Daly et al., "Effect of Dietary Protein and Amino Acids on Immune Function," *Critical Care Medicine*, Vol. 18, No. 2 (1990): p. S87.

18. Florence Fabricant, "The Geography of Taste," *The New York Times Magazine*, March 10, 1996, p. 40.

19. Samuel S. Epstein, op. cit.

20. Ibid.

21. Ralph Golan, *Optimal Wellness* (New York: Ballantine Books, 1995), p. 86.

22. Andrew Weil, *Spontaneous Healing* (New York: Alfred A. Knopf, 1995), p. 149.

23. Thomas B. Clarkson et al., "Estrogenic Soybean, Isoflavones and Chronic Disease Risks and Benefits," *Trends in Endocrinology and Metabolism*, Vol. 6 (1995): pp. 11–16.

24. Carole Bullock, "Soy Protein Has Profound Effect on Lipid Levels," *Medical Tribune*, June 8, 1995, p. 14.

25. Jon Kaiser, *Immune Power: A Comprehensive Treatment Program for HIV* (New York: St. Martin's Press, 1993), p. 29.

26. Ibid.

27. Patrick Quillin with Noreen Quillin, op. cit., p. 122.

28. Roger B. McDonald, "Influence of Dietary Sucrose and Biological Aging," *American Journal of Clinical Nutrition*, Vol. 62 (Suppl.)(1995): pp. 284S–293S.

29. Jeffrey A. Lowell, "Dietary Immunomodulation: Beneficial Effects of Oncogenesis and Tumor Growth," *Critical Care Medicine*, Vol. 18, No. 2 (1990): p. S145.

30. John E. Kinsella and Belur Lokesh, "Dietary Lipids, Eicosanoids, and the Immune System," *Critical Care Medicine*, Vol. 18, No. 2 (1990): p. S98.

31. Ibid., p. S96.

32. Ralph Golan, op. cit., p. 49.

33. Robert M. Russell, "Nutrition: Review of 1994," *The Journal of the American Medical Association*, Vol. 273, No. 21 (1995): pp. 1699–1700.

34. Artemis P. Simopoulos, "Omega-3 Fatty Acids in Health and Disease and in Growth and Development," *American Journal of Clinical Nutrition*, Vol. 54 (1991): p. 444.

35. Ibid., p. 439.

36. Ibid., p. 441.

37. Joseph R. Hibbeln and Norman Salem, Jr., "Dietary Polyunsaturated Fatty Acids and Depression," *American Journal of Clinical Nutrition*, Vol. 62 (1995): pp. 1–9.

38. Artemis P. Simopoulos, op. cit., p. 441.

39. Anastasios Salachas, "Effects of a Low-Dose Fish Oil Concentrate on Angina, Exercise Tolerance Time, Serum Triglycerides and Platelet Function," *Angiology: The Journal of Vascular Diseases*, Vol. 45, No. 12 (1994): pp. 1023–1031.

40. Mark Percival, "Fish Oil, Omega-3 Fatty Acids and Vitamin E," *Nutritional Pearls*, Vol. 29 (1995): p. 1.

41. Joel M. Kremer et al., "Dietary Fish Oil and Olive Oil Supplementation in Patients with Rheumatoid Arthritis," *Arthritis and Rheumatism*, Vol. 33, No. 6 (1990): p. 810.

42. Olle Haglund et al., "The Effects of Fish Oil on Triglycerides, Cholesterol, Fibrinogen, and Malondialdehyde in Humans Supplemented with Vitamin E," *Journal of Nutrition*, Vol. 121, No. 2 (1991): p. 165.

43. Jon Kaiser, op. cit., p. 27.

44. ———, "Kitchen Notes," *Health*, March/April 1996, p. 128.

45. Bob Condor, "Overcooked Foods Lose Vitamin C Punch," *Reporter Dispatch* (Gannett Suburban Newspapers, Westchester, NY), February 7, 1996.

46. Debra Lynn Dadd, *Nontoxic, Natural and Earthwise: How to Protect Yourself and Your Family from Harmful Products and Live in Harmony with the Earth* (Los Angeles: Jeremy P. Tarcher, 1990), p. 77.

47. ———, "New Coffees: Are You Going Caffeine Crazy?" *Health*, September 1995, p. 30.

CHAPTER 6

1. Michael Janson, *The Vitamin Revolution in Health Care* (Greenville, N.H.: Arcadia Press, 1996), p. 201.

2. Quentin Myrvik, "Immunology and Nutrition," *Modern Nutrition in Health and Disease*, 8th ed. (Lea and Febiger, 1994), p. 657.

3. Patrick Quillin with Noreen Quillin, *Beating Cancer with Nutrition* (Tulsa: Nutrition Times Press, 1994), p. 78.

4. John D. Bogden, "Micronutrient Nutrition and Immunity: Part 2," *Nutrition Report*, Vol. 9 (1995): p. 16.

5. Morris W. Cohn, "Miracle Pills" (letter), *Arizona Highways*, August 1996, p. 48.

6. C. J. Bates, "Vitamin A," *Lancet*, January 7, 1995, p. 33.

7. Jane Brody, "Researchers Question Beta Carotene's Value," *The New York Times*, February 21, 1995.

8. Adrianne Bendich, "A Role for Carotenoids in Immune Function," *Clinical Nutrition*, Vol. 7, No. 3 (1988): p. 117.

9. Norman Krinsky, "The Evidence for the Role of Carotenes in Preventive Health," *Clinical Nutrition*, Vol. 7, No. 3 (1988): p. 110.

10. Ibid., p. 112.

11. Gina Kolata, "Studies Find Beta Carotene, Used by Millions, Doesn't Forestall Cancer or Heart Disease," *The New York Times*, January 19, 1996.

12. Michael T. Murray, "A Comprehensive Review of Vitamin C," *American Journal of Natural Medicine*, Vol. 3, No. 6 (1996): p. 11.

13. Parris M. Kidd and Wolfgang Huber, *Living with the AIDS Virus: A Strategy for Long-Term Survival* (Berkeley: HK Biomedical, 1990), p. 116.

14. Ewan Cameron et al., "Ascorbic Acid and Cancer: A Review," *Cancer Research*, Vol. 39 (1979): pp. 663–681.

15. Aristo Vojdani and Mamdooh Ghoeneum, "In Vivo Effect of Ascorbic Acid on Enhancement of Human Natural Killer Cell Action," *Nutrition Research*, Vol. 13 (1993): p. 753.

16. Catherine Gale, "Vitamin C and Risk of Death from Stroke and Coronary Heart Disease," *British Medical Journal*, Vol. 310 (1995): pp. 1563–1566.

17. Patrick Quillin with Noreen Quillin, op. cit., p. 39.

18. Harri Hemila, "Does Vitamin C Alleviate the Symptoms of the Common Cold? A Review of Current Evidence," *Scandinavian Journal of Infectious Diseases*, Vol. 26 (1994): p. 4.

19. Jane Brody, "Vitamin C: Is Anyone Right on Dose?" *The New York Times*, April 16, 1996.

20. D. R. Fraser, "Vitamin D," *Lancet*, January 14, 1995, p. 105.

21. Mohsen Meydani, "Vitamin E," *Lancet*, January 21, 1995, p. 170.

22. Natalie Angier, "Vitamins Win Support as Potent Agents of Health," *The New York Times*, March 10, 1992.

23. Mohsen Meydani, op. cit., p. 173.

24. Ranjit K. Chandra and Shamim Tejpar, "Diet and Immunocompetence," *International Journal of Immunopharmacology*, Vol. 5, No. 3 (1983): p. 179.

25. Ranjit K. Chandra, "Trace Elements and Immune Response," *Clinical Nutrition*, Vol. 6, No. 3 (1987): p. 121.

26. Michael Janson, op. cit., p. 83.

27. Ananda Prasad, "Zinc: An Overview," *Nutrition*, Vol. 11 (1995): pp. 93–99.

28. Quentin Myrvik, op. cit., p. 648.

29. Melvyn R. Werbach, "Alkylglycerols and Cancer," *Journal of Orthomolecular Medicine*, Vol. 9, No. 2 (1994): pp. 95–100.

30. Mary Sano et al., "Double-Blind Parallel Design Pilot Study of Acetyl Levocarnitine in Patients with Alzheimer's Disease," *Archives of Neurology*, Vol. 49 (1992): p. 1137.

31. Eric R. Braverman and Carl C. Pfeiffer, *The Healing Nutrients Within* (New Canaan, Conn.: Keats Publishing, 1987), p. 87.

32. Judy Shabert with Nancy Ehrlich, *The Ultimate Nutrient, Glutamine* (Garden City Park, N.Y.: Avery Publishing Group, 1994), p. 58.

33. J. E. Cheshier et al., "Immunomodulation by Pycnogenol in Retrovirus-Infected or Ethanol-Fed Mice," *Life Science*, Vol. 58 (1996): pp. 87–96.

34. John F. Prudden, *Summary of Bovine Tracheal Cartilage Research Programs*, 1993.

35. Alan R. Gaby, "The Role of Coenzyme Q10 in Clinical Medicine: Part I," *Alternative Medicine Review*, Vol. 1, No. 1 (1996): p. 12.

36. Knud Lockwood et al., "Partial and Complete Regression of Breast Cancer in Patients in Relation to Dosage of Coenzyme Q10," *Biochemical and Biophysical Research Communication*, Vol. 199, No. 3 (1994): pp. 1504–1508.

37. Parris M. Kidd and Wolfgang Huber, op. cit., p. 138.

38. Ralph Golan, *Optimal Wellness* (New York: Ballantine Books, 1995), p. 451.

39. Parris M. Kidd and Wolfgang Huber, op. cit., p. 134.

40. Peter D'Adamo, "Larch Arabinogalactan Is a Novel Immune Modulator," *Journal of Naturopathic Medicine*, Vol. 6, No. 1 (1996): pp. 33–37.

41. H. Naik et al., "Inhibition of In Vitro Tumor Cell-Endothelial Adhesion by Modified Citrus Pectin," *Proceedings of the Annual Meeting of the American Association of Cancer Research* (1995): Vol. 36: p. A377.

42. Lester Packer et al., "Alpha-Lipoic Acid as a Biological Antioxidant," *Free Radical Biology and Medicine*, Vol. 19, No. 2 (1995): pp. 227–250.

43. Jeffrey Bland, conducting an interview with Burton Berkson, *Preventive Medicine Update*, June 1996.

44. Lester Packer, op. cit., p. 244.

CHAPTER 7

1. Oscar Janiger and Philip Goldberg, *A Different Kind of Healing* (New York: G. P. Putnam's Sons, 1994), p. 31.

2. David Eisenberg et al., "Unconventional Medicine in the United States," *The New England Journal of Medicine*, Vol. 328, No. 4 (1993): p. 246.

3. S. Andersson and T. Lundeberg, "Acupuncture: From Empiricism to Science: Functional Background to Acupuncture Effects in Pain and Disease," *Medical Hypotheses*, Vol. 45, No. 3 (1995): pp. 271–281.

4. J. Hyvarinen and M. Karlsson, "Low-Resistance Skin Points That May Coincide with Acupuncture Loci," *Medical Biology*, Vol. 55 (1977): pp. 88–94.

5. Lixing Lao, "Efficacy of Chinese Acupuncture on Postoperative Oral Surgery Pain," *Oral Surgery, Oral Medicine, Oral Pathology* (1995): pp. 423–428.

6. The Burton Goldberg Group, *Alternative Medicine: The Definitive Guide* (Puyallup, Wash.: Future Medicine Publishing, 1994), p. 37.

7. Jon Kaiser, *Immune Power: A Comprehensive Treatment Program for HIV* (New York: St. Martin's Press, 1993), p. 47.

8. Ibid., p. 67.

9. Paul Bergner, "Botanical Medicine," *The Nutrition and Dietary Consultant*, April 1988, p. 4.

10. Subhuti Dharmananda, "A New Herbal Combination for the Treatment of Immunodeficiency Syndromes," *Pacific Journal of Oriental Medicine*, Vol. 3, No. 1 (1986): pp. 20–29.

11. Da-Tong Chu et al., "Immunotherapy with Chinese Medicinal Herbs I," *Journal of Clinical and Laboratory Immunology*, Vol. 25 (1988): pp. 119–123.

12. Da-Tong Chu et al., "Immunotherapy with Chinese Medicinal Herbs II," *Journal of Clinical and Laboratory Immunology*, Vol. 25 (1988): pp. 125–129.

13. Subhuti Dharmananda, *Chinese Herbal Therapies for Immune Disorders* (Portland, Ore.: Institute for Traditional Medicine and Preventive Health Care, 1988), p. 30.

14. Andrew Weil, *Optimal Wellness* (New York: Ballantine Books, 1995), p. 180.

15. Jon Kaiser, op. cit., p. 65.

16. The Burton Goldberg Group, op. cit., p. 272.

17. David Taylor Reilly et al., "Is Homeopathy a Placebo Response?" *Lancet*, October 18, 1986, pp. 881–885.

18. Jennifer Jacobs et al., "Treatment of Acute Childhood Diarrhea with Homeopathic Medicine: A Randomized Clinical Trial in Nicaragua," *Pediatrics*, Vol. 93, No. 5 (1994): pp. 719–725.

19. David Reilly et al., "Is Evidence for Homeopathy Reproducible?" *Lancet*, December 10, 1994, pp. 1601–1606.

20. Victor Herbert, letter to *The New England Journal of Medicine*, October 14, 1993, p. 1204.

21. David Taylor Reilly, op. cit., p. 885.

CHAPTER 8

1. Joan Borysenko and Myrin Borysenko, "On Psychoneuroimmunology: How the Mind Influences Health and Disease . . . And How to Make the Influence Beneficial," *Executive Health*, Vol. 19, No. 10 (1983): p. 218.

2. George P. Chrousos and Phillip W. Gold, "The Concepts of Stress and Stress System Disorders," *The Journal of the American Medical Association*, Vol. 267, No. 9 (1992): p. 1249.

3. David Goleman, *Emotional Intelligence* (New York: Bantam Books, 1995), p. 173.

4. Paul Grossman, "What Feeds the Heart Feeds the Mind," *Lown Forum*, Winter 1995, pp. 10–11.

5. Daniel Goleman, "Severe Trauma May Damage the Brain as Well as the Psyche," *The New York Times*, August 1, 1995.

6. Leonard A. Sagan, *The Health of Nations: True Causes of Sickness and Well-Being* (New York: Basic Books, 1987), pp. 187–188.

7. Ernest Lawrence Rossi, *The Psychobiology of Mind-Body Healing: New Concepts of Therapeutic Hypnosis* (New York: W. W. Norton and Co., 1986), p. 18.

8. The Institute of Noetic Sciences with William Poole, *The Heart of Healing* (Atlanta: Turner Publishing, 1993), p. 33.

9. Bernie S. Siegel, *Peace, Love and Healing* (New York: Harper and Row, 1989), p. 95.

10. The Institute of Noetic Sciences with William Poole, op. cit., p. 34.

11. Bill Moyers, *Healing and the Mind* (New York: Doubleday, 1993), p. 82.

12. J. Edwin Blalock, "The Immune System as a Sensory Organ," *Journal of Immunology*, Vol. 132 (1984): pp. 1067–1070.

13. Bill Moyers, op. cit., p. 214.

14. Ibid., p. 174.

15. Bernie S. Siegel, op. cit., p. 36.

16. Leonard A. Sagan, op. cit., p. 185.

17. Janice K. Kiecolt-Glaser et al., "Modulation of Cellular Immunity in Medical Students," *Journal of Behavioral Medicine*, Vol. 9, No. 1 (1986): p. 19.

18. Steven J. Schleifer et al., "Suppression of Lymphocyte Stimulation Following Bereavement," *The Journal of the American Medical Association*, Vol. 250, No. 3 (1983): pp. 374–377.

19. Janice K. Kiecolt-Glaser et al., op. cit.

20. Arthur A. Stone et al., "Evidence That Secretory IgA Antibody Is Associated with Daily Mood," *Journal of Personality and Social Psychology*, Vol. 52, No. 5 (1987): pp. 988–993.

21. Robert Ader et al., "Psychoneuroimmunology: Interactions Between the Nervous System and the Immune System," *Lancet*, January 14, 1995, pp. 988–993.

22. Bill Moyers, op. cit., p. 173.

23. Claudia Wallis, "Faith and Healing," *Time*, June 24, 1996, p. 61.

24. Janice K. Kiecolt-Glaser et al., op. cit., p. 17.

25. Ibid., p. 6.

26. Joan Borysenko, *Minding the Body, Mending the Mind* (New York: Bantam Books, 1988), p. 97.

27. David Goleman, op. cit., p. 170.

28. Joan Borysenko, op. cit., p. 64.

29. Claudia Wallis, op. cit., p. 60.

30. Ibid.

31. David Goleman, op. cit., p. 179.

32. Institute of Noetic Sciences with William Poole, op. cit., p. 10.

33. Mitchel L. Zoler, "Psychosocial Elements Add to CAD Risk: Behavioral Medicine May Extend Survival After Myocardial Infarction," *Family Practice News*, Vol. 24, No. 24 (1994): pp. 1, 15.

34. Bente K. Pedersen and Helle Bruunsgaard, "How Physical Exercise Influences Establishment of Infections," *Sports Medicine*, Vol. 19, No. 6 (1995): pp. 393–400.

35. Stanley Fisher with James Ellison, *Discovering the Power of Self-Hypnosis* (New York: Harper Collins, 1991), p. 13.

36. The Burton Goldberg Group, *Alternative Medicine: The Definitive Guide* (Puyallup, Wash.: Future Medicine Publishing, 1994), p. 471.

37. Joan Borysenko, op. cit., p. 36.

38. Ibid., p. 51.

39. Bill Moyers, op. cit., p. 142.

CHAPTER 9

1. Gary W. Elmer et al., "Biotherapeutic Agents: A Neglected Modality for the Treatment and Prevention of Selected Intestinal and Vaginal Infections," *The Journal of the American Medical Association*, Vol. 275, No. 11 (1996): p. 870.

2. Sandra Blakeslee, "Genes Tell Story of Why Some Get Cancer While Others Don't," *The New York Times*, May 17, 1994.

3. Tomotari Mitsuoka, "Bifidobacteria and Their Role in Human Health," *Journal of Industrial Microbiology*, Vol. 6 (1990): p. 264.

4. Philip A. Mackowiak, "The Normal Microbial Flora," *The New England Journal of Medicine*, Vol. 307, No. 2 (1982): p. 85.

5. Glenn R. Gibson and Marcel B. Roberfroid, "Dietary Manipulation of Human Colonic Microbiota: Introducing the Concept of Prebiotics," *Journal of Nutrition*, Vol. 125 (1995): pp. 1401–1412.

6. Michael Kirsch, "Bacterial Overgrowth," *American Journal of Gastroenterology*, Vol. 85, No. 3 (1990): p. 231.

7. R. K. Robinson, ed., *Therapeutic Properties of Fermented Milk* (London: Elsevier Science, 1991), p. 104.

8. Sherwood L. Gorbach, "Lactic Acid Bacteria and Human Health," *Annals of Medicine*, Vol. 22 (1990): pp. 37–41.

9. Leo Galland, "The Effects of Intestinal Microbes on Systemic Immunity," *Post-Viral Fatigue Syndrome* (New York: John Wiley and Sons, 1991), p. 406.

10. Christina M. Surawicz et al., "Prevention of Antibiotic-Associated Diarrhea by *Saccharomyces boulardii*: A Prospective Study," *Gastroenterology*, Vol. 96 (1989): pp. 981–988.

11. Jean-Paul Buts et al., "Stimulation of Secretory IgA and Secretory Component of Immunoglobulins in Small Intestine of Rats Treated with *Saccharomyces Boulardii*," *Digestive Diseases and Sciences*, Vol. 35, No. 2 (1990): pp. 251–256.

12. Richard L. Gregory, "The Biological Role and Clinical Implications of IgA," *Laboratory Medicine*, Vol. 25, No. 11 (1994): p. 725.

13. Edwin A. Deitch et al., "Bacterial Translocation from the Gut Impairs Systemic Immunity," *Surgery*, Vol. 109, No. 3 (1991): pp. 269–276.

14. Samuel M. Behar and Steven A. Porcelli, "Mechanisms of Autoimmune Disease Induction," *Arthritis and Rheumatism*, Vol. 38, No. 4 (1995): pp. 458–476.

15. Leo Galland, op. cit., p. 412.

16. Samuel M. Behar and Steven A. Porcelli, op. cit., p. 464.

17. David W. Riddington et al., "Intestinal Permeability, Gastric Intramucosal pH, and Systemic Endotoxemia in Patients Undergoing Cardiopulmonary Bypass," *The Journal of the American Medical Association*, Vol. 275, No. 13 (1996): p. 1007.

18. John C. Alverdy, "Effects of Glutamine-Supplemented Diets on Immunology of the Gut," *Journal of Parenteral and Enteral Nutrition*, Vol. 14, No. 4, Supplement (1990): p. 111S.

19. Gary W. Elmer et al., op. cit., p. 871.

20. Leo Galland, op. cit., p. 415.

21. Eileen Hilton et al., "Ingestion of Yogurt Containing *Lactobacillus acidophilus* as Prophylaxis for Candidal Vaginitis," *Annals of Internal Medicine*, Vol. 116, No. 5 (1992): p. 353.

CHAPTER 10

1. Howard S. Gold, "Antimicrobial-Drug Resistance," *The New England Journal of Medicine*, Vol. 335, No. 19 (1996): p. 1446.

2. Broda O. Barnes, *Hypothyroidism: The Unsuspected Illness* (New York: Harper Collins, New York, 1976).

3. W. M. Jefferies, "Cortisol and Immunity," *Medical Hypotheses*, Vol. 34 (1991): p. 203.

4. Wolfgang Oelkers, "Adrenal Insuffiency," *The New England Journal of Medicine*, Vol. 335, No. 16 (1996): p. 1206.

5. W. M. Jefferies, op. cit., p. 202.

6. J. Herbert, "The Age of Dehydroepiandrosterone," *Lancet*, May 13, 1995, pp. 1193–1194.

7. Benedict Carey, "Hooked on Youth," *Health*, November/December 1995, p. 70.

8. Saul Kent, "DHEA: 'Miracle' Drug?" *Geriatrics*, Vol. 37, No. 7 (1982): p. 157.

9. R. F. Van Vollenhoven et al., "An Open Study of Dehydroepiandrosterone in Systemic Lupus Erythematosus," *Arthritis and Rheumatism*, Vol. 37 (1994): pp. 1305–1310.

10. Eileen Hoffman, *Our Health, Our Lives: A Revolutionary Approach to Total Health Care for Women* (New York: Pocket Books, 1995), p. 257.

11. Maurizio Cutolo et al., "Androgen Replacement Therapy in Male Patients with Rheumatoid Arthritis," *Arthritis and Rheumatism*, Vol. 34, No. 1 (1991): p. 4.

12. Virginia Morell, "Zeroing In on How Hormones Affect the Immune System," *Science*, August 11, 1995, pp. 773–775.

13. M. Provinciali, "Relationship Between 17-Beta-Estradiol and Prolactin in the Regulation of Natural Killer Cell Activity During Progression of Endometriosis," *Journal of Endocrinological Investigation*, Vol. 18, No. 8 (1995): pp. 645–652.

14. Henry M. Lemon, "Reduced Estriol Excretion in Patients with Breast Cancer Prior to Endocrine Therapy," *The Journal of the American Medical Association*, Vol. 196, No. 13 (1966): p. 1128.

15. M. Cutolo et al., "Androgen and Estrogen Receptors Are Present in Primary Cultures of Human Synovial Macrophages," *Journal of Clinical Endocrinology and Metabolism*, Vol. 81, No. 2 (1996): pp. 820–827.

16. The Burton Goldberg Group, *Alternative Medicine: The Definitive Guide* (Puyallup, Wash.: Future Medicine Publishing, 1994), p. 777.

17. Jane Brody, "Restoring Ebbing Hormones May Slow Aging," *The New York Times*, July 18, 1995.

18. Maurizio Cutolo et al., "Androgen Replacement Therapy . . . ," op. cit., p. 1.

19. Serafino Fazio, "A Preliminary Study of Growth Hormone in the Treatment of Dilated Cardiomyopathy," *The New England Journal of Medicine*, Vol. 334, No. 13 (1996): pp. 809–814.

20. Jane Brody, "Restoring Ebbing Hormones . . . ," op. cit.

21. G. Mardh et al., "Growth Hormone Replacement Therapy in Adult Hypopituitary Patients with Growth Hormone Deficiency: Combined Data from 12 European Placebo-Controlled Clinical Trials," *Endocrinology and Metabolism*, Vol. 1, Supplement A (1994): pp. 43–49.

22. Ky Ho and J. D. Veldhuis, "Diagnosis of Growth Hormone Deficiency in Adults," Workshop Report, *Endocrinology and Metabolism*, Vol. 1, Supplement A (1994): pp. 61–63.

23. Steve Harakeh et al., "Suppression of Human Immunodeficiency Virus Replication by Ascorbate in Chronically and Acutely Infected Cells," *Proceedings of the National Academy of Sciences*, USA 87 (1990): pp. 7245–7249.

24. Robert F. Cathcart, "Vitamin C, Titrating to Bowel Tolerance, Anascorbemia, and Acute Induced Scurvy," *Medical Hypotheses*, Vol. 7 (1981): pp. 1359–1376.

25. Irwin Stone, *The Healing Factor* (New York: Grosset and Dunlap, 1972), p. 160.

26. Allan Campbell et al., "Reticulum Cell Carcinoma: Two Complete 'Spontaneous' Regressions in Response to High-Dose Ascorbic Acid," *Oncology*, Vol. 48 (1991): pp. 495–497.

27. Aurel Lupulescu, "Vitamin C Inhibits DNA, RNA and Protein Synthesis in Epithelial Neoplastic Cells," *International Journal for Vitamin and Nutrition Research*, Vol. 61 (1991): pp. 125–129.

28. Stanley Bram, "Vitamin C Preferential Toxicity for Malignant Melanoma Cells," *Nature*, Vol. 284 (1980): pp. 629–631.

29. N. H. Riordan, "Intravenous Ascorbate as a Tumor Cytotoxic Chemotherapeutic Agent," *Medical Hypotheses*, Vol. 44 (1995): pp. 207–213.

30. Joseph Egger et al., "Controlled Trial of Hyposensitisation in Children with Food-Induced Hyperkinetic Syndrome," *Lancet*, May 9, 1992, pp. 1150–1153.

31. Gordon L. Sussman and Waldemar Pruzanski, "Treatment of Inflammatory Myopathy with Intravenous Gamma Globulin," *Current Opinion in Rheumatology*, Vol. 7 (1995): pp. 510–515.

32. Chau-Ching Liu et al., "Lymphocyte-Mediated Cytolysis and Disease," *The New England Journal of Medicine*, Vol. 335, No. 22 (1996): pp. 1651–1658.

33. Malcolm Gladwell, "The New Age of Man," *The New Yorker*, September 30, 1996, p. 62.

34. The Burton Goldberg Group, op. cit., p. 299.

35. Richard Gerber, *Vibrational Medicine: New Choices for Healing Ourselves* (Santa Fe: Bear and Company, 1988), p. 308.

36. Reuven Sandyk, "Electromagnetic Fields for Treatment of Multiple Sclerosis," *International Journal of Neuroscience*, Vol. 87 (1996): pp. 1–4.

CHAPTER 11

1. Nathaniel Altman, *Oxygen Healing Therapies* (Rochester, Vt.: Healing Arts Press, 1995), p. 1.

2. I. Bjarnason and T. J. Peters, "Influence of Anti-Rheumatic Drugs on Gut Permeability and on the Gut Associated Lymphoid Tissue," *Baillieres Clinical Rheumatology*, Vol. 10, No. 1 (1996): pp. 165–176.

3. Jeffrey S. Bland, "Oxidants and Antioxidants in Clinical Medicine: Past, Present and Future Potential," *Journal of Nutritional and Environmental Medicine*, Vol. 5 (1995): p. 270.

4. Ibid., p. 263.

5. Patrick M. Tibbles and John S. Edelsberg, "Hyperbaric-Oxygen Therapy," *The New England Journal of Medicine*, Vol. 334, No. 25 (1996): pp. 1642–1648.

6. T. H. Oliver et al., "Influenzal Pneumonia: The Intravenous Injection of Hydrogen Peroxide," *Lancet*, February 21, 1920, pp. 432–433.

7. Nathaniel Altman, op. cit., p. 29.

8. Keith H. Wells et al., "Inactivation of Human Immunodeficiency Virus Type I by Ozone In Vitro," *Blood*, Vol. 78, No. 7 (1991): p. 1882.

9. Robert Jay Rowen, "Ultraviolet Blood Irradiation Therapy (Photo-Oxidation): The Cure That Time Forgot," in press 1996. Taken from original article, pp. 11–12.

10. Lida H. Mattman, *Cell Wall Deficient Forms: Stealth Pathogens* (Boca Raton: CRC Press, 1993), preface.

11. Otto Warburg, "The Prime Cause and Prevention of Cancer," lecture at the meeting of the Nobel Laureates on June 30, 1966. English edition by Dean Burk, National Cancer Institute, Bethesda, Md.

12. Robert Jay Rowen, op. cit., p. 10.

13. Renate Viebahn, *The Use of Ozone in Medicine* (Heidelberg: Karl F. Haug Publishers, English edition, 1987), pp. 44–47.

14. V. Bocci, "Ozonization of Blood for the Therapy of Viral Diseases and Immunodeficiencies: A Hypothesis," *Medical Hypotheses*, Vol. 39 (1992): p. 31.

15. William Campbell Douglass, *Into the Light* (Dunwoody, Ga.: Second Opinion Publishing, 1993), p. 22.

16. Ibid., p. 43.

17. Robert Jay Rowen, op. cit., p. 12.

18. Ibid., p. 2.

CHAPTER 12

1. Bernie S. Siegel, *Peace, Love and Healing* (New York: Harper and Row, 1989), p. 140.

2. Ibid., p. 144.

3. Don Bakken et al., "Performance of 45 Laboratories Participating in a Proficiency Testing Program for Lyme Disease Serology," *The Journal of the American Medical Association*, Vol. 268, No. 7 (1992): p. 891.

CHAPTER 13

1. Patrick Quillin with Noreen Quillin, *Beating Cancer with Nutrition* (Tulsa: Nutrition Times Press, 1994), p. 125.

2. Jeanne Achterberg et al., *Rituals of Healing: Using Imagery for Health and Wellness* (New York: Bantam Books, 1994), p. 243.

3. Ernest Lawrence Rossi, *The Psychobiology of Mind-Body Healing: New Concepts of Therapeutic Hypnosis* (New York: W. W. Norton and Co., 1986), pp. 4–5.

4. Bill Moyers, *Healing and the Mind* (New York: Doubleday, 1993), p. 68.

Resources

❦

Recently when I was in New York City walking up a typically crowded street to an appointment, I found myself looking at the hundreds of New Yorkers and thinking, *Every one of them has a different story.*

You, too, have your own story, and you will have unique needs as you set out on your journey to vitality and immune system health. I hope this book has given you new ideas and new avenues to pursue, and I hope the resources that follow will help you find what you need, whether it's an alternative treatment or a holistic physician or a particular nutrient.

If you are in need of supplements, you can check your local health food store, contact your nutritionally oriented physician/health care practitioner, or you can contact Rhinebeck Health Nutrients at (888) 616-6590 to have particular formulas shipped to you. Over the years, I have found certain types and brands of nutrients to be more helpful than others. We stock these high-quality, high-potency balanced supplements in our health centers so they are readily available to our patients. In addition, I have developed specific formulas and packs for use in particular clinical situations. For example, we have different formulas to support patients with arthritis, premenstrual syndrome, CFIDS, executive stress, and more. We also have an immune support pack to help strengthen and balance the immune system, a Lyme disease support pack, various support packs for patients with cancer, and a probiotic supplement called Co-Biotic, "the antibiotic companion," for use when antibiotics are required. If you'd like to know more about a product or nutrient that is mentioned in this book, either in the text or in the case studies, you can obtain information by calling the number above.

You also can reach my offices at:

Rhinebeck Health Center
108 Montgomery Street
Rhinebeck, NY 12572
(914) 876-7082

Center for Progressive Medicine
Pinnacle Place
Suite 210
10 McKown Road
Albany, NY 12203
(518) 435-0082

OTHER ORGANIZATIONS

ACUPUNCTURE

American Academy of Medical Acupuncture
5820 Wilshire Boulevard
Suite 500
Los Angeles, CA 90036
(213) 937-5514

American Association of Acupuncture and Oriental Medicine
433 Front Street
Catasauqua, PA 18032
(610) 433-2448

National Commission for the Certification of Acupuncturists
1424 16th Street NW
Suite 501
Washington, DC 20036
(202) 232-1404

AYURVEDIC MEDICINE

American School of Ayurvedic Sciences
2115 112 Avenue NE
Bellevue, WA 98004
(206) 453-8022

BIOFEEDBACK

Biofeedback Certification Institute of America
10200 West 44th Avenue
Suite 304
Wheat Ridge, CO 80033
(303) 420-2902

CANDIDA/YEAST

The International Health Foundation
P.O. Box 3494
Jackson, TN 38303
(901) 427-8100

CHIROPRACTIC

American Chiropractic Association
1701 Clarendon Boulevard
Arlington, VA 22209
(703) 276-8800

International Chiropractors Association
1110 North Glebe Road
Suite 1000
Arlington, VA 22201
(703) 528-5000

ENERGETIC HEALING

Barbara Brennan School of Healing
P.O. Box 2005
East Hampton, NY 11937
(516) 329-0951

ENVIRONMENTAL MEDICINE, ALLERGY, AND CLINICAL IMMUNOLOGY

AAEM (American Academy of Environmental Medicine)
P.O. Box CN1001-8001
New Hope, PA 18938
(215) 862-4544

ENZYME-POTENTIATED DESENSITIZATION (EPD)

American EPD Society
141 Paseo de Peralta
Santa Fe, NM 87501
(505) 983-8890

GUIDED IMAGERY THERAPY

Academy for Guided Imagery
P.O. Box 2070
Mill Valley, CA 94942
(415) 389-9324

HERBAL MEDICINE

American Herbalists Guild
P.O. Box 746555
Arvada, CA 80006
(303) 423-8800

Herb Research Foundation
1007 Pearl Street
Suite 200
Boulder, CO 80302
(303) 449-2265

HOMEOPATHY

British Institute of Homeopathy and College of Homeopathy
520 Washington Boulevard
Suite 423
Marina Del Rey, CA 90292
(310) 306-5408
(800) 494-9790

Homeopathic Educational Services
2124 Kitredge Street
Berkeley, CA 94704
(510) 649-0294

National Center for Homeopathy
801 North Fairfax Street
Suite 306
Alexandria, VA 22314
(703) 548-7790

HYPNOTHERAPY

National Guild of Hypnotists
P.O. Box 308
Merrimack, NH 03054
(603) 429-9438

LYME DISEASE

The Lyme Disease Foundation
1 Financial Plaza
Hartford, CT 06103
(800) 886-LYME

MEDITATION AND STRESS MANAGEMENT

Institute of Noetic Sciences
P.O. Box 909
Sausalito, CA 94966
(415) 331-5650

NATUROPATHIC MEDICINE

American Association of Naturopathic Physicians
2366 Eastlake Avenue East
Suite 322
Seattle, WA 98102
(206) 323-7610

National College of Naturopathic Medicine
049 Southwest Porter Avenue
Portland, OR 97201
(503) 499-4343

ORGANIC PRODUCE

Eden Acres, Inc.
12100 Lima Center Road
Clinton, MI 49236
(517) 456-4288

Mothers & Others for a Livable Planet
40 West 20th Street
New York, NY 10011
(212) 242-0010

OSTEOPATHY

American Academy of Osteopathy
3500 DePauw Boulevard
Suite 1080
Indianapolis, IN 46268
(317) 879-1881

American Osteopathic Association
142 East Ontario Street
Chicago, IL 60611
(312) 280-5800

OXIDATIVE MEDICINE

IOMA (International Oxidative Medical Association)
P.O. Box 890910
Oklahoma City, OK 73189
(405) 634-1310
FAX: (405) 634-7320

PERSONAL GROWTH

The Pathwork Center
P.O. Box 66
375 Pantherkill Road
Phoenicia, NY 12464
(914) 688-2211

PHYSICIANS

Nutritional, preventive, and holistic medicine; chelation therapy

ACAM (American College for Advancement in Medicine)
23121 Verdugo Drive
Suite 204
Laguna Hills, CA 92653
(800) 532-3688

YOGA

International Association of Yoga Therapists
109 Hillside Avenue
Mill Valley, CA 94941
(415) 383-4587

Index